Gift of Drexel U.
to me May 2015

Clarence Ruth MD.
1953 - 1957 at
Hahnemann Med
College

I always enjoyed
Dr. Di Palma's lectures on pharmacology
(Medicine,
Drugs)

DECANUS
MAXIMUS

Born 1917·
1937

at 2015,

DECANUS MAXIMUS

The Life and Times of a Medical School Dean

Joseph R. DiPalma, M.D.

Library of Congress Number: 2004090467
ISBN :   Hardcover   1-4134-4690-6
                    Softcover   1-4134-4689-2

To order additional copies of this book, contact:
Xlibris Corporation
1-888-795-4274
www.Xlibris.com
Orders@Xlibris.com
23904

CONTENTS

PREFACE

I started this autobiographical work with the simple idea that it might amuse me and perhaps others. As I reviewed the first few chapters, I soon realized how boring this must be to most casual readers. Who might imagine that a dean, especially one of a medical school, could have an exciting, adventurous life full of rewards and failures? I'd had derogatory concepts of deaning, and I vigorously resisted becoming one. Yet when I had completed just two years at the job, the position grew upon me. My imagination soared. Consonant with the present understanding of evolution and genetic expression, I conceived a chimerical figure that had the proper body organs and mental equipment to function as a medical school dean. I expressed these ideas as an oil painting that I named *Decanus Maximus*, or simply *Big Dean*.

The central figure of the painting is the classical medical caduceus of a bundle of sticks encircled by the body of a snake. Instead of the usual snake's head, this fiend has the head of an owl with penetrating eyes, a superior brain, and most important the ability to rotate 180 degrees so it can protect against attack from the back. I incorporated the adaptable body of an octopus whose eight arms afford a mechanism to devote special attention to the major functions of deaning. Seven of the arms are each equipped to manage finances, education, research, construction of facilities, conduct of medical practice, maintenance of justice, and adjudication of arguments. The eighth arm, which handles relations with the faculty and discretionary funds, is wounded and bleeding. This indicates the vulnerable spot of the dean's existence. He can never make the entire faculty and all the students happy and satisfied all the time. A sturdy pelvis and strong legs keep the dean upright, while camel's feet provide stability in the mass of paper generated by correspondence, committee reports, and minutes of meetings. Big Dean is pictured in the appropriate setting of his medical school campus, surrounded by associate deans (dodo birds) who take care of additional functions like student health and affairs, affiliations, and continuing education. Other creatures represented by rats and snakes serve minor functions. Despite the power of Big Dean he is only middle management. A shrewd owl (the provost) in the upper right hand corner is ready to pounce upon any creature who gets out of line, while an eagle (the president) in the opposite corner surveys all with the intent of raising money.

During most of my tenure as dean, the painting hung in a prominent place behind my desk. It served the useful purpose of breaking the ice with some people I interviewed. Others were adversely affected. I had the notion that they were wondering what kind of a crackpot this dean was.

An autobiography should reveal the intimate character of the writer. Some imagery and drama should lend motion to a sometimes dull subject. Perhaps the painting portrays more of me than the written word. That is why I have named the book after the painting.

As I progressed towards the later chapters, many of my personal goals had been achieved. Environmental changes now seemed to dominate my life. One had to adapt to computers and increasing technology that made possible automation of all operations. Commercialization of medicine and education led to financial inflation. Steep rises in tuition became the mandatory and agonizing decision of the dean. Valuable data and methodology were abandoned in favor of new gadgets and systems. Professors who were obsolete (those who did not get grants) were eliminated. Tenure was no longer honored. This was especially the case when takeover by the freely spending Allegheny Health Education Research Foundation led to even greater changes in operations. New concepts of molecular biology and genetics dominated all research in science. Insurance companies dominated healthcare: those that insured patients for medical care and those that protected the physician and hospital from damage suits. Attorneys made hay of both. Education was put on the back burner by most institutions, although many would deny this.

As I was already retired when these major changes took place, they did not affect my position materially. What was hurt was my ego. It was disheartening to see all the carefully constructed projects and plans become dissipated like dust in a storm. Yet, if what had been accomplished before had not happened, what happened later could not have eventuated. If an ambitious, commercially oriented president had not managed to finance the construction of the fine, modern Hahnemann Hospital, the institution might not have been attractive for takeover by Allegheny and later by Tenet. Certainly what the dean had helped to accomplish—the organization of a modern university of the health sciences with its various schools and tremendous research potential—must have been attractive to Drexel University. Consequently, the last chapters of this book concentrate on the changes in medical education, healthcare delivery, and research rather than the involvement of the life of the author.

CHAPTER I

The Early Years and College

1916-1935

"The sons and daughters of emigrants, barbers, small businessmen, and journeymen make the best doctors."

Rupert Black, M.D.

Having reached an age well beyond threescore and ten, and feeling the infirmaries that accompany such antiquity, I have determined to set down some account of my life. It will be of interest to some, perhaps of no interest to others. But I must confess that my own ego dictates that it has been a fascinating trip thus far.

I have read many autobiographies and compared the adventures of my life with others. Some have recounted lush, amorous adventures, great voyages of exploration, fabulous business deals, glorious battles, and all the sins of Dante's Inferno. My life has been devoid of these opportunities. It may seem like a dull, ordinary existence. Yet even in the grinding away of an ordinary life, countless chances arise for intrigue and adventure. After many years of self-analysis, I am convinced that only intellectual pursuits bring the greatest pleasure. The height of self-gratification is the formulation of a new thought or the discovery of the most minor of a new fact or principal. The most magnificent adventure may be locked in the confines of the calvarium (the dome of the skull), as may the most dreadful despair.

Notwithstanding, I have been greatly involved in the affairs of men. Only by holding positions of responsibility can the entire value of a personality be judged. Only service to fellow man successfully achieved can bring ultimate satisfaction. All this sounds rather pedantic, but only you the reader can judge.

I was born at home, like most babies of my day, and delivered by my first cousin Salvatore, a young doctor later to become an obstetrician and gynecologist. The month was March, the first day of spring 1916, the third year of World War I. I'm told that the day was dreary and cold. Snow fell lightly. Despite my mother's advanced age of forty-four, baby and mother did well. I was my mother's third child, but only the second by her present husband.

I was much younger than my siblings. At the time of my birth, my sister Catherine was seven years old and my stepsister Aurora was fourteen. Two stepbrothers—Frank, thirteen, and Albert, fourteen—were my father's sons by a previous marriage. Father was fifty-four when I was born. I give these statistics to emphasize that I was the late-born child of a marriage of convenience to older parents. I wouldn't characterize myself as an unwanted child, but my birth certainly had none of the planning and anticipation of a first born. In fact and in deed, I was much loved and cherished by my parents and older brothers and sisters.

We lived in a tenement house on 27th Street and 7th Avenue in the borough of Manhattan, New York City. My father had a grocery store nearby in a neighborhood occupied largely by French immigrants. As a consequence of having French customers, my brother Albert learned to speak some practical French while working in the store. However, my family spoke mostly Italian at home—specifically, the Neapolitan dialect. My brothers and sisters spoke English as well, so I was exposed to both languages. I think I must have learned Italian first because, though my English is not accented, it retains some Italian taint.

My earliest memory is of the tenement cold-water flat on the third floor of 619 Lexington Avenue, where we moved about 1920.

My father had moved his grocery store to the corner of 54th Street and Lexington Avenue. Our family moved nearby to a railroad flat, so-called because of its design. The kitchen was at one end, followed in a straight line by dining room, bedrooms, and parlor at the other end.

In winter we huddled around the wood-fueled kitchen stove that served as a heating and cooking unit. A kerosene burner provided additional heat during the evening when everyone was at home. We slept under heavy quilts in the unheated bedrooms. It was common for females to sleep together for additional warmth as it was for males. In the large families of those days, single beds and private bedrooms were impractical except for the very rich. As a young boy, I remember sleeping in the middle between my mother and my older sister. It was very cozy, but since I slept with my head toward the foot of the bed, I smelled feet all night.

The apartment grew very warm in summer because we were on the top floor just underneath the roof. There were windows only at the front and the back of the apartment. They were kept open in the hopes of getting a flow of air through the flat. On really hot days, when the air was still and quite torrid, we used to sleep on the roof.

Given the living conditions of those days, we were comfortable. We considered ourselves lucky indeed to have a toilet right in the apartment. Some tenements had one toilet on the floor shared by several occupants. Even worse was the arrangement of a single outhouse in the backyard. Residents of those flats made sure to have a pisspot under the bed to avoid having to go outdoors in the middle of the night.

The parlor end of the flat faced Lexington Avenue. I remember spending many hours just looking down at the traffic below. The rear view was a backyard filled with clotheslines stretched between various buildings. The only vegetation was a single allantus tree. The uninspiring view was not enhanced by the many window boxes, including our own, that served as refrigerators in wintertime. On very cold days, milk froze and pushed the cream up and out of the top of the bottle. This frozen plug was highly prized by children as a substitute for ice cream. The adults were left with low fat milk by this simple extraction process. Some tenements had fire escapes that served as crude balconies where people grew various potted plants and flowers.

Both my parents were of Italian peasant stock born in Vico Equense, a small town on the Bay of Naples not far from Sorento. Vico was a beautiful place, but the people were poor because there was little industry. Vico did not attract the tourists as did the more popular Sorento and Castile a Mare. My father was born in 1865, the youngest of eleven children. Their schooling was primitive, but he did receive the equivalent of what would be four or five years of elementary school today. He could read and write Italian and do arithmetic. When my father was eleven years old, an uncle who was a sailor got him a job as a cabin boy on a schooner that transported lumber to African ports. With this and other odd jobs, he was able to book passage to America when he was about eighteen. Like many young men of that era, when Italy was just unified and building an active army, he was likely to be drafted. He'd heard stories of easy money to be made in America, so his choice to immigrate was easy. He had every intention to return when he made his fortune and the danger of being drafted was less. He did return to Italy about five years later but only to find a wife in his hometown of Vico Equense. Once married, he took his young wife to America—never to return to the country of his birth.

The keys to my father's business success were his native shrewdness, common sense, and a great willingness to work hard. He was also blessed with the ability to work with his hands. He started in the grocery business by using scrap lumber to build an enclosed fruit stand on a street corner. To economize and guard his wares, he slept in his stand at night. Even today, when I pass a fruit stand run by an immigrant, it reminds me that my father started his career in this fashion. He earned and saved enough money to rent a store and start a more enterprising grocery business. The fruit and vegetable display was always his first love, even when he had a large establishment complete with a butcher's department and as many as twenty-five employees.

Nevertheless, my father had his wild moments. When he was a young man with two young sons, he grew disgusted with city life and decided to sell his business and go into farming. His older brother had a farm in Vineland, New Jersey, and my father bought a farm next to his brother's. This farming fling lasted only one year. He grew a fine crop of watermelons and brought them to market only to learn that there was an abundance of melons that year. When he found that his fine crop would bring in only a few dollars, he refused to sell them. On his way home he came to a bridge, overturned his wagon, and dumped all the melons into the stream below.

Back in New York City, he started a grocery business again. His older brother John, who had more education and had completed merchant marine school although never actually sailed, also decided to immigrate to America. My father took him in and made him a partner in the grocery business. They made a good pair. Uncle John knew how to keep books and accounts—a tedious task for my father. Their families got along quite well, probably because their wives were sisters, but that changed after my father's first wife died. When my father married my mother, her family and my uncle's did not get along as well. Yet the brothers' business partnership carried on and the two families lived close together. When we moved to Lexington Avenue, my Uncle John's family lived in the apartment directly underneath ours. Their family also consisted of five siblings: Salvatore, the doctor, and four girls. The girls were even older than my sisters, while the youngest was my age. I can remember playing on occasion with this one, but I had very little contact with the rest of the family.

My mother had even less education than my father. Although she spoke little English, she was fluent in Italian. Despite little formal schooling, she was an intelligent woman capable of intricate thought and fully competent about making sensible decisions. She was very good with her hands and made all the clothes for our family. When I was ready to start school, she tailored an entire suit for me from one of the legs of my father's pants. A short man of only five feet, two inches, he weighed about 300 pounds at this time.

I started school at age seven. Children began in the first grade because kindergarten instruction was uncommon in those days. The parochial school was run by the priests of St. Patrick's Cathedral in a small building on 50th Street between Lexington and Park Avenues. About two or three hundred students, all boys, were in classes of about twenty-five students. The school was strictly run with rigid attention to reading, writing, arithmetic, and, of course, catechism.

No one was promoted unless he made the grade. One unfortunate fourteen-year-old was in my first grade class. Brother Henry, whom the lay teacher would summon when a misdemeanor occurred, strictly enforced discipline. Punishment consisted of being called to the front of the class and slapped on the hand an appropriate number of times by Brother Henry who used a long flat ruler that he struck with force and obvious pleasure. Despite what psychiatrists now claim about such primitive methods, I can attest that it was very effective. I have never observed more orderly classroom sessions.

The majority of the boys was Irish and called "Micks." The few Italian boys were "Wops." Constant fistfights broke out over small matters such as this name-calling. Since I was rather small compared to some of the bruisers, I suffered many a physical insult. I stayed to myself and ran home as soon as school was over. There was no lunchroom or gymnasium or any semblance of recreational area or activity. I was fortunately able to walk home for lunch because the school was only a few blocks away. During the four years that I attended that school, I didn't make a single friend.

I grew up a child amid adults. At this stage of my life, I had very little contact with children my age. Not that my family was unkind or lacking in sympathy for a child's desires, but their lives were hard and they were busy with their own pursuits. My father worked seven days a week. At least two of these days he went to market at five o'clock in the morning to purchase the week's supply of fruits and vegetables. He worked half a day on Sundays arranging the vegetable and fruit stands. In the afternoon, he would often entertain relatives in the grocery business. They sat around and told stories of little interest to a child. They drank wine and smoked and became quite boisterous.

My mother worked very hard to keep a large family in running order. She devoted two days a week to washing by hand with a washtub and scrub board. She spent another two days ironing with flat irons that were heated on the stove. Then there was the daily cooking and cleaning, making beds and general housework. We had practically no upholstered furniture and no rugs. All the floors were wood, except for the kitchen and dining areas, both covered with linoleum. At least once a week, she scrubbed them on her hands and knees with a brush.

All my brothers and sisters either worked or went to school and had little time for me. So I learned to entertain myself. My memory is dim about what I actually did. I had some toys, of course. I was particularly enamored of an erector set with miniature girders of various sizes and curves that fit cleverly into each other. With the aid of nuts and bolts, I could make a semblance of many objects like bridges and cranes. An assortment of wheels, pulleys, and axles could also be used to make models of cars and trains. My set was quite advanced because it even had a small battery-powered electric motor that allowed some models to be working ones. All this took a considerable amount of imagination. I spent countless hours unwittingly learning about levers, cantilevers, mechanical advantage, and other physical principles that I did not appreciate until many years later when I studied physics.

The erector set required considerable manual dexterity that I acquired and which many youths who concentrate on sports don't have. I never was too graceful at catching a ball or even such simple things as running and jumping. Going out in the street and playing stickball with the boys was unthinkable in that neighborhood. Even in those days Lexington Avenue was a major traffic artery. There was no schoolyard or park nearby. But the major reason I stayed close to home was the "Gashouse Gang" from Second and Third Avenues who would pulverize a young lad like me.

When my mother could break free of her many tasks and the weather was nice, she would take me to Central Park, which was within walking distance. We would sit awhile at the fountain in front of the Plaza Hotel. I would splash my hand in the water and float small objects. Almost sixty-five years later on the occasion of an overnight stay at the Plaza, I noticed that the fountain hadn't changed a bit and a picture flashed upon my mind's eye of a small boy playing at its rim.

Mother and I would enter the park and walk to the lake, sit on a bench, and watch the ducks and swans. She would buy me a box of Cracker Jack, and I would feed some to the ducks. If we had enough time, we would visit the zoo. I learned at an early age to name all the animals, which made my mother very proud, but the word *hippopotamus* was too much for me. I ended up calling this monstrous creature a "mamous." This was apparently funny to my family because I was teased with remarks such as "Did you see the mamous today?"

Even before I went to school, I had learned to read some words. I don't think I was more advanced for my age than children who go to kindergarten today. But I was an avid reader, thanks largely to my sister Catherine. She loved to read and went to the public library at least once a week, sometimes more often. When she took me along, I'd browse in a children's section that had a good selection of fairy-tale books. Soon I had read every book. My mind was full of kings and queens, fairies and elves, dwarfs and giants—even witches and devils.

In those days before movies, television, or even radios, children read or heard stories from their parents. Even the newspapers had few if any cartoons for children. One day I was a bold Knight who slew dragons and rescued fair damsels; the next I was a Merlin who brewed strange mixtures and could exert magical events. Then I was Sinbad on a wild trip of adventure, or I found an old corked bottle that contained a genie.

My father's business prospered in the mid-1920's, and he was finally able to buy a private home in Jackson Heights, Queens, just off Roosevelt Avenue on 76th Street. This meant a separation from my uncle's family and a distinct rise in our living standard. I gained the most from this move. For the first time, I could go outdoors to play and have neighborhood friends my own age. Jackson Heights had many open spaces and an abandoned farm nearby. Our street was unpaved like most others that weren't main arteries. Little traffic meant kids could play ball and other games with no interference. The local public school a few blocks away had a large paved playground. We adopted some adjacent empty lots to form a baseball diamond. I now had freedom of activity that was beyond my fondest dreams. Modern children cannot realize how tough life could be living in the middle of the city in a cold-water flat.

In Manhattan, I had managed to get through the fourth grade in the parochial school. But when I enrolled in the Queens public school, my parents were told that the Catholic schools' teaching was notoriously bad and not equivalent to that of public schools. I was forced to repeat fourth grade. This was a severe shock to me, and I suppose I worked very hard to excel. As it turned out, I was far more advanced than my classmates and was soon moved into my rightful fifth grade. School was rather boring. I seemed to be able to latch on to the material with minimum effort, so I developed lazy and deficient study habits. Educators at the time believed that children should have a minimum of homework so they could develop sports and hobbies.

In 1927, Charles Lindbergh made his historic solo flight across the Atlantic Ocean. Like all eleven-year-old boys of that generation, I was greatly inspired by this adventure. Aviators were my great heroes. I was sure that I would become an aviator of outstanding merit. Making and flying model airplanes became a practical outlet for this desire. Hobby stores appeared overnight to answer this craze. My first real friends were boys who built and flew model airplanes—flimsy structures of balsa wood and Japanese tissue paper. They had to be as light as possible because they were powered only by rubber bands. A great deal of skill and patience was required to construct a model that consistently flew well. Local clubs formed. Even national organizations sponsored contests. There were various divisions for indoor models, outdoor models, longest airborne time, speed contests, novelty aircraft, and flying scale models.

I built model planes with my pals Jimmy McPheat and Henry

Struck. We became quite skilled, competed with each other, and flew our aircraft on a regular basis. Fortunately there were some large fields within walking or biking distance where we could fly our craft without interference from buildings and trees. We learned a good deal about weather and wind, updrafts and downdrafts. A favorite place was Holmes Airport, a small local airfield used mostly by barnstorming pilots who put on weekend air shows to attract crowds and sell local air rides to adventurous onlookers. The planes were mostly open cockpit biplanes of post-World War I vintage. There was a small amount of commercial flying with a Stinson cabin monoplane. Flying lessons were available, but neither my friends nor I could afford them. Besides, we were considered too young. By befriending the aviators and doing odd jobs, however, we would get an occasional free ride. I even managed to save enough money to take one lesson in an OX5 Swallow, an open cockpit biplane with an inline engine. It was quite thrilling. I was confident that I would eventually become an aviator.

My family took a very dim view of my aircraft activities. None of them thought becoming an aviator was a decent or even a slightly meritorious goal. To them, flying was a dangerous sport and a frivolous adventure fit for the rich and crazy. No one foresaw that aviation was the travel avenue of the future and would become one of the most important arms of modern warfare. My father pointed out that when an engine failed in a boat, it could still float and people could be rescued, but if the engine stopped in an airplane there was no choice but to fall to the ground and be killed. Actually, my father hoped that I would go into the grocery business. And my brother Albert didn't want me to do anything that would outshine his accomplishments. My mother and sisters wanted me to get as much education as possible and become a physician. If my Uncle John's family had a physician, why not ours?

Despite much discouragement, I continued my intense interest in aviation. I read every book and magazine on the subject that I could get my hands on. My hero was Igor Sikorsky who built and flew the first multimotored plane in 1913 and later designed the helicopter. One great day I had a chance to meet him when he made a minor excursion to North Beach Airport, later to become LaGuardia Airport. I had a camera and asked if I could take his picture. He consented even though he saw that I was only a young lad. How I prized that picture! Sikorsky and me standing in front his latest plane design.

My time was completely occupied with airplane modeling activities. I hardly noticed that I was going to school. I can't remember doing any homework. While in class, I dreamed of fantastic plane designs. Yet I must have done well because, on completing the sixth grade, my teachers recommended that I go to junior high school where superior students were allowed to complete the seventh and eighth grades in one year followed by the first year of high school. In this way, a student could save a whole year of schooling and be permitted to enter the second year of high school.

That's how I got to Junior High School 125 in Astoria. This was a great adventure because I had to take the subway to get there. The teaching was not as vigorous as it should have been. Although I did relatively well, this showed up in my later education. I did minimal homework and learned little in subjects like French, much to my detriment later.

Art was one subject I did well in and enjoyed. The art teacher took a shine to me, and I was able to do special projects like making posters for school events. She encouraged me to apply for a scholarship to the Leonardo DaVinci School of Art. I received the scholarship, but my family dissuaded me from this direction, too. Besides, my main ambition still was aviation. However my skills in art came in very handy later.

Our family life was very strict. Each child had his and her duties. Mine was to do the dusting and rug cleaning, which I did religiously every Saturday with my sister Catherine. I remember scrubbing the floor on my knees a few times. My older sister Aurora worked as a secretary in an insurance firm on Wall Street. Brother Albert had occasional jobs as a bookkeeper. My other brother Frank was the "bad sheep" of the family. My parents gave him money to enroll in a business school. Instead of matriculating, he played hooky. Frank pretended to go to school each day but actually wandered the streets and parks until it was time to go home. When my father found out, there was a big fuss. Frank was ordered to work in the grocery store. He never was a reliable worker, but he did learn to drive the horse and wagon and make deliveries. He later drove the truck that replaced the horse-drawn wagon. He was the only one in the family who went out evenings after work. We didn't know where he went or what he did, but there was a strong suspicion that he hung out with bad company. In some ways, I think Frank was more human and more with the times than the rest of our family.

I don't think my father paid Frank a salary, but he did give him a small allowance. My father started a bank account for him that accumulated about $4,000 dollars—a fair amount of money for those days. Frank disappeared one day, and so did the bank account. We eventually found out that he had eloped with a girl from Vineland, New Jersey. This made him an outcast. The family was not allowed to see or talk to him. Poor Frank didn't do well at marriage, and his wife divorced him after a few years. They had one child, a boy, whom none of us ever saw. I remember that his wife came to our door one day and asked to become acquainted with us, but my mother chased her away. I was very young at the time, but it struck me that one must avoid bad relations. It was also difficult for me to align my mother's behavior with our Catholic indoctrination, and it was the first suspicion of incongruous actions of religious persons. In any event, I didn't have contact with Frank until many years later.

My brother Albert it was a different story. He was one of the most naturally intelligent persons I have ever met. It was impossible to outdo him in a calculation or memory exercise. His intellect, however, was combined with a weak personality. He lacked aggressiveness and drive and was very clumsy with his hands. He stuck close to the house and never married. He had few or no friends. Being the oldest he was allowed to have music lessons. The violin was his instrument of choice, and he practiced to the irritation of all. He repeated the same tune incessantly—a Grieg piece that I can still hear to this day. After nine years of lessons, he could play moderately well, but it was obvious that he was never going to be a musician. The rest of us were denied music lessons because Al had received them, not that I had even the most remote interest in music at that time.

Because Albert was intelligent and made a good appearance, he got jobs easily but after a few weeks got fired. This pattern was attributed to laziness and a hypochondriac personality. Twice in his adolescence, Albert had lobar pneumonia and almost died both times. Pneumonia was a very serious disease then, with no cure other than supportive care. Cousin Salvatore, the doctor, took care of him. Each time Albert was sick for a month, followed by a six-month convalescent period. He was babied because the family feared he would succumb again to some fatal illness. As a result, Albert got away with doing no household chores. He mooned away time at home and avoided outside encounters. My mother finally got fed up and chased him out of the house with a broom one day. Albert gradually recovered and got a job with the city by getting a very high mark on a competitive examination. He could not be fired from this civil service job, but he never did his share of physical work around the house.

At this point of my young life, Albert was more like a father to me than a big brother because our difference in age was so great. I recall eating a hotdog and riding the roller coaster when he took me to Coney Island. Another summer, we went to Coney Island to swim. We changed into bathing suits in a bathhouse. When we went back to change out of our wet suits, my brother discovered that his wallet had been stolen. He became quite hysterical because we did not know how we could get home. The kindly woman clerk at the change booth lent us ten cents to pay the subway fare home. Funny, but I have no recollection of romping in the surf of the mighty Atlantic, but I remember the subway ride as more exciting than the bathing.

Perhaps the greatest adventure of my early childhood happened during the two-week summer vacation when I accompanied Albert to the Catskill Mountains. The fresh mountain air was expected to do him good since he was always so sickly. I was sent along, not because I needed or merited a vacation, but to keep my brother company, or perhaps to give him a sense of responsibility that might prevent him from doing anything rash, such as meet a girl he might fancy. We would take walks in the mornings and go bathing in a nearby stream. I even managed to learn to float and swim a little. In the afternoons, Albert would go to sleep in a convenient hammock while I would play around the barn. There were no farm animals, but I remember numerous cats and kittens. Meals were quite different from what we had at home. I suppose one would call it American cooking. To me, it was rather bland and monotonous. I never got to like warm milk directly from the cow. This was the only vacation I experienced until many years later. In fact, no one was allowed a vacation in those years. I can't remember my father, mother, or sisters ever taking a vacation. If you had any time off from work, you went to help out in the store.

My sister Aurora (We really called her Mary.) was in her twenties and should have been socializing to find a husband. She was not allowed to go out, however, even though she was working and earning decent wages. Money was handled simply in our family—my father handled it all. Everything the children earned was immediately handed over to Father. He took care of all the expenses. Each morning, he would hand out any carfare and lunch money needed by any of us. He carried such an enormous amount of change that it wore holes in his pocket. He did all the banking. All transactions were in cash. He carried a large roll of bills in a special pocket sewn into his vest. At the end of the day, he took the money from the store's cash register and brought it home. On the days he went to the wholesale grocery market, he paid cash for all the produce he bought. All this may seem strange today, but there were no credit cards then, and relatively few people held bank checking accounts. There was—at least in my family—no such thing as a weekly allowance. Whenever we needed anything, we had to ask my father. Very few, if any, luxury or frivolous items were ever purchased. My father was not stingy or unfair—we simply were economical. Many families, particularly those of European origin, followed the same rules.

We were never hungry. Every day my father sent a clerk home with a basket of fruits and vegetables and other staples like boxed or canned goods. Many of the fruits and vegetables were a little on the rotten side and could not be sold; however, they were quite edible. We got to eat some fancy items like prickly pears, kumquats, watercress, and Belgian endive that I'm sure most families in our class never heard of. We had meat at least three times a week and, of course, always a chicken on Sunday and fish on Fridays.

A distant relative whom we called Uncle Louie worked for my father until he went off on his own to establish a fish market. Though he was quite a character with many weird stories about his own prowess, no one ever doubted his ability as a fisherman. Every time he visited us, he brought an enormous lobster or some other fish delicacy. In season, he brought fillet of shad. Shad is a great delicacy but has so many bones that it is virtually impossible to fillet. Uncle Louie had devised a set of special knives that he used to produce a satisfactory fillet. In fact, he made a decent living just by selling fillet of shad to fancy restaurants.

All the childhood diseases were visited upon me. I had measles when I was only two, then chicken pox at four, followed by the mumps. The disease I remember best was scarlet fever, which I had at about age twelve. This was considered a very serious communicable disease and required strict quarantine. I had to be kept in a separate room with a sign from the health department pasted on the closed door. I was sick for a month, or what today would better be described as the period of quarantine. Only the doctor and my mother were allowed in the room. Several evil tasting medicines were forced upon me, which I'm certain did no good. I recovered with no serious complications in spite of their horrendous taste. I spent my time sneaking out of bed to peak out the window and see what the other kids were doing outdoors.

When I finished junior high school, I enrolled in Newtown High School in Elmhurst about two miles from my home. There was no public transportation, and it was well before the age of school buses. The walk was in some ways interesting and adventurous. My friends and I devised cross-country routes across backyards and open fields. One of these routes involved crossing the Long Island Railroad tracks. It was simply good luck that none of us were killed because it was a commuter line with a lot of traffic. Sometimes I rode my bike and, for five cents a day, parked it at a local store. I was allowed ten cents for lunch.

High school was a shock to me academically. The teaching was at a much higher level than what I had been used to in junior high school. Classmates were older, more mature, and had better study habits. I continued my lazy study routine, expecting to skin by as I had in the past. Since I was supposed to have had a year of French in junior high school, they put me in second-year French, which unfortunately had some of the brightest students in the school. I flunked French and did poorly in other subjects. My report card got me holy hell at home. I decided to make up for this by going to summer school to repeat French and also take trigonometry. My sister Catherine was a substitute French teacher so she was in an excellent position to coach me. I did very well and passed the third year New York State Regents Exam, which enabled me to skip a whole term of French. This achievement, plus another session of summer school, allowed me to skip a year of high school so I was ready for college at age sixteen. I thought I had turned a bad situation to my advantage, only later to regret my immaturity compared to my college classmates.

Meanwhile our family situation turned drastically worse. My father's grocery had flourished thanks to a high-class Park Avenue clientele, but it was in a very vulnerable position in 1929 when the stock market crashed. By 1932—the third year of the Great Depression—the business fell away to practically nothing. Unfortunately my father was stuck with three more years of lease. He had to keep running the store even though it was losing money. He lost practically all of his life savings. Our family managed to survive only because Mary kept her job and Albert had his city job from which he could not be fired.

Although my father was now sixty-five and without much capital, he was anxious to open another store in a cheaper neighborhood in the hopes of again making a successful living. He had his eye on me to help him in this undertaking. He had no intention of my going to college. Most families of our station did not consider college necessary for a successful career in almost anything, especially business. One climbed the ladder of fortune by hard work and native skills. Brother Albert, who had no desire to have a sibling acquire more education than he had, sided with my father against my mother and two sisters. I would have liked to help my father, but I really had no interest in the grocery business. Neither was I that anxious to go to college. I still would have liked to get into some aspect of aviation—my first love—even perhaps as a mechanic.

While the arguments flew back and forth, I proceeded to take college entrance exams and apply to a few local colleges, though my marks were quite average except for chemistry and math. It was unthinkable that I could afford to go away to college. I was restricted to local colleges where I could live at home and commute. This left City College of New York, which had free tuition, Columbia University, New York University, and Fordham University.

My mother and sisters won the argument on the dubious reasoning that, since my uncle's family had a son who was a doctor (Cousin Salvatore), then our family should have one too! So it was decided that I should go to college as a prerequisite for medical school. Incidentally, Salvatore never went to college. In his day, one could enter medical school directly from high school.

Only City College accepted me. Columbia University offered me the opportunity to go to Seth Low Junior College, a new endeavor located in the Borough Hall section of Brooklyn and housed in part of the Brooklyn Law School building. I was assured that the education at Seth Low Junior College was the equivalent of that of Columbia, and that university professors would teach the courses. Moreover, my degree would be from Columbia University, and I would have access to all the library facilities and other courses of the University.

It sounded like a good deal to me, although my family probably would have preferred City College where tuition was free. I convinced them that it was very difficult to get into medical school from City College. After some further arguments, I was allowed to enroll in Seth Low Junior College's premedical curriculum, which I soon discovered was a liberal arts education peppered with a heavy dose of science. I was pleased to learn that Seth Low was the distinguished former president of Columbia University and was even more impressed with the Seth Low Library on the main campus. The tuition was about $400 a semester, a pittance today but a great burden to my family in the 1930s.

In the summer of 1932, just before I entered college, an unusual event changed my perspective on careers. *The Daily Mirror*, a prominent New York City tabloid, announced a national model airplane contest to be held at Roosevelt Field in Valley Stream, Long Island. There were various categories such as longest duration of flight, greatest speed, novelty of design for a flying model, and scale models that did not need to be capable of flight. My boyhood friends, Jimmy and Henry, and I decided to enter this contest. For much of the summer we three were busy constructing and testing models.

When the great day arrived, it turned out to be a bright and sunny with some cumulus clouds, which meant that there would be hot air rises that favor long duration flights. At best, the rubber band motors could last maybe ten minutes, and then the plane would glide to the ground. If you could catch a riser, much longer flights were possible. If the model caught a lateral breeze, however, it would soon disappear from sight.

With this in mind, I held off flying my model until late in the morning when the risers were active. Fortuitously my model caught a riser. After about thirty minutes of flight, it was starting to disappear in the clouds. My good friend Jimmy had a pair of binoculars and kept yelling to the judge with the stopwatch, "I still see it! I still see it!" or later "See it—it's just at the tip of that cloud!" The judge was in no position to argue because he had no glasses. My flight was timed at sixty-seven minutes—and captured first place! I won second place in the speed contest for my twin pusher canard model. And to cap it all, my novelty model of a roller wing plane also won first place. For the highest overall average, I was awarded the silver loving cup with my name inscribed on it. My friends did not win anything but shared in my elation as if we were a team, which in reality we were. I could not have won without their support. As a postscript, I must add that I was quite chagrined to learn later that the handsome cup cost only $17.

One would imagine that my success in this contest would strengthen my resolve to enter the field of aviation. For reasons that I do not understand to this day, I put away my models and other paraphernalia and never touched them again. Perhaps it was just a phase of growing up or a matter of "I came, I saw, I conquered." In a moment of truth, I perceived that I had achieved my full potential in this endeavor. I also realized that my nearsighted right eye prevented me from having satisfactory binocular vision that would deny me access to the Army Air Force Academy.

My interests turned in other directions. Photography had always been a side hobby. A gift of some cash from my sister Mary enabled me to buy a 9-by-12 centimeter plate camera from a pawnshop. A Voightlander with a 4.5 Schneider lens with an iris shutter capable of speeds of one second to 1/400th of a second, it was capable of doing quite good technical work. I constructed a darkroom in the basement complete with a homebuilt enlarger. I now had an outlet for my slender artistic skills.

About this time, Albert bought a second-hand 1928 Chevrolet Coupe for fifty dollars. A cute little car with a rumble seat. The engine and the drive train had seen their best days, however, as we soon found out. My brother was too scared to drive it, so it fell upon me to do the honors. I'd learned to drive when I was about fourteen. The driver of my father's grocery truck took a shine to me and let me drive the truck home at night from the store. I quickly picked up the skills of clutching and shifting, as I guess most kids would. Of course, I did not have a license and was lucky never to have been stopped by a cop. Traffic and auto rules were much more lax in those days.

When Albert bought the old Chevy, I was over sixteen so I was able to get a license with minimum effort. My brother never did drive this car. I drove the family on Sunday excursions and had to be chief mechanic as well. The carburetor was fickle, and the engine stalled either because of flooding or being starved of gas. I took the gas supply system apart numerous times. The clutch plate soon had to be replaced. The weak drive train showed up as a broken axle and later a cracked drive shaft. Most of these breakdowns happened on family trips. Soon no one wanted to ride in Albert's car.

I learned automobile mechanics the hard way. I found my way to auto junk shops to locate used parts. Cars in those days were comparatively easy to work on. There was plenty of room under the hood, and most parts could be taken apart and reassembled with a few tools. The owner's manual showed all the parts in skeletal detail, which enabled anyone with some mechanical skill to do most repair work. When I finally got the Chevy in good enough shape to drive again, the family decided to buy a new car.

We acquired a black 1933 Dodge for about $800 by turning in the Chevy and my father's truck, which wasn't needed after he retired. It had two spare tires with covers, one on each fender that swept gracefully into the running boards. A four-door sedan with a trunk rack in the back, it handily accommodated five people. Now the family could take a comfortable, secure ride on Sundays. We usually traveled to some point on Long Island or more distant beaches such as the Rockaways and Jacob Riis Park.

I was the willing driver on these trips until brother Albert finally went to driving school. The Dodge stayed in the family for at least a dozen years, and many exciting experiences were associated with its use. Once we started out on a long trip to Vineland, New Jersey, to visit my father's brother, the one who had established himself as a farmer. On a rainy spring morning, we all packed into the car—me as driver, brother Al, Father, and Mother. To get to New Jersey from Queens, we had to cross the 59th Street Bridge to Manhattan and then travel through the Holland Tunnel. The surface of the bridge was composed of wooden blocks that had been tarred over; consequently the roadway became very slippery in wet weather. Old trolley car tracks were also in the center of the roadway.

In the middle of the bridge, I decided to overtake a slow-moving truck by swinging to the left and accelerating. Suddenly the front wheel caught in the trolley car tracks while car's rear skidded to the left. We made two rapid circles, ended up aside the guardrail of the opposite lane, and faced on-coming traffic head on. The miracle of it all was that no cars were in the way when our Dodge made the involuntary gyrations. No one was hurt. I calmly waited for a break in the traffic and slithered into the correct lane, driving very gingerly. This close call with sudden death happened so quickly and unexpectedly that no one made a comment. We continued quite sedately on our way. I'm sure my family had less confidence in me as a driver, however, after this episode. That accident made a great impression on me. Even after all these years, when I pass a truck in wet weather, that scene on the 59th Street Bridge flashes through my mind.

College classes started in the fall of 1932. Most of my courses were in the liberal arts: English composition, French, and contemporary civilization. The last was a required course devised by Columbia University professors. It was really just history from antiquity to the present, all contained in one gigantic volume with small print. I never bought the book because I was confident that what I'd learned before and what I heard in class would carry me through with ease. What a mistake! The professor turned out to be extremely dull and was obviously uncomfortable before the class. I also did not take into consideration that all my classmates were a select group of very bright students. The level of education was much higher than what I had been used to in high school. The result? I barely squeezed by with a C minus—a remarkable achievement considering that I never read the book and never listened in class.

English composition was another matter. The professor was an interesting character who made the subject come alive. We had no exams, but our grades depended upon a number of assigned written exercises. One was to write the first chapter of a novel. We were warned that plagiarism would earn us an F. It was well known that the way to get an A was to copy from a pulp magazine or to find a former student willing to sell his prize paper. Like the naive fool I was, I took the professor at his word—that he could distinguish a copy from an original—and I struggled to write a completely original chapter. The result was a well-earned C. My new friend Dave found an obscure pulp novel, copied the first chapter word for word, not even changing the names of the characters, and got an A.

My extra study in high school made French a snap. The professor was a short, stocky Italian by the name of Brunetti. All the students liked him because he was a self-proclaimed authority on "feminism," which I guess today would be called "sex." He invited groups of students to his Greenwich Village apartment for Italian dinners. But most of all his students loved him because he rarely gave less than a B in his courses.

A Professor Elfman taught biology at Columbia's Morningside Campus. I enjoyed it because it had a lot of lab work. One of the experiments was the dissection of a dogfish. Sharks have no bones, only cartilage, and it was possible to cut into the skull to the inner ear. I was quite proud of myself because I was the only one in the class to dissect out the semicircular canals. It did not help me too much, though, as I only got a B in the course while my friends, Dave and Sol, who did rather sloppy dissections, got A's.

Chemistry in the venerable Havermeyer Laboratory at the Columbia Campus was more difficult than I expected. With a prodigious effort against stiff competition, however, I managed to get a B. I soon discovered that premed students are a greasy lot who would murder their mothers to get a good grade, especially in the sciences. About 90 percent of my classmates were Jewish and knew that their chances of getting into medical school were slim because most, if not all, schools had quotas on how many of that race were admitted at that time. Catholics were also not easily admitted, yet there was not the same pressure that my Jewish classmates felt.

We also had to take gym, which I did not appreciate at all. The college had the philosophy that all students had to participate in intramural sports. I reluctantly chose wrestling because it looked relatively easy. Surprisingly, it turned out to be very strenuous. I had my big nose rubbed in the mat and my back badly twisted. Despite this, I have to admit that I rather enjoyed the sport. At the least I learned how to fall without getting hurt. But I was glad when in the later years of college gym was not required.

Social life was non-existent for me at college. Not only did I have to commute two hours each day on the crowded New York subways—and it was rare to get a seat, especially during rush hours—but also my spending money was limited. I was allowed twenty cents a day: ten cents for carfare and ten cents for a meager lunch. I made friends with two other students who seemed to have similar outlooks to my own. Dave was a couple of years older than I and considerably better off financially. Dave was cheerful, alert, and worldly-wise. I never quite understood why he had come to junior college when he obviously could have been at an Ivy League college in residence at a fraternity. Perhaps it was because he was partially Middle Eastern or because his father's chemical business was probably doing poorly during the Depression. My other close friend Sol was short in stature and Jewish. He was by far the brightest and most scholastic student of our group. He always got an A in every course and, unlike his classmates, was not a greasy grind. He was generous with his knowledge, and we leaned heavily on him during cramming sessions.

The three of us stuck together, along with Carmine who joined us on occasion. Carmine was about ten years older and had had his own business as a furrier. When the Depression hit him badly, he decided to sell his business and go back to college to become a physician, which he had always wanted to do. He had to work part-time as a furrier to pay his tuition and living expenses. Carmine was wiser in some ways than the rest of us, but had to struggle with the course work because of the long lapse in his education.

The rest of the students were mostly very bright, seriously inclined, and came from lower middle-class families. There were no dorms so all the students lived at home. Each was determined to outdo the others to get into medical school. We did not mix with the Columbia College students because their classes were completely separate. We were, in effect, Columbia University extension course students organized as an integral group of primarily premed students. I also suspect that this arrangement gave some starving faculty a chance to make a living during hard times.

From the comments and interpretations given to students, it became obvious that many if not most of the Columbia faculty at that time were either communists or had strong communist leanings. None of them openly declared it, but their criticism of capitalists and their praise of communists gave away their true feelings. I suppose this was the result of the Depression, which they blamed on the capitalist system. I was rather amused because they were radicals making a living from us poor capitalists who wanted to become doctors so we could make a better living than our parents! Yet Columbia undoubtedly had some of the best minds in government and economics. In fact, President Franklin Roosevelt leaned heavily upon them in constructing a New Deal. As I look back, it was a time of movement toward socialism with the intent of equalizing opportunities for the underprivileged and deprived. This was all to the good, but it took many years—and World War II—to finally end the Depression and institute the social changes we enjoy today.

Fredrick Allen, our Dean, was a typical WASP characteristic of educators of that period. I do not say this disparagingly. While they controlled education, WASPs must be given credit for starting and maintaining most of the educational institutions of this country. Allen took a personal interest in his students and made it his business to become acquainted with each. When I had almost finished the first year, he called me into his office one day. I concluded that he probably was going to give me a dressing-down, as I had a miserable record compared to the other premeds. Instead, he was sympathetic and agreed that my long commute and my youth compared to the other students made study more difficult for me. Then he gave me a big boost by telling me that my I.Q. indicated that I was capable of getting better marks. He probably told this to all the students, but it had a salutary effect on me. I studied more and put more effort into every course but to no avail. My immaturity and previous poor preparation were handicaps that could not prevail against the competition. I was lucky to end up with an average of C plus.

An event that inordinately depressed me was the suicide of my histology professor. He was a very intense, dedicated, but shy person who always conveyed an impression of being uncomfortable. It seemed such a great loss to end life at a young age, especially because he was so intelligent and capable. I never learned if there was a precipitating cause, such as a lost love affair or failure to achieve a goal. I compared myself to him—for no good reason—and questioned whether working so hard to get into medical school was worth the effort. Suppose, as it seemed likely, I didn't get in? My family, who had skimped to put me through college, would be so disappointed.

For myself, I cared little. I'd become convinced that medicine was not such a great a profession. It wasn't really my personal goal. I probably would have been secretly pleased if I was not accepted into medical school. Several of my classmates swore that they would end their lives if they did not get in to some school. This attitude amused me because most of the students had no intention of becoming physicians to help their fellow man. They wanted the prestige and the supposedly better income of the profession.

As I look back, the more plausible reason that the professor's suicide made such an impression on me was because I had suicidal thoughts myself. Adolescence is fraught with frustration. At such a tender age, a young person feels the weight of realizing his full potential but isn't yet able to express it. The most depressed people I have known are high achievers. To have great ambitions, to fantasize wonderful accomplishments, and yet be unable to realize them is traumatic to youth who have not yet been beaten into the pulp of normal existence. The best protection, I've found, is an innate sense of humor. What is sad is also comical. Fortunately, I have always been able to see the humor in my own frustrations as well as those of others.

Physics for the premeds was the course that separated the men from the mice. The course was taught in a large lecture hall accommodating at least 200 students. The professor, who shall remain nameless, was a tall, trim fellow with a mustache—later described as a Hitler type. All he lacked was horns to portray a devil. His deep voice penetrated your gut. There was no doubt that he would flunk half the class that made it impossible, of course, to get into medical school. The grading was so tough that even the weasels were glad to settle for Cs. Our grades were determined strictly by the mathematical average of the dreaded weekly written exam. The test consisted of three problems that had to be solved in fifteen minutes. No matter how hard we studied the week's work, the questions were cleverly designed to stump us. Even my bright friends Dave and Sol had difficulty answering them.

Dave met me in the hall one day and whispered in my ear, "I have a copy of this week's physics exam."

"You're kidding? How did you get it?" I replied.

Dave had made friends with an extension student who took the course at night. For some scheduling reason, the night course was one week ahead of our course, so the extension student already had the correct solutions to the problems. I could not really believe that the brilliant physics professor could be so naive as to give the same exam. The next day, however, when we sat for our exam, it turned out to be identical. My hands began to tremble and sweat so that I could hardly write. I felt everyone in the room looking at me. Barely managing to put down the solutions, I made sure to make a few minor mistakes so that I would not get a perfect score. Dave, on the other hand, was perfectly calm and smiling—clearly enjoying his ingenuity. Despite my misgivings, we were not caught. This was one of the few exams in which I received a near perfect score. Nevertheless, call it stupidity or just plain cowardice I refused to cheat again. At the end of the course, I was happy to get a hard earned C. Dave got an A, and so did Sol who was not in on the exam deal.

Quantitative chemistry turned out to be quite a bore. It was one of the few courses in which our grades depended on a series of quantitative experiments to determine the amount of a product with an accuracy of a tenth of a milligram. First we had to calibrate a swing balance, which took all day. In his usual fashion, Dave slopped over this part in contrast to my meticulous application of the recommended procedures. One of the unknowns consisted of determining the water of hydration of a certain metallic salt. It required weighting a small crucible containing a known amount of the chemical, then heating the crucible and its contents to a red heat, followed by another accurate weighing after the crucible had cooled. I did the experiment in perfect order and felt confident that I must have a perfect result. Dave had the misfortune of dropping the hot crucible on the dirty stone bench top. This ruined the experiment, but that didn't faze Dave. Instead of wasting another day repeating the experiment, he devised an ingenious plan. He went around the class obtaining everyone's results. Arranging these in the alphabetical order of students' names, he was able to interpolate his intended result. Guess what? Dave got an A. And I—for all my fastidiously accurate work—got a B.

Organic chemistry was the next backbreaker for the premeds. Like physics, if we flunked this course we forgot our desire to get into medical school. Only 10 or 15 percent of the class flunked because the less able students had already been eliminated by the physics course. Even so, the grading was excessively tough. Out of a class of about thirty students, Professor Clauson would allow three A's, about five B's, and the rest would be either C's or flunks. I actually liked this course because it involved structural formulas. With a good visual memory, I had no trouble visualizing formulas as did some students. I also enjoyed the lab work that involved the synthesis of new compounds. Our marks depended on the purity and yield of the synthesized compound, given a certain amount of base chemicals. One of the required experiments was the synthesis of an organic liquid using a Grignard Reagent. It involved a complex distillation that had to be delicately done by first applying heat and then actually cooling the flask once the reaction started. Otherwise the contents of the flask would spill over, and one would not get the water clear and uncontaminated product. I carefully did the tedious experiment and obtained a good yield. My good friend Dave botched the whole thing. I thought to myself, "How is he going to get out of this one?" No problem for Dave. He simply ordered the chemical expressly delivered from one of his father's suppliers. The only trouble was that the liquid had a distinct pink color. So Dave put the liquid in an amber-colored bottle hoping that the instructor would be lazy and not check. Apparently the ruse worked because Dave got an A in the course, while I was happy to get a hard earned B.

As a science major in biology, like most premeds, I took all the required courses including histology, genetics, and comparative anatomy. All were excellent courses, and I performed fairly well in them. They also were substantial background for the work in medical school. However, I needed credit points in another science to qualify for the degree. I felt quite confident in chemistry, so I decided to round out this requirement in this subject. What a mistake! I selected physical chemistry that was given in the evenings. It turned out to be a course designed for engineering graduate students and dealt mainly with gas laws involving calculus calculations. My calculus was extremely weak, and the evening work turned out to be sleeping time for me, especially since I could not comprehend what the instructor was saying. I should have dropped this course. I foolishly continued, hoping somehow to skin through. I flunked every exam except the final. I only passed that because some kindly soul whose name I never knew saw my dilemma and kindly passed me his exam paper to copy. After the exam I went to the professor and told him that if he would be kind enough to pass me, I would promise never to go into chemistry. On this sour note, so ended my formal premedical training in science.

Credits in the liberal arts were also requirements, though the premeds called them "crap courses." I thoroughly enjoyed a Shakespeare class taught by a Professor Lyons whom students liked for his dramatic flair and antics. Several of Shakespeare's most important plays were analyzed in class by interaction between student and instructor. There was considerable recitation for which I frequently volunteered. My good voice and sense of timing, as well as a sense of the dramatic, stood me in good stead. This experience encouraged me to believe that I might be talented in acting. I joined the Dramatic Society of Columbia University and acted in several plays. I particularly remember "The Importance of Being Earnest" in which I played the Reverend Dr. Chasabule, DD. The dramatic coach called me aside one day and told me that I ought seriously to consider entering an acting career. This intrigued me. I gave it serious consideration, even though I was sure my family certainly would not favor this prospect. Even after all these years, I often wonder what my life would have been like had I failed to get into medical school and had drifted into an acting career.

I took public speaking as an elective course. Two or three students debated current news items as subjects while the rest of the class served as audience, critic, and judge. I can't claim to have been a great debater, but I did learn to stand up and speak coherently and logically. In some ways, this course was a most useful preparation for what I was eventually to become.

We were required to take philosophy. Most premeds thought this was a waste of time. Many of them cut class and only crammed for the final exam, which was a snap for anyone who had access to lecture notes and last year's exam questions. We were supposed to do a lot of outside reading of the great philosophers' works, but hardly anyone did. I'm sorry to reveal that I did not read them either. My young mind was not attuned to this rather stuffy and inane thinking, yet later in life I found pleasure and profundity in the works of Spinosa, Kant, Montaigne, and others. The section on epistemology made a lasting impression on me. The ways of seeking knowledge and the analysis of the veracity of the beliefs we acquire was a revelation to me. It made me question my thinking on any subject and made me adopt a modus operandi of logical thought, a reliable asset throughout my life.

Another required course was psychology, which I liked because the professor was a very practical character who used a common sense approach. The field of psychology can become quite esoteric in the hands of some individuals. Our professor fortunately did not seem to suffer from any phobias or neurosis that seem to afflict so many who profess to be psychologists. In those days, sex was not a subject that was discussed in society, not even in college classes. This class was an exception. We had open discussions about sex and its problems.

At first this was embarrassing to me, as I had been brought up in complete ignorance of sex. It certainly was never mentioned at home or at school. Naturally I had streetwise sex experiences. The local street gang used to meet in one of the member's cellars, where boys showed off their penises and sometimes even masturbated together. One of the gang had the largest and most perfectly shaped organ that I had ever seen. He was greatly admired and was the only one who had a girlfriend with whom he had intercourse. The others, including myself, never even had a date. We hardly had any money, and it was considered highly improper for boys our age to have dates with girls. So I had relatively little to discuss with our professor. I remember one thing he said that seemed profound at the time and has stuck with me ever since. He pointed out that the act of sex was a gut reaction analogous to defecation. Both acts involve the passage of an object through a body orifice. Both are partially autonomic, that is involuntary, once they have been initiated by the systemic nervous system. And both are accompanied by a feeling of pleasure followed by a sense of relief. This explanation did little to relieve the sexual stimulation on seeing a pretty girl, but it did seem to enhance my enjoyment of a good bowel movement. Anyhow, for no good reason, I got a much needed A in this course.

I managed to participate in one other extracurricular activity, the Camera Club of the University. My interest in photography persisted, and I found much pleasure in the company of other enthusiasts. We had lectures by famous photographers and field trips where we competed to take the most interesting photographs. Some of the members later became professional photographers for *Life* magazine and *The Daily News*. For me, photography was just a hobby and a way to develop what artistic instincts I possessed.

Strangely, this involvement with photography led to a

friendship with a young German professor. I don't remember how we happened to meet since I never took German. Frederick Auhagen was quite different from the other faculty. He was far more affluent, had a fancy car, and made frequent trips to Germany. He also gave lectures for a fee to German-speaking organizations like the Bund. His subject was usually the advances that the New German Republic was making under its new leader, Adolph Hitler. It rather amused me that most of his students were Jewish because they seemed to be the only ones who studied German. He had some of the finest cameras of that era. He was married to a lovely German girl and lived with her family in Elmhurst, not far from where I lived in Jackson Heights. He also maintained an apartment in Manhattan where he had a completely equipped darkroom. On occasion I developed his films there when he was too busy to do it himself. Once we went to Minsky's Burlesque and sneaked in his fast lens Lieca in the hopes of filming the strip tease acts. As photography was strictly forbidden, we had to sit in the back to avoid detection. As a result, the images—especially on 35-mm film—were too small for decent enlargement. The modern telephoto lens and fast film of today would make that project a snap. Nevertheless, we had a good time thinking that we could sneak out some risque pictures. When I consider the easy availability of pornography today, our little excursion seems tame indeed. But at that time it was a daring and adventurous episode.

I genuinely liked Auhagen and looked up to him as a role model of a forward-looking, energetic young man who did what he wanted and carried himself with grace and ease. His tall good looks and attractiveness to women were a source of envy and attempted emulation. After I left college, I lost track of him, except for some small news items about his orations concerning the glories of Germany. After the United States had declared war against Germany, I read in the newspaper that Auhagen had been apprehended and put in jail while attempting to escape to a neutral country. The charge against him was carrying pornographic pictures, but I surmised that Auhagen had all along been an agent and perhaps a spy of the German government. This would have explained his affluence and his many trips to Germany. I never did find out what ultimately happened to him, but in all probability he was interned during the war and then deported to Germany. Through friends of the wife's family, I learned that she divorced him. Thus ended in disillusionment my admiration for Professor Auhagen. This episode taught me not to judge people by appearances.

My concern at this stage was to try to get into medical school at the end of my third year of college. It was possible to do this and still be awarded the bachelor's degree after the first year of medical school. This tactic had the great attraction of saving a year's tuition as well as a year's time. My advisor, no less than Dr. Allen, the Dean, told my academic record and me not to waste my time and money because I was too young not good enough to get accepted after the third year. I should have taken his advice, but I went ahead and applied to several local New York City medical schools. So did my friends Dave and Sol. Much to my disappointment I soon received rejections without even the courtesy of an interview. Despite a straight A record and excellent recommendations, Sol got the same treatment. Dave the rascal got into the famous College of Physicians and Surgeons of Columbia University. This was an astounding development because no one from Seth Low had ever been accepted into this prestigious medical school. We found out later that Dave had an uncle who had, for unknown reasons, considerable influence at P and S. Although happy for Dave, I was inordinately depressed. I did not look forward to another year of college and felt my prospects of getting into medical school even then were slim. I had serious thoughts of quitting college and going into something else.

Just as I was sinking more into a depressed mood, a lucky break came along. Summer jobs were scarce for college students. Since my father no longer had the store, I was looking forward to a fruitless vacation. A passing acquaintance and fellow Seth Low student asked me if I would like to be a counselor at a summer camp in Vermont. I would get transportation, room and board, and enough time off to enjoy activities like tennis, swimming, boating, and horseback riding. No pay—but a bonus of $75 at the end of the season. For once, my family did not have serious objections, so I jumped at the chance to spend the summer away from home. I soon found myself at Grand Central Station, surrounded by the other counselors, directors, a doctor, a nurse, and about 100 screaming kids. Considerable misgivings crept into my mind about my ability to live with so many monsters. However, the trip to St. Johnsbury, Vermont was relatively uneventful.

The camp was set on a hillside that descended into a broad field with a lake, or more accurately a pond, at its edge. The view of the mountains on both sides was exhilarating. After supper I was assigned to one of the individual cabins on the hillside. The cabin accommodated four campers and a counselor. My four campers turned out to be first graders—nice kids but definitely not high achievers. Most could not dress themselves or tie their shoelaces. I learned quickly that parents sent their kids to camp so that they could be taught how to be self-reliant and less clumsy. Other parents simply wanted to get rid of their kids so they could have a decent vacation themselves. I also discovered that only the nurse and I were Gentiles. As I became more experienced in the camping business, I found out that at least Jews owned 90 percent of the camps scattered throughout New England. The campers were also Jewish and came mostly from large cities like Boston or New York. Most were reformed Jews, and I suppose I was picked to be a counselor because they liked their children to be exposed to some Gentiles. This was no problem for me because I had no racial prejudices and had many Jewish friends.

Each counselor had a specialty, mostly of an athletic type such as tennis or swimming. I was relegated to be the craft counselor. This turned out to be mostly basket weaving and other simplistic crafts. The camp had a well-equipped shop, and some advanced carpentry and metal work could be done. I soon discovered that I was also in charge of making the scenery sets for the annual dramatic performance. On rainy days everyone wanted to take crafts. Otherwise only the little ones and the athletic duffers frequented the crafts shop.

Camping was such a new experience for me that I enjoyed all the activities as much or more than the campers did. I learned to swim tolerably well, taught myself to handle a canoe expertly, and even did some horseback riding. They must have had confidence in me for I was chosen to set off the fireworks on the 4th of July. On occasion I was even allowed to chauffeur the campers into town. The camp owned a Model-A Ford station wagon that was a lot of fun to drive. On our single day off, Freddie Schiff, a fellow counselor and Seth Low College student, and I were allowed to drive the Ford to nearby New Hampshire and visit Dr. Allen at his summer home. One of the rare liberal arts students and a great athlete, Freddie was loved by all the kids. He had coached Dr. Allen's children, and we had a cordial visit with Dr. Allen and his family. It did not do me any harm, of course, to be seen in a favorable light by the Dean.

I had a great summer and returned home in late August in much better mental and physical shape. I proudly turned over to my father the $75 dollars I had earned. Now I was ready to go back to college and make a determined effort to get into medical school. The only science course I took was genetics. My other courses were all liberal arts subjects. In many ways, the last year of college was a maturing one for me. I began to fit more into the social structure of my environment. I became editor of the college yearbook. Sol was the assistant editor, and we made a good team working together. I did all the photography and artwork, while Sol took care of any writing that needed to be done. We were assigned a small room as an office, which gave us a place to hang out. It wasn't much of a book as the finances were meager, but then few yearbooks are. Our main task was to get all the pictures of the graduates in, plus some candid shots of the faculty and student activities. Some jokes and trite sayings usually rounded out the whole.

The main social event of the year was the Senior Prom. I had carefully avoided going to the Junior Prom the year before, but peer pressure forced me to go to this one. Since I had never dated a girl, much less had any female acquaintance, I faced a serious problem. My family came to my rescue with a suggestion. They asked a schoolteacher, a busybody who lived across the street, if she knew a nice girl my age who might consent to go to the prom with me.

"Oh yes!" was her enthusiastic reply. "I know just the girl for Joe."

When the night of the Prom arrived, I went forth in my best and only suit, with small corsage in my hand, to the address I'd been given. To my astonishment, it turned out to be a funeral parlor. My impulse was to turn and flee. After much hesitation, I timidly rang the bell. The mother answered the door and escorted me upstairs. I was introduced to a very shy, ordinary looking girl who was clearly even more nervous than I. As an undertaker's daughter, she had some social privations herself, I guess. The evening was dismal. We didn't have much to talk about because she had not been to college and didn't seem to be interested in anything. I couldn't ask her what it felt like to live above some corpses in the cellar. I was an extremely poor dancer, and she wasn't great either. The evening dragged on. I was much relieved when it was over. I never saw her again and don't even remember her name.

I concentrated on applying to medical schools. Through one grapevine or another, I determined that my chances of getting into a prestigious school were nil in view of my unimpressive academic record. My family discouraged using my cousin Salvatore as a source of advice and possible recommendation. By then he was a Clinical Assistant Professor of Obstetrics and Gynecology at Columbia's P and S and might have been of considerable help, but our families were severely estranged and were not talking.

I settled on applying to two medical schools out of town and two in New York City. To my surprise, I was accepted at Marquette Medical School in Wisconsin and the University of Maryland School of Medicine in Baltimore—without even an interview. Since they were out of town, which meant substantial extra financing, I held out for local schools. I got a flat rejection from New York University School of Medicine, which did not surprise me because they accepted only students with superior academic records. I had almost given up hope when Long Island College of Medicine called me for an interview.

As luck would have it, just before my interview I'd been experimenting with photographic flash powder trying to make an electrical device to set off the powder in synchrony with the shutter. Ordinarily it was set off by hand with a flint sparker with the shutter open. This did not allow for candid shots that I wished to take. I concocted a device that worked erratically at best. This time it failed to fire, so I leaned over the pan containing the powder to see why the electrodes had not worked. Flash! The damn device went off, burned my right hand, and neatly removed my eyelashes and my eyebrows. At my interview the next day, I had to present myself with a bandaged hand and a bald face.

To be honest, I was not too nervous going in because I had already been accepted by two schools. I also harbored a secret wish to be turned down so that I might have some excuse not to attend any medical school. But when I entered the interview room, I got the shakes. I was facing four middle-aged doctors. There's an inherent fear of doctors who are purveyors of ominous news. Naturally, their first question was, "What happened to you?" I thought of some bizarre story about an explosion of the gas cooking stove, but I ended up telling them the truth. This didn't impress them much, and they probably thought that I was a clumsy goof.

They wanted to know if I had any experience in medicine. Did I have any associations with practicing doctors? I said I did not except when I had childhood illnesses. My mother had diabetes, and I usually accompanied her when she visited her physician, I added. This did not seem to impress them. Then they asked the question all premeds fear, "Why do you want to become a doctor?" Can you tell them, "It's mainly because my parents really want me to . . ." or answer, "It's a prestigious profession and doctors make a very good living?" Neither are wise answers, although they may be the primary reasons in most cases.

After some hesitation I answered that I genuinely liked people, it satisfied me to do things for my fellow man, and I felt that I had the potential in brains and skills to do this if given the opportunity.

This was a white lie because I actually was a shy person who didn't socialize well and, if the truth were told, I had little concern for my fellow man at this time in my life. With that, the interview ended. I felt that I had done rather badly. Yet, two weeks later, I received an acceptance in the mail. Now my fate was sealed. I had no excuse to avoid going to medical school.

My good buddy Sol had an interview at the same time. Unfortunately, he was short in stature and had a facial tic that became worse when he became excited or nervous. He had a brilliant academic record, however, and we all thought that if anyone should get in, it should be Sol. But he did not get into any medical school. We attributed this to the fact that Sol was Jewish because it was generally conceded that there was a Jewish quota in every school. Several other Jewish students got into Long Island and other medical schools who had good academic records, but not matching Sol's. He was proud and deeply hurt. He did not take graduate work and apply again, as did many unlucky students. Medicine thereby lost a potentially fine and dedicated physician. When I later met some medical students who were in every way unqualified, I had occasion to rue Sol's sad fate and question the fairness of it all.

When the spring term of my senior college year ended, I did not even bother to attend the graduation ceremonies. I collected my diploma from the registrar's office after paying the requisite $25 fee. The diploma was a big sheet of parchment paper bearing the seal of Columbia University and signed by Nicholas Murray Butler, president of the University. At the time, I thought it was just a ticket to medical school. I did not realize the considerable mental and personal development that the last four years had wrought.

The intense competition of the premeds had hardened me and made me more cynical. Although I had spent the first four years of my schooling in a Catholic grammar school, indeed almost becoming an altar boy at St Patrick's Cathedral, I had drifted away from religion by the time I was fifteen. College further convinced me of the fallacies of religion, and it wasn't long before I became an agnostic. I was now twenty years old, hadn't even a glimmer of a love affair, and I faced another four years of grueling medical study.

The Depression wore on, and summer jobs of any kind were hard to find. I decided to be a camp counselor again. Now that I had some experience, I could be more demanding. Through a fellow Seth Low College student whose father ran a summer camp, I got myself a crafts counselor job at the magnificent salary of $150 for the summer. The student, Cy, had serious hearing and sight problems resulting from a middle ear infection in childhood. I mention this because I was expected to be a companion to Cy, which I didn't mind at all because he was a brilliant scholar and had an excellent sense of humor.

The camp was in Lunenberg, Vermont; about fifteen miles north of St. Johnsbury, quite near the Canadian border. A group of six counselors was to go to camp two weeks before it opened to prepare cabins and other buildings for the campers' arrival. The owners had bought a ten-year-old Nash touring sedan for the trip and general use around camp. It was near the end of its useful life but was a great fun car because it was open on all sides. We had a terrific sense of speed even though the greatest acceleration it was capable of was forty miles per hour—downhill. We started toward Vermont on the ancient Boston Post Road that went through every little town as well as the cities. We took turns driving. When we were well into Vermont, the motor began to stall so that we could only travel about ten miles per hour. We stopped at a gas station, where adjustments were made to the carburetor and improved its performance somewhat. We staggered into St. Johnsbury at about eleven o'clock at night, just as the engine quit completely. We were able to push the vehicle to a garage. A sleepy mechanic told us that he would have to take the whole engine apart to find out what was wrong. Calling in to the camp, we found that the resident carpenter had a car and could pick us up. We finally arrived at camp about 1 a.m. Exhausted and extremely cold, we found unmade beds in empty cabins. All we had were mattresses, so we slept in our clothes between two mattresses. I have never been so cold, and I can still remember the shivering and the teeth chattering.

Next morning we had a good hot breakfast and a chance to survey what we had to do to prepare for the camp's opening. As arts and crafts counselor, I had the task of helping the carpenter. About twenty-five cabins were built on piers on a rather steep hillside. Every winter the heavy Vermont snows slid some of them off their supports. Our job was to jack them back up and restore their piers. Some cabins also needed siding replacement as well as repairs to the doors and windows. I enjoyed this work and learned some practical carpentry. Eddie the carpenter was quite a rough and ready character from Brooklyn who liked to work in isolated spots to escape a former wife, a Native American. She would track him down and sit on his doorstep until he escaped to another location. Now he lived in Lunenburg for the summer and shacked up with a woman who had a young child. We were all in on this secret, so we weren't surprised one day when a stoic squaw showed up at camp. Eddie made a quick exit, and eventually his squaw disappeared. Fortunately, we had made all the necessary repairs and preparation and were ready to receive the campers on the first of July.

Camp Winneshewauke was much more substantial than my previous camp experience. It was situated on Miles Pond about seven miles from Lancaster, New Hampshire, a fairly typical New England town that had seen better days when its sweater factory was active. Now it relied on tourism to eke out a living. I found it charming and in sharp contrast to life in the big city.

This summer I was counselor for four boys aged eight or nine who were quite bright and at least knew how to tie their shoelaces. They could even dress themselves, which made life easier for me. I still had bed wetters duty, though. Two counselors took turns staying up late (about midnight; bedtime was nine o'clock), went from cabin to cabin, and woke up the bed wetters so they could urinate and not wet the bed. It was surprising how many bed wetters went to camp. We wondered if parents sent them to camp so as to be rid of them at least for the summer.

The craft shop was well equipped. We had more senior campers who wanted to do more serious projects. Since we didn't have any sailboats, two seniors wanted to install a sail on a canoe. I remembered some plans I had seen in *Popular Mechanics*, and we went ahead on this project. A canoe is inherently unstable so it took considerable improvising to accomplish this. All the parts, including the mast, had to be clamped on because we didn't wish to destroy the canoe. After much work, which I largely did, the sailing canoe was ready. On the big tryout, one of the boys and I paddled out to the middle of the pond. Even without the sail raised, the heavy mast made the canoe very tipsy. It was obvious that the leeboards that I'd attached to the sides of the canoe were too small. Urged on by hecklers on shore, we nevertheless bravely raised the makeshift sail made from old bed sheets. For a moment all seemed well, but the first puff of wind tipped the canoe over completely and dumped us into the pond. We heard the horselaughs as we swam back to shallow water. The canoe could not be righted because the sail gripped the water. After we installed larger leeboards, the sailing canoe functioned to some degree, but I don't recommend putting a sail on a canoe.

I made several trips with the campers that summer. We went to Mount Washington and The Old Man of the Mountain. I was surprised to see a good layer of snow in Tuckerman's Ravine. One counselor even went skiing there on his day off. On one of my free days, I took a solo hike to the top of Mount Moran, which is only slightly lower in altitude than Mount Washington. It can be more or less walked up, but the only difficulty is crossing some rocky fields. I was quite proud to reach the fire tower on top. I had the top of the mountain and the exquisite view all to myself, except for some nosy jackrabbits. Now I understood why some people go to such extremes to climb mountains.

Another trip that sticks in my mind is one I took with two fellow counselors to Maidstone Lake in Vermont. Situated in a basin at the top of the surrounding mountains, it was unspoiled by humans because it was a steep two-mile hike from the highway. The water was absolutely clear, the surrounding scenery breathtaking. Although the water was icy cold, the skinny dip we took was memorable. When I revisited this lake years later, summer cottages and a passable road had been built. I was disappointed because I could not capture the spirit of the past. My children and my wife were still very much impressed, but I wish they could have seen it in its maiden state, appropriate of its name.

The summer passed pleasantly and without any untoward events. I rode the train back to the city with the campers. I didn't volunteer to stay and shut down the camp, as did some of the counselors. The thought of starting medical school made me nervous, and I was anxious to make a good start. I knew that I had to buy a good microscope, so I asked my father if I could use the money I had earned at camp. Through a friend of the family, I learned that I could get a discount if I purchased the scope directly from the Fischer Scientific Company that had an outlet on Third Avenue in downtown Manhattan. The microscope, a Bausch and Lomb monocular with 5x and 10x eyepieces and objectives up to oil emersion complete with mechanical stage and a carrying case, cost all of $125, almost all of my summer earnings. I proudly carried it home with the feeling that I had already arrived at some significant point in my career.

CHAPTER II

Adventures at Medical School

1936-1941

*"There are late bloomers, but most talented physicians show
their mettle early on in medical school."*

Rupert Black, M.D.

Opening day of medical school arrived soon enough. We
freshmen assembled in Long Island College of Medicine's Polhemus
Building amphitheater, a semicircular lecture hall where the floor
was set at an angle of forty-five degrees so that viewers could easily
see into the pit below. At floor level, the pit had a separate entrance
from which patients or demonstration anatomical specimens were
brought in. A mounted skeleton resided in one corner, a movable
blackboard at the rear.

Five distinguished looking portly gentlemen walked in and sat
down. A hushed silence swept over the audience in sharp contrast
to the considerable buzz that had filled the hall a moment earlier.
The man on the end rose and walked to the center of the pit. He
was a rather handsome fellow of medium height, about fifty years
old, with a full head of gray hair and meticulously dressed in
obviously expensive clothes. He introduced himself as Wade Oliver,
the acting Dean and Chairman of the Department of Bacteriology.
After congratulating us for choosing one of the three honored
professions (I later found out that the other two were law and
theology), he smiled sardonically and said, "Look to each side of

you. In six months the fellow next to you may no longer be present."
I was amused to see that every student actually looked to each side
and shuttered a bit.

After this ominous statement, he warned us that professional
behavior was required at all times. We were to be dressed in business
suits with white shirt and tie. Our hair was to be kept trim and
our fingernails clean. We had to wear clean gowns in the
laboratories. Then he smiled and wished us good fortune in our
work in medical school. After this illuminating talk, the other
professors walked out with their accustomed decorum. The buzz
of conversation resumed, this time quite solemn in texture. All I
could think of was how hard and uncomfortable the seats were. In
subsequent lectures I noticed that many of the students had
acquired inflatable doughnuts to sit on.

A buxom fair-haired anatomy secretary then instructed us to
walk up the steps to the top floor (seven or eight stories). The
building had an ancient, rickety elevator operated by a hydraulic
piston that ran from the basement to the top floor. An ancient,
grumpy elevator man operated it. Students were not allowed to
use the elevator so there was much traffic on the stairs. Gradually
we arrived at the top floor and entered a large, well lit room filled
with row upon row of marble tables that each held the unmistakable
outline of a human corpse covered by a well-used tarpaulin. A pail
hung at one end of each table to catch the drippings. We were
handed a paper that gave us our table assignments—four students
to a corpse.

Two students were assigned to one side of the table so that
both sides of the cadaver could be dissected simultaneously. My
partner was a tall bespectacled young man, Dick Dodge, whom I
soon learned was a New Englander who'd gone to Dartmouth. He
had a sense of humor and was not too anxious to hog all the
dissection. The other two were more local residents. One was a
New Jersey lad who had attended Union College. The other was
an Italian from Brooklyn who had gone to LaSalle. I could see
from the start that our table partners were not going to get along
with each other. Both were too anxious to do all the dissection. I

was glad that they had their side of the body all to themselves. At this time the smell of formalin and human fat was not too bad, as the bodies were covered and still intact. How different after a few hours when the students were at work. Many students could not tolerate it and had allergic attacks, yet they persisted. Fortunately the odors or the bodies did not bother me excessively.

Dr. Congdon, chairman of anatomy, came in and began rapping a table with a pointer to indicate that we should all gather around him. I soon learned that he had a habit of giving short talks during which we all had to stand at attention. He explained that we were to get bone boxes that would contain a skull and selected long bones, including the bones of the wrist and the foot. He warned us to treat these bones with great respect, as they were once a living person. He asked us not to expose them to general view, as one student did when he took out the skull and began to study it on the subway. A stiff fine would be imposed if the bones were not returned in good shape at the end of the semester. We were then given general directions about how to dissect the arm and axilla. We also had to purchase a dissecting kit consisting of a scalpel, scissors, and fine forceps.

That afternoon we started our first session of dissection. When we entered the anatomy laboratory this time, the eerie sight of nude cadavers lying row upon row greeted us. Strangely, when the room filled with students, it did not look too bad, as if the living balanced out the dead. The bodies were partly covered with cheesecloth that had to be wetted with formalin solution to prevent the tissues from drying out. The pungent, irritating odor was overpowering. Today formalin is considered a powerful carcinogen and modern medical students probably use some odorless preservative instead. In those days, we were ignorant of this so we gaily plunged in. My partner and I flipped a coin to see who would make the first cut. I won. We cut into the skin deeply and then stripped it back so as to expose the fat layer, muscles, and superficial veins. It was relatively easy to cut if your scalpel was sharp and if you made decisive cuts. We stripped away the skin with the blunt end of the knife or forceps. An expert dissector can strip an arm in a minute, while the inept student pecks and diddles for an hour. I had it half done in about ten minutes, so I turned the arm over to my partner. Getting out our anatomy text—Cunningham's and not the famous Gray's—I began to compare the pictures with the actual muscles in the cadaver to learn the origins, insertion, and functions of the various muscles. Moving each finger individually also helps to identify the tendons that belong to each muscle. The arm is really a marvelous mechanical contrivance.

Across the table, the other half of our quartet was having trouble. Both were so anxious to dissect that each tried to work at the same time. It took them all afternoon to expose the arm. They never looked at the book to learn what they had to cover in the day's assignment. Dr. Congdon rapped his pointer, and we dropped our instruments and gathered around him for one of his small talks. He apparently was the world authority on *fascia,* or connective tissue. The *fascia* divides the organs of the body into various planes and compartments and forms a natural cleavage for the surgeon when operating. These *fascia* planes are not easy to see, especially in the embalmed body. They are not even shown, in fact, in most anatomy textbooks. Congdon had given them names and wanted us to appreciate this special knowledge. Most students grumbled because they felt this was simply useless knowledge that would never be asked on licensing exams. We wanted to know about bone and muscle, nerve and brain, heart and lungs, and other vital structures. We listened attentively, however, because Congdon was such an intense, sincere man, and the students respected him. He had spent much of his professional career in the Far East in places like Siam (Thailand, today), where he had acquired tropical sprue. He had the pale, gaunt features characteristic of this syndrome. He might have indeed been one of the cadavers raised from the dead.

The gross anatomy course ground on and on. We finished the arm and the axilla, moved on to the leg and pelvis, then to the neck. I did as little dissection as possible and studied the book and an anatomy atlas, *Spalteholtz.* I walked about the room frequently, looking at everyone else's dissection, noting differences and relationships. One wall of the laboratory had a series of what looked like a ship's portholes with cross-sections of the body inside. These were most useful to visualize relationships of parts of the body that were difficult to interpret from dissection or diagrams in a book. I knew that a major portion of our grade was determined by our performance on practical exams that were horrendous to most students. A series of tables were lined up around the lab, each containing several dissected portions of the body. Each had a tag attached to a nerve, artery, or other structure that we had to identify. Under the pressure of the exam, the dissection always looked different from anything we had seen before.

The way the exam was conducted also created pressure. After filing in, each student stood before a specimen. A gong would then sound—a Siamese gong that Congdon had imported. Its sonorous sound was itself daunting. At the sound, we were allowed ten seconds to identify the structure. We were not allowed to touch or move the specimen. The dreaded gong would ring again, and we had to move on to the next specimen. After missing the identification of one or two specimens, the student degenerated into a dazed and confused state that rendered him incapable of performance. I was fortunately able to do very well on these practical exams because I had a visual memory and had spent time looking at everyone's dissection. My partner Dick did fairly well, but the other two of our quartet did dismally.

The assistant professor of anatomy was an unusual character named George Paff. Thin, of medium height, with sharp and decisive features, the students either liked him or hated him. There was no indifference about Doctor Paff. He made it his business to know each student personally and soon learned who the would-be smart alecks were. If he took a liking to you, you could do no wrong. I got on his right side early by identifying the bones of the wrist when they were put into my hand held behind my back. He claimed this was a feat first performed by Vesalious, the famous anatomist of Renaissance fame. We also became friendly because we both had a habit of being late in the mornings and sneaking in the laboratory when Congdon started one of his short talks. (More about Paff later as he had a great influence on my career in medicine.)

In the fall semester we were required to take histology. We were issued a box of fifty slides that were sections of the various organs of the body. The histology lab consisted of long rows of benches set at a convenient height for microscope work. We were assigned lockers where we stored our microscope. The instructor was Doctor Sharp, a kind, elderly man who probably would never flunk a medical student if he could avoid it. The students knew this and took advantage of his good nature. He walked around the lab and looked at the drawings of the slides we were required to make. Students asked him obvious questions, which pleased him because he could answer them so easily. Unfortunately the practical exam in histology involved of a row of microscopes with unknown slides that had to be identified. For some diabolical reason, the unknown slides of organ sections never looked the same as those we had studied. Most students, including myself, found histology difficult. I realized I would never be a pathologist.

Three students dropped out of school after the first week of anatomy. They decided that medicine was not for them and that life would be more pleasant in their father's business or some other profession. By the end of the semester, four more students were asked to leave because of academic failure. No allowance was made for repetition of the course or a make-up exam. Of the original 90 students admitted, seven had already been eliminated. I thought about my good friend Sol and what a shame it was that he was refused admission. He could have done the academic work of medical school with ease. My two partners from the opposite side of the dissecting table were dropped. They were nice young men who came from weak colleges, had mediocre records, and were obviously poorly prepared. It was unfair to admit them to medical school when there were better candidates. I noticed that the brightest students generally came from modest income families, often first generation Americans who had gone to City College of New York or some large university. Although critical of the admission committee's judgment, I was grateful that they had admitted me with my rather average record. I found that the work in medical school was indeed easier than my college science courses. I no longer had doubts that I wanted to be a physician. The fact that I finished the first semester easily in the top percentile of the class probably aided this decision.

In the second semester, we had two major courses, physiology and biochemistry, plus a minor course in neuroanatomy. The chairman of physiology was George B. Ray, a tall, heavy man recently imported from Western Reserve University School of Medicine. His major work was spectroscopy of hemoglobin and its variants. He had been associated with C. J. Wiggers, a world famous cardiovascular physiologist. Not surprisingly, Ray had recruited two members of the department from Western Reserve, J. Raymond Johnson, assistant professor and a cardiovascular physiologist, and S.R.M. Reynolds, associate professor and an endocrinologist.

I include these details because my fortune at the Long Island College of Medicine was tied to the Department of Physiology. From the first exposure, I felt akin to the subject. The physiological approach to the normal as well as the abnormal functioning of the body seemed to me to be the most sensible approach. I also liked the laboratory exercises that consisted of animal and human experiments. I even liked to smoke kymograph drums, which most students hated. (These instruments had moving surfaces on which a pin recorded information; the surface had to be "smoked" first for the pin to make an imprint.) I did well in the subject. Students were grouped in quartets at each experiment. We were supposed to take turns as surgeon, technician, note taker, and recorder, but my partners let me do all the work because they saw that I had natural skills and usually could make the experiment work. Once the experiment got under way, they liked to sneak off and play pool in the recreational house next door. Despite this, our group had some of the best experimental records of the entire class.

Biochemistry was an entirely different kettle of fish. Matthew Steel, the chairman, a red-faced individual with a mop of gray hair, laughed easily at his own jokes, which we thought were pointless. His ruddy face, it was rumored, was attributed to the bottle of whiskey he kept underneath his desk. Dr. Steel had written a text of biochemistry that we had to use because the course consisted only of excerpts from his book. His uninspiring text lacked discussion of biochemical theory and consisted simply of detailed methods of biochemical analysis of blood and urine. Most students thought that it was directly plagiarized from Hawk and Bergheim, a well-respected laboratory manual in biochemistry. Our laboratory followed the text closely for it simply consisted of determinations of blood sugar, blood urea, and other common substances in blood and urine. While this was handy information, it was hardly challenging. We received no information about the Emden-Meyerhoff Cycle, which was already known at that time. It was one of the few courses in which we had conferences, but these were mainly quizzes on the details of the chemical determinations that we had to memorize. I suppose there was some merit to this. As an intern later, I could do a blood sugar in an emergency in the middle of the night.

Students were allowed to do a research project on their own time. It was completely voluntary and did not count toward our grades. Most students avoided this, but foolish me undertook a project. I selected the experimental production of rickets. I was assigned a cage of three rats that I had to take care of for six weeks, and I had to devise a vitamin D deficient diet. The cage had to be kept well shaded because mammals can synthesize vitamin D in skin exposed to sunlight. I faithfully did the experiment, and the rats were sacrificed at the end of the period. I was amazed when silver stain of the epiphyseal junction of the tibia showed the typical findings described for rickets.

Dr. Haley, a rather kindly biochemist, told me it was the first time in his memory that a student had made this experiment successful. I had the impression that my instructors were beginning to spot me as a "researcher type." I wasn't too happy with this possibility because there was an unofficial axiom that researcher types generally made poor clinicians, so I made a silent determination to suppress this researcher tendency and concentrate on practical clinical approaches.

The minor course in neuroanatomy turned out to be not so minor. Dr. Novak, the main instructor, was a tall thin young man, trained at Columbia University, who was supposed to be very bright. He was, however, a poor lecturer in a subject that wasn't interesting to most students. Mostly from an atlas, we learned the various nervous tracts and ganglionic connections of the brain and spinal cord. Fortunately another lecturer, Dr. Perkins who was chief of the neurological service, gave us some vivid clinical pictures of various syndromes of lesions of the brain and spinal cord. By actually acting out the gait of a Parkinson patient, or one with syphilitic atrophy of the spinal cord, he made the subject interesting. The exams were made out by Novak and consisted of detailed questions of the structure and functions of the nervous system.

I was quite pleased when my first year of medical school ended because I had passed all subjects and landed in the top percentile of the class. Although I had worked hard, the time flew by swiftly. It seemed to me that the subject matter was distinctly easier than my college courses. The volume of work was greater, but the level of abstract thought was lower.

I contemplated going to camp again as a counselor. But it was still the period of the Great Depression and one of President Roosevelt's projects was helping college students earn tuition money by working in an educational environment. Various departments could hire students to do research or help in teaching. The federal government would pay about $20 a week for such work. One job offer was a research assistant to Dr. Johnson in physiology. This seemed like a good deal to me so I applied and got the job. This was my start in what was to be a long series of research endeavors.

Johnson was a young man, probably about thirty-five, of average height, a narrow face, and a good stock of jet-black hair. He had earned his Ph.D. degree under Dr. Wiggers, who was famous for his cardiovascular research. Johnson's thesis had been on coronary circulation, and he still had an interest in this area. He had an idea that he could dissect under the anterior descendens branch of the coronaries in the anesthetized cat and thus be able to measure pressure and perhaps flow. One of the current items of discussion was whether at peak of systole (cardiac contraction) the internal cardiac muscle pressure was great enough to impede the flow of blood in the coronaries. Wiggers and his coworkers had already worked out in detail the coronary flow curve throughout the cardiac cycle in relationship to aortic blood pressure, but this detailed point was still in argument.

My job was simply to come in early in the morning, get a cat from the animal holding area, anesthetize it with an interperitoneal injection, then operate to open the chest and establish a pericardial cradle. This would properly expose the heart. Artificial respiration was established with the aid of a tracheal cannula. The animals were adequately anesthetized and felt no pain. I loved cats and made certain about this. Blood pressure was measured crudely, even for those days, with a mercury manometer recording on a smoked drum and a mechanical kymograph.

Johnson came in about 11 a.m., sleepy-eyed and rather grumpy. He was married with two children and another on the way. Salaries in those days were at starvation level (about $2,500 a year), and he could not afford help. I suspected that he did the wash and took care of the children while his wife rested. He also left early because he had to do the shopping and cooking. As a result, he diddled about, and the experiment never succeeding in the coronary dissection. It was soon obvious that we were getting nowhere.

In a rare moment of insight, I conceived a different approach to the problem. Why not just sew a section of blood vessel through the myocardium and measure either flow or pressure throughout the cardiac cycle? Johnson thought this was a good idea, but we did not have the proper equipment or the funds to purchase what we needed. Optical manometers, invented by a physiologist named Hamilton, were state-of-the-art then for measuring accurate blood pressure with respect to time. We didn't have one, but this did not faze me at all. Working evenings at home in my cellar workshop with a small lathe; I turned out a couple of manometers from some copper and lead tubing, plus a few other odds and ends. Each manometer had a swivel joint so it could be aimed accurately at an optical kymograph. The only problem was that we did not have an optical kymograph. I was able to rescue an ancient one from a discarded quartz wire electrocardiograph machine. It had only one speed, but it was fortuitously the right one for the cardiac cycle. An old inner tube from a car supplied the necessary rubber membranes.

Johnson happened to have some small front surface optical mirrors of the appropriate diopters. A pinpoint light source supply, scavenged from some other equipment, completed what we needed to proceed. I spent some happy hours calibrating the manometers and adjusting the apparatus to make sure that everything was working efficiently. To our delight, the first experiment was a decided success. We were able to sew a section of carotid vessel obtained from the same cat through the wall of the left ventricle, measure the pressure developed in this vessel, and compare it to that in the aorta throughout the cardiac cycle.

In repeated experiments on a dozen cats, we were able to show that there was a distinct relationship between aortic blood pressure and the tension, or intramyocardial, pressure. With normal aortic blood pressure, the intramyocardial pressure never develops to a higher level than that during systole in the aorta. On the other hand, when aortic blood pressure is raised, the intramyocardial pressure, especially in the inner layers of the heart, does exceed aortic systolic pressure. In the outer layer of the left ventricular wall, intramyocardial pressure never exceeds aortic systolic pressure so that continuous flow is possible. These experiments helped to interpret the increased myocardial ischemia in hypertensive patients and explain why myocardial infarction occurs most frequently in the inner layers of the ventricular wall.

With the data now well in hand and most of the summer gone, I perceived that Johnson was not about to start writing a formal article on our findings, so I proceeded to write it myself. I charted all the pertinent graphs and figures and wrote the text. I handed it to Johnson for review, and he made some minor changes. G. B. Ray, the chairman, also read the paper and thought it was very good. He advised us, however, to wait a few weeks before submitting it because C. J. Wiggers was about to visit the department. Ray would ask Wiggers to review the paper. It would help get it accepted for publication if we could say it had been gone over by this eminent cardiovascular physiologist. Sure enough, Wiggers arrived one day and agreed to review the paper. A large man with an expansive face and ready smile, he smoked a big cigar and delicately tapped the ashes in a convenient beaker. He leaned over a lab table and carefully scanned the paper. I was sure that he was going to tear it apart. Instead, he seemed quite pleased although he made some corrections. He felt that it could be submitted to the prestigious *American Journal of Physiology*.

In all versions of the paper, I had never listed the authors. I assumed that Johnson would discuss this with me because I had done 90 percent of the work and the original idea was mine. I naively assumed that he would put my name first. Although I was pleased when the paper appeared in print in the *Journal*, I was deeply disappointed that Johnson appeared as the senior author. This was petty on Johnson's part, and I determined that I would never collaborate with him in the future. I also resolved that, if I ever did more research with a collaborator, I would always place the younger man's name first whenever possible. I was pleased to observe that in subsequent years Johnson never wrote another paper of the merit of this one. This paper definitely established my reputation as a researcher. I was one of the very few medical students who could claim to have published a paper in a world-class journal while still in his early years in medical school.

Things looked good for me at the end of that summer. I had not only earned some money, but I had actually distinguished myself in research. I handed the money over to my father with considerable pride as I felt that I had earned at least part of my tuition. When I rejoined my classmates in the fall, I discovered that many had summer jobs that paid much more money. One was an ice cream salesman running a small wagon and hawking his wares on suburban streets. Another worked for the Long Island Railroad as a conductor, a job he held throughout the school year by working the night shift. How he managed to study and still

attend school was a mystery. The resources of energy and drive
that most medical students demonstrate will always be a source of
astonishment to me.

In the fall term of the second year, we studied applied
physiology and applied anatomy, which were supposed to correlate
with actual clinical medicine. Much of it was repetition, but we
had some interesting clinical conferences in which patients were
demonstrated before the whole class. This was supposed to make
us feel that we were really going to be doctors. We actually had
somewhat more time off, which I spent in physiology working on
some minor projects. Having done so well, I was accepted almost
as a faculty member in the department.

Pharmacology and pathology followed these courses. In the
1930s, there was no separate department of pharmacology. It was
combined with physiology. Johnson taught the course with the
help of two clinicians, J. Hamilton Crawford, a Scotsman with a
decided brogue that made understanding him difficult, particularly
when he lectured, and George Roberts, a really handsome man
who should have been in the movies. He was esteemed as a clinician,
but it was obvious that he was no pharmacologist. The course
would have been extremely dull except that we had a number of
laboratory experiments that showed the action of drugs in a vivid
manner. We conducted some of the experiments on ourselves, such
as injections of epinephrine or sublingual nitroglycerin, in which
we would self-measure our own blood pressure, pulse, respiration,
and on occasion even basal metabolism. In modern times, such
experiments on animals and humans are not done. Animals cannot
be used for this purpose because of the expense and the objection
of antivivisectionists. Administration of drugs to medical students
for experimental purposes is not done because of informed consent;
if a student had a reaction, the medical school would be certain to
be sued. In this respect, medical education has degenerated to just
ordinary lecture material.

When I took the course in 1937, there were no decent
textbooks of pharmacology. We used Cushney's text, which left
much to be desired because it was mainly material medica rather

than what was later considered pharmacology. Johnson had little or no interest in the subject, and his lectures were merely paragraphs read from the book. Our clinical lectures were just that—lectures about what pill was good for what, spiced with a few clinical anecdotes. On the final exam, one of the main questions concerned the effect of drugs on the coronary circulation. I enthusiastically attacked this question because I thought I had a superior knowledge from my work the previous summer. It was an essay exam, as were all exams in those days. I scribbled away in the blue book and made the fatal mistake of answering more than the question asked for. When J. Hamilton Crawford marked my exam, he took one look and promptly gave me a zero on the basis that he couldn't read my handwriting. Johnson interceded for me and convinced Crawford that it was actually a good answer. Crawford, however, would not allow more than a passing grade of 75. This hurt me deeply because I knew down deep that I had a better knowledge of the subject than most of my classmates who got higher grades. I learned the bitter lesson so important in essay exams: Don't answer more than the question asks and always write as clearly as possible. As fate would have it, I was to have more intrigue with the wily Dr. Crawford.

Pathology was entirely different from pharmacology. Its other name, morbid anatomy, explains that it has a strictly morphological approach rather than an interpretation of principles. In recent years this has changed, but when I took the course it was strictly about structure, with some interpretation of how the change from normal architecture altered function. Jean Oliver, the department chairman, gave all the lectures. He was a tall, thin man with a bald pate and a moustache that he twitched from side to side as he talked. The rest of the faculty looked up to him because he had a worldwide reputation. His fame rested on his fastidious dissection of the renal nephron in health and disease. His lectures were quite good, but he was a terrible speller. He wrote a word on the blackboard and then decided to change the spelling, which he did by rubbing it out with his hand instead of the board eraser. This made the students nervous because they wanted to laugh but didn't dare. Our labs consisted of the examining fresh specimens of organs removed during recent autopsies. We also had an assigned set of histological slides of various disease entities. The assigned textbook was MacCallum, a lengthy, dull tome. Like most students, I got a secondhand copy of Boyd's text that was brief and readable. The course dragged on its weary way, and I managed to get through all the exams without failure, but without any honor either.

Dr. Oliver, the acting Dean, taught the next course, bacteriology. He gave most of the lectures, which were good except for his frequent mention of the Rockefeller Institute and the work he did in foreign countries. The real fun was in the lab where we made culture media, grew cultures in petri dishes and test tubes, and of course made endless slides of bacteria using Gram stain. Arnold Eggert, a real character, was the main lab instructor. A chubby, bent-over, teddy bear-like individual, he had a wry smile and a twinkle in his eye. It was rumored that he was the prototype for the bacteriologist in the famous novel *Arrowsmith*. He was adored by the students but was actually quite strict and didn't let anyone off from doing his work.

An interesting episode involving one of my classmates, a perky young fellow named DiGrady, occurred in the bacteriology laboratory. DiGrady worked next to me because we were arranged alphabetically. He ran excitedly to Eggert one day and pointed out that his culture dish, which was contaminated with fungi, showed a zone inhibiting bacterial growth surrounding each colony of fungi.

Eggert smiled and said, "There's a fellow by the name of Fleming in England who thinks that the fungi produce a chemical that kills bacteria." DiGrady had made the same observation that led Fleming to the development of penicillin. The rest of us non-observant students hid or discarded our contaminated culture plates because it showed poor technique. The moral of this is that discovery depends upon an observant eye and an open but prepared mind. It also requires drive to follow through on the observation. Thousands of bacteriologists, students, and technicians must have made the same observation, but only Fleming followed through to give the world penicillin and the wholly new field of antibiotics.

Up to this point in medical school, most of us still felt like undergraduate college students. But that all changed when we were required to purchase short white jackets, stethoscopes, ophthalmoscopes, otoscopes, reflex hammers, and pocket flashlights. These made us feel that we had arrived into the real world of doctoring, and we happily made these purchases. Wealthier students naturally bought fancy expensive models, while most of us made do with more staple items. The stethoscope had to fold so that it draped noticeably out of the left-hand jacket pocket. The flashlight and wooden tongue depressors were inserted in the chest pocket, while the ophthalmoscope and blood pressure machine were carried in a small doctor's bag. This was all for a course called, in those days, "Physical Diagnosis," a series of short lectures that briefly outlined how to take a medical history and perform a physical examination.

The practical part of the course involved of small groups of students with an individual instructor. For the first couple of weeks, we spent our time examining each other. We had a great deal of fun in our group when we found that one student had a tiny cockroach stuck in the wax of his ear canal. The poor fellow had to suffer the jibes of his classmates for the rest of his career in medical school. We learned to percuss and ascultate, to listen to heart sounds and breath sounds. Quite a few students were surprised to discover that they had abnormalities like high blood pressure, heart murmurs, and extra systoles. Real patients came next. We were assigned to examine patients individually on the wards of the Long Island College Hospital, Kings County Hospital, and Brooklyn Hospital. I was assigned to Kings County Hospital.

My first exposure to the wards was quite a shocker. It was still the Depression; destitute people would claim serious illness just to be put to bed and get clean sheets, shelter, and three square meals a day. Most had chronic conditions that could have been treated at home. They were interspersed with seriously ill patients because a city ordinance dictated that no one could be refused admission to city hospitals. Kings County was a 2,000-bed hospital, but at any time there were at least 3,000 patients in residence. Wards that were supposed to hold thirty-five patients held sixty or seventy. Beds were lined up in the halls and in the middle of the wards, creating a general pandemonium—not to mention an extreme fire hazard because many patients insisted on smoking. Some patients were coughing, some spitting, some in obvious respiratory distress, and many just moaning.

There were only two private rooms to a ward, and they were used to isolate only the most dangerous communicable diseases. Cases of pneumonia, tuberculosis, and syphilis were interspersed on the open ward. None of us wore masks or gloves, nor did we take any other precautions to avoid being infected. One classmate, who never entered a hospital without carefully putting on a facemask and gloves, was considered to be psychotic. He was probably a victim of obsessive-compulsive behavior because he also washed his hands at least thirty times a day. Actually, he wasn't so dumb because many doctors and nurses who were exposed to patients did become infected with tuberculosis and other diseases. Medicine as a profession had its inherent dangers.

I liked physical diagnosis and energetically went around taking histories and doing physicals. Using our assigned text, which was Major's, I soon found examples of most of the illustrations in the book, such as disorders of gait and posture, various facies, and abnormalities of the skeleton. As I rode the New York subways two hours every day, I recognized that the most varied clinical material in the world was right before my eyes. The facies of disease were the most interesting, and I collected cases of acromegaly, hypothyroidism, hydrocephalus, Down and Marfan syndromes, and many others.

We also had a course called Introduction to Medicine, which consisted of assigned reading in Cecil's textbook, followed by quizzes. By the end of the term, we had a pretty good idea of the standard disease syndromes. We also had a lecture course in obstetrics given by the famous professor and chairman, Alfred Beck himself. The Long Island College of Medicine prided itself on its history of excellent obstetrical services headed by a series of distinguished obstetricians. Beck was obviously a Prussian and strict disciplinarian. He assigned seats alphabetically and by number. He called on individual students to recite assigned reading from a text that he wrote. Beck tolerated no absences, which he noted by simply marking down the number of the empty seat. That's how we discovered that we had a student whom no one had ever seen in the class. Apparently he never attended classes but had friends who supplied him with lecture notes. He just came in, took exams, and believe it or not, did graduate. That is, not before he had to make up his absences in Beck's class.

Despite the rigidity of the course, we learned in detail the physical diagnosis of pregnancy, its stages, and all aspects of the actual delivery. Although most of us were not interested in obstetrics, it was excellent training for our assignment of delivering at least fifteen babies in our clinical years.

As a result of my research work the previous summer, I was allowed to hang around the physiology department. I even managed to do a little research and publish two short technical papers in *Science*. But this activity cut in to my study time, and consequently I didn't do as well academically as I had done the first year of medical school. Still, I was in the upper third of the class and in some ways ahead of my classmates who did nothing but concentrate on their work. When the next summer arrived, I could have worked in physiology again or returned to summer camp as a counselor. I was anxious to improve my clinical skills, however, so like many of my classmates I sought a summer externship at a hospital. With two of my classmates, I was pleased to secure a position at the State Tuberculosis Sanatorium at Oneida, New York. Early in July we set out for Oneida. We were quite happy with our choice because we were treated as if we were already physicians. The food was excellent, and we had quite handsome private rooms. The work was leisurely as befits a sanatorium. We really had to do nothing but observe and learn. The patients were mostly ambulatory. It was difficult to realize the extent of their disease until we saw their x-rays and visualized the cavitation and destruction of their lungs. We soon realized that the doctors and nurses also had arrested tuberculosis and many worked there because they were unable to withstand the rigors of private practice. Few people today can realize the deadly scourge of tuberculosis and the burden of morbidity and mortality it inflicted on the population. At that time, tuberculosis was a far greater problem than is AIDS today. Doctors and nurses, because of frequency of exposure and their strenuous lifestyle, were ready victims. As many as 10 percent of a graduating class of physicians or nurses would eventually acquire tuberculosis. I found this out by firsthand experience.

All newcomers to Oneida were required to have a physical examination and a chest x-ray. My classmates and I were no exception. After taking the tests, two days later I was called to the front office to confront a grim-faced staff physician.

"Young man, you have tuberculosis!"

He raised my x-ray to the light box and pointed out an abnormal shadow about the size of a half-dollar in the upper lobe of my right lung. A shiver went down my spine, and a lump developed in the pit of my stomach.

"But I have no symptoms, no cough, no sputum, no fever," I replied.

He shook his head. "That doesn't matter. The lesion is typical, and if you do not receive treatment you will go on to cavitation and open tuberculosis in a few weeks."

"What do I have to do?" I asked.

"You have to be on complete bed rest for at least a year. I strongly urge you to go home immediately and start treatment."

I left Oneida and arrived home completely devastated. My folks were equally upset and went into the usual harangues about keeping late hours and not eating properly. I went to see the Chairman of Medicine, Dr. Tasker Howard, a kindly man in his early sixties. Looking at the x-ray, he confirmed the diagnosis but admitted that on physical signs alone, the presence of the tuberculosis infection could not be made. He arranged for me to be admitted to the tuberculosis ward of the Long Island College Hospital for a complete workup.

The tuberculosis ward was a solarium on the top floor of the hospital where windows were kept open, even in wintertime, because fresh air and sunshine were considered beneficial. About fifteen beds were occupied by severe open cases of tuberculosis. It might have been silly, but I felt I might get additional infection and kept my mouth under the covers most of the time. Dr. Howard assigned a young pulmonary specialist, Alfred Ingegno, to take care of me. Everyone was most solicitous, especially the student nurses. After a month of complete bed rest, my sputum remained negative, and by x-ray the lesion in my right lung appeared stable. I was discharged to continue complete bed rest at home for six months. No medications were of any value. If the natural defenses of the body could not heal the disease, you were doomed to a slow death. The complete bed rest theory—and this means lying flat most of the time—was that the upper lobes of the lung, where tuberculosis most often started, were relatively starved of blood when in an upright position. The horizontal posture was beneficial because it improved the blood supply to these parts. No one ever proved this scientifically, but it appeared reasonable and I followed the routine faithfully. Images of x-rays of patients with far advanced tuberculosis were always in the back of my mind; along with the thought that it was impossible to recover once the disease had advanced to a certain point.

Endless hours flat on my back allowed more than ample time to think about my future. I lay completely helpless at the age of twenty-three when I should have been with my classmates doing the clinical work of the third year of medical school Whether I would continue in medical school or turn to a less demanding occupation depended on the degree of recovery. Even if I recovered to the satisfaction of my physicians and returned to my medical studies, I wondered whether I should concentrate on a research career rather than the more strenuous practice of medicine. I could choose a specialty like pathology or radiology that were pretty much sit-down professions with little legwork or patient contact. I decided to play it by ear, but deep down my desire was to practice, particularly internal medicine. I'd had enough contact with patients already to feel that I could relate to them, and I believed I had the ability to diagnose and treat disease skillfully. The daily drama of contact with sick patients and the mysteries of disease were far more interesting than the monotonous collection of data that serious inquiry requires. The monetary rewards were, then as now, much less in a research career. Intellectual rewards were much greater in an academic following, and I could not put that aside lightly. I knew that my family, who had given me so much support, would be disappointed if I did not practice medicine.

Despite all my misgivings, I realized that fate would decide my destiny. I might just as well sit back and enjoy the unfolding of my future. After six dreary months went by, I was finally allowed to dangle my legs off the edge of the bed. I began to walk again a few days later. A chest x-ray showed considerable healing, and I had no other symptoms. It was decided that I could be ambulatory, but that I must lead a very quiet life for at least six more months with regular hours and bed rest for two hours each afternoon.

George Ray, the chairman of physiology, who had been so impressed with my research work, offered me a part-time teaching job in the department. I was to help in the laboratory by teaching physiology studies. I plunged into this opportunity with great enthusiasm because it allowed me to undertake research that might have more direct and immediate clinical application. An associate professor, Sam R.M. Reynolds, was an endocrinologist in a then rapidly growing field of research. A short, stocky man with an energetic attitude, he had a commendable reputation as an outstanding researcher. He was able to relate his work to clinical problems and was much sought after by clinicians, particularly gynecologists and obstetricians who had need of endocrine answers to their problems. More importantly, he had grants to fund his research. This support was a rare event in the days before National Institute of Health grants. Reynolds was envied by the less fortunate faculty and was considered to be too aggressive and opportunist. He could afford to have his own technician and travel to meetings, an added source of jealousy to the rest of the faculty. I had a strong feeling that Ray and Johnson didn't like him but tolerated him because he was such a capable scientist. Despite their feelings, I decided to latch onto him because he represented a better chance for productive research. I approached him and boldly asked if he had a research problem that I could assist him in possibly solving. He looked at me with a twinkle in his eye and a smile. "Yes. I do have a problem that I think you can help me with, but it will take a lot of ingenuity."

Reynolds had been working on the effect of estrogens on bleeding tendencies in women. At the height of the menstrual cycle when blood estrogen is at its highest level, some women tend to have petechia (tiny hemorrhages in the skin) or even nose bleeds. He had access to a group of post menopausal women who were receiving estrogen injections. Reynolds had been researching their bleeding tendency by measuring skin capillary fragility, which was done by a negative pressure to a given area of skin for a determined time and then by counting the number of petechii that formed. The method proved to be inconsistent and insensitive, so he needed to find a better index.

"I wonder if, by applying the observations of Sir Thomas Lewis on the blood vessels of the human skin, we can come up with a better method?" he asked me.

"I'll look into it." I was elated that Reynolds thought enough of me to give me a problem that he had been unable to solve. I was also pleased that this work involved human subjects and was a clinical problem.

I started by a careful reading of Sir Thomas's monograph entitled, "The Responses of the Smallest Blood Vessels of the Human Skin." The prose was precise and most readable, so typical of English authors. The observations were all direct and subjective without the use of any apparatus, but nevertheless all valid. I read and reread about the "triple response" of the skin blood vessels to injury. This consisted of the local red response that occurred only in the exact area where the injury was applied, the flare that occurred in the surrounding area, and the swelling or edema that occurred later. Try as I might, I could not seem to get an idea that would advance our knowledge so that the "triple response" could be used to determine the effects of estrogen or, for that matter, any other drug. I knew I had to devise a method for measurement, but I couldn't figure out what or how.

I sat on the toilet one day and took a long time thinking about this problem. I happened to glance in the mirror when I got up. Sure enough, there was a ring of red where the toilet seat had pressed against my buttocks. The solution to the problem struck me like a flash. The weight of my body on the toilet seat had caused a compression of the skin blood vessels, or a period of oxygen deprivation, which medical people call ischemia. When the compression was relieved, the blood vessels dilated, presumably to make up for the period of ischemia—hence the redness of the skin. Other investigators had described this phenomenon and called it reactive hyperemia. But none had thought how it might be applied to other problems.

I hurriedly raced to the lab, turned out rubber rings with a surface area of five square centimeters, and cemented them to 500 gram lead weights. Some calculations assured me that, when applied to the weight loading of 100 grams per square centimeter, the apparatus would definitely occlude the skin blood vessels. I applied three weights evenly and firmly to the skin of the forearm by a special device that I also created. The three weights could be raised separately at appropriate times and the resultant hyperemia interpreted. I found that at room temperature the average subject would require a period of ten to fifteen seconds to develop a ring of even hyperemia. Lesser times would result in uneven or mottled redness, while longer times would cause a flare of redness beyond the area of application of the weight. It was therefore possible to produce a threshold response dependent on the length of time the weight was applied. Other experiments showed that the threshold time depended on the state of tone of the small blood vessels of the skin. I also found that the time it took for the threshold hyperemia to disappear completely was related to the rate of blood flow in the skin. This was called the clearing time.

I felt that I now had measurements that could be used to detect physiological and biological variables of the small blood vessels of the skin. When I showed the apparatus and preliminary results to Reynolds, he was enthusiastic and offered me the part-time services of his technician, Frances Foster, an intelligent young lady. I taught her the methodology, and she became quite sufficient. We decided to do a large number of normal subjects over a long period of time to establish accurate figures for comparison with abnormal conditions and the effects of drugs on them. With the help of Ms. Foster and many student volunteers as subjects, we collected data over the period of a year. This study resulted in a fine paper on the hyperemia ring test, individual and seasonal variations, which was published in the *American Heart Journal*. This time my name was listed first, for Reynolds was a fairer and more generous person than Johnson. I was pleased to receive many requests for reprints. I was even bold enough to send a reprint to Sir Thomas Lewis along with a letter thanking him for the inspiration of his work on the "triple response." He replied with a gracious letter that I greatly treasured. Imagine me—a mere medical student—being praised for my research work by such an eminent clinician and scientist!

Meanwhile I did not neglect my teaching duties that I enjoyed very much. I was about the same age as the students, so I could empathize with their feelings quite easily. I helped several of them get over difficult interpretations in physiology, which helped me because I usually ended up learning more than they did. Ray seemed pleased with my work and asked me to make a working model of the human respiratory rib cage, illustrating the movements of inspiration and expiration. Paff helped me salvage an old but usable human rib cage that I mounted on a ring stand and articulated so that the respiratory movements could easily be visualized. Paff loved the model, and after this we became closer friends.

The spring semester passed quickly, and I worked through the summer to complete and extend the reactive hyperemia research. My health fortunately remained good. I was careful to include two extra hours of bed rest every day and to eat a nutritious diet. My medical advisors felt that I now could enter the third year of medical school. So in September of 1939, I happily rejoined the Class of 1941.

My junior year turned out to be three morning hours of lectures, plus attendance at ambulatory clinics each day. The lectures were boring, but everyone religiously attended. The rubber doughnut (for my rear) came in very handy as we listened to various clinicians expound on their various specialties. I particularly remember those given by the ophthalmologist John Evans who'd had poliomyelitis and walked with crutches. An excellent clinician and researcher, he had a laboratory next to Reynolds that I had occasionally visited. Evans was kind enough to explain to me his work on flicker-fusion, a specialized test of eye function.

The work in the clinics was practical but not very challenging. Most patients were old timers who had been coming to the clinics for years. Their charts bulged with notes and lab reports and numerous histories and physicals taken by generations of medical students. Many of them spoke a foreign language, and it was impossible to find out why they came to the clinic. On the whole, it was a good experience because it resembled a crosscut of medical practice that we would probably be exposed to later. With the specialty clinics like otolaryngology, ophthalmology, gynecology, and urology, we learned to be familiar with these specialties. Our education was designed for general practice, and we really needed no further instruction to be quite competent in this field. I managed to get by this year without major incident.

The fourth year began on the first of July with rotations in medicine, surgery, pediatrics, obstetrics and gynecology. My rotations started with obstetrics and gynecology, split into four weeks each, at two different hospitals. The first was Methodist Hospital, a private church hospital that catered to the middle class. The women demanded absolutely painless childbirth, and they got what they wanted. Each childbirth was an exercise in anesthesia—heavy preliminary sedation followed by chloroform. As a result, there was much use of forceps and difficulty in getting the baby to breathe spontaneously. Students seldom got to do much, but we had to stand by and watch every step. We were on call every third night and usually got a few hours sleep on a stretcher. The nurses were old battleaxes who loved to hassle med students.

There was a strict pecking order. On Sundays the attending physicians made rounds in frock coats. When they entered the ward, the nurses stood up at attention. Needless to say, I didn't learn very much, either practically or theoretically.

My next experience at Greenpoint Hospital was in marked contrast. At this large public hospital in the poorest section of Brooklyn, interns and residents did all the deliveries. Seldom did a night pass with fewer than ten births. No sedation or anesthesia was used. Unlike at Methodist's sedate birthing rooms, plenty of yelling and screaming was heard all night long. Interns were fed up with doing so many deliveries and let the students do as much as possible with the help of nurses. I easily got in my fifteen required deliveries. I even got to do a couple of episiotomies, although I never got to use forceps. Though it was an interesting experience, I knew that I would never have a deep attachment to obstetrics or to gynecology.

Pediatrics, for the most part, was interesting because we visited various hospitals and children's services, which I had no idea even existed. The infectious disease hospital in Brooklyn was the most fascinating. Here we saw cases of diphtheria, typhoid, and even leprosy, as well as the usual childhood diseases like measles, chicken pox, and scarlet fever, but in their most severe forms. The thing that perhaps impressed me most was the character of the pediatricians. They were always kind, concerned people who represented an atmosphere of youth themselves. Some even had cherub-like features. I wondered if they were that way to begin with or whether it was acquired from their association with children.

Medicine was the longest rotation—16 weeks. Part of this time, however, was spent in psychiatry and neurology. I was assigned to Kings County Hospital for the entire time, which turned out to be a lucky break because Philip Kendall chose me, one of the residents, to be his student. Phil was shrewd. He managed to pick students who were industrious and bright so that he could exploit them and make his own work easier. In return, if he liked the student, he was a very good instructor and allowed the student to do procedures ordinarily done only by interns. He would also sneak us in to the house staff dining room for free meals, and even let us use the dormitory so that we could sleep in a bed on our nights on call rather than on a stretcher in a back hall.

The price we had to pay for these favors was to do all the blood counts and urine analysis on his patients. It was actually a good deal because I soon found out that we didn't learn much from the attending physicians. Phil treated us as equals, but that did not stop him from being sharply critical of our mistakes. There was plenty of clinical material and we made rounds twice a day. I learned all the practical tricks of history taking and physical diagnosis, and I perfected my skills. Phil even let me do spinal taps, chest taps, and paracentesis. I was able to do bone marrow biopsies and a colonoscopy. I particularly liked admissions duty because I got to work up a patient fresh and come to my own conclusion about diagnosis and therapy.

About this time, students applied for internships. The majority of students did graduate work before they went into practice. Most did only a year or two at the most. A rotating internship provided experience in medicine, surgery, pediatrics, obstetrics and gynecology, plus a few specialties like otolaryngology, which was the most popular. This adequately prepared us for general practice, which at least 60 percent of the class preferred. Internships and residencies were not salaried. The only recompense for working long hours, seven days a week, was room and board and uniforms in some cases. If a student was married and the hospital found out, the student never got the internship.

There were more applicants for the more desirable internships than there were positions. Competition was very keen for internships at the major academic center hospitals like Columbia, Cornell, or New York University. Large private charity hospitals like Lenox Hill, Mount Sinai, and St. Vincent's were also very desirable. City hospitals, like Bellevue and Kings County, were least favored because there was less teaching and more work.

Restricted services were assigned to the medical school for teaching purposes and were highly sought after. This is what I sought at Kings County Hospital so that I could be with my favorite preceptor, Philip Kendall, but I knew it wouldn't be easy because my history of tuberculosis would put me at the bottom of any list. Chiefs of service wanted not only the brightest but also the most robust students who would do the most work. My ambitions soon cooled because my physicians and advisors insisted that it would be wisest to delay my internship at least a year to allow my tubercular lesion to heal completely. This was most depressing news. To lose another year after so many years of study and devoted effort was a severe blow.

What could I do to change this decision? Nothing. So I decided to make the best of it and not waste the year in leisurely activities. Fortunately, Dr. Ray came to my rescue again and offered me a job as instructor in physiology and pharmacology at the handsome salary of $1,800 dollars a year. That gave me a base of operations as well as an opportunity to pay my family back for some of the many expenses they had incurred for my education. Sam Reynolds also confided that he was leaving to take a Guggenheim fellowship with Dr. Corner, a famous embryologist and endocrinologist, at the Carnegie Institute of Research in Baltimore. He was willing to leave his laboratory and some useful equipment for my use. More importantly, he set up an interview for me with Dr. Frank Fremont-Smith, then chief officer of the Josiah Macy Foundation, which supported medical research. Sam wisely advised me to apply for a research project that would use our reactive hyperemia ring test to develop better diagnostic and prognostic criteria for traumatic and surgical shock. Although the United States was not at war that spring of 1941, war clouds were developing, and scientists were beginning to concentrate attention to medical problems of warfare. Circulatory shock was a prime target.

My interview at Josiah Macy Foundation, located in an impressive mansion between Park and Madison Avenues, was a success despite my extreme nervousness. I never did find out, but I suspect Sam urged Gregory Pincus, an advisor to the foundation, to put in a good word for me. Pincus later achieved great fame as the originator of oral contraceptives. Whatever the circumstances, Fremont-Smith offered me a grant of $3,000 dollars, which was more than adequate to allow me to hire a research assistant and pay all expenses for the year's research. He had one special request of me. Before I started the work, he asked that I visit Walter Bradford Cannon for guidance and advice. Cannon could truly be said to be the father of physiology in the United States. He had just retired as chairman of the physiology department at Harvard Medical School and was now a visiting scientist at the New York University College of Medicine.

I rode the IRT subway at Lexington Avenue and walked east to First Avenue, where I found the old red brick Victorian building that housed the physiology department. I walked up to the third floor and spotted an older lady who directed me to a room at the end of a long, dark corridor. Through the open door I could see an elderly man sitting at an old oak desk next to a huge window. This was apparently an old laboratory with wooden benches but no other appurtenances—no books, no papers, or other paraphernalia common to professors' offices. A musty smell pervaded the air. Cannon noticed me and without getting up, motioned me to a chair beside the desk facing him. He was rather on the short, stocky side with a square face and kindly eyes decorated with steel rimmed glasses. On the smooth desk surface, little white flakes looked like dandruff. I immediately saw that they came from a scaly rash on his hands. From time to time he would scratch his thigh, suggesting that the rash covered other parts of his body. This made me uncomfortable, and I felt itchy myself. I could not help but think what a sad twilight for one of the country's greatest scientists. I did not know it at the time, but Cannon had mycoides fungoides, a form of skin cancer acquired from working with unshielded x-rays early in his career. He was the first to study the movements of the human stomach using fluoroscopy.

"I read your paper and research proposal with interest and I believe that you may have a useful contribution," he said as he looked at me whimsically. "You know that I was head of a commission to study circulatory shock for the military in World War I. The main problem they wanted solved was to distinguish recoverable shock from irreversible shock. This was important for triage officers in the field because only so many could be saved, and quickly picking the salvageable ones would actually save lives. Although blood pressure and pulse were the main indicators, they often proved to be poor predictors. Perhaps your method of assaying reactive hyperemia might turn out to be a better index."

Naturally I agreed and indicated my willingness to work in his suggested direction. Cannon went on to say, "I also recommend that you send apparatus and directions to these prominent scientists working on shock so that you may have comparisons with their results." He then handed me a list of six people with their addresses. I agreed to do this, but I really didn't like the idea of letting someone else get ahead of me by using my invention. We parted without shaking hands, presumably because of his rash. He wished me good luck with the research, and I expressed the desire that he continue to advise me as work progressed.

My next stumbling block was the new dean of the medical school, Jean Alonzo Curran. He had arrived the previous year and was still trying to prove himself to the faculty and the Board of Trustees. Curran was about as genuine a WASP as could be found. A graduate of Harvard Medical School, he had never practiced medicine but had gone from one administrative position to another. The Rockefeller Foundation had sent him to Peking University in China, which was the right track to be on for a deanship at that time. His one claim to fame was a monograph of a survey of U. S. internships and graduate medical training. I shuddered when I got a call to see him. A lowly medical student finishing his senior year is always likely to feel that it's bad news when the dean wants to see you.

My heart sank as Miss McNamara, the portly secretary of countless prior deans, motioned me toward the heavy oak door on the second floor of the Polhemus Building. When I entered the room, the impressive wood paneling, an enormous mahogany desk, oil paintings of imposing former faculty, and thick carpeting struck me. Curran was no less imposing. He was about average height with a broad brow above thick eyebrows and deep set piercing blue eyes. He motioned me to a chair.

"Young man, don't you know that you put me in a very embarrassing position by applying for a grant from the Josiah Macy Foundation without going through proper channels? You should have at least informed me before applying. Now the faculty thinks I helped you, a mere medical student, get a grant instead of representing one of them."

I thought that if I had I gone through proper channels, they probably would insist that some low achiever like J. Raymond Johnson would have to be assigned as principal investigator. However, I simply replied, "Sir, I am sorry I put you in a bad position, but in my enthusiasm I plunged ahead to secure a grant that would bring honor to the Long Island College of Medicine. Also, you must know that I will be a member of your faculty in July."

Curran softened a bit. "I don't understand how you, a son of a grocer with a modest academic record, could be such an active researcher."

What he meant was "How could someone of Italian background from a lower-income family have acquired the motivation and inspiration to do high class science?" He himself, who had been to Harvard and the Rockefeller Institute, had never written a scientific paper.

I said humbly, "Sir, I had an excellent education at Columbia University and, though my overall average was poor, I did relatively well in science."

Could I tell him that the real reason was that I spent my youth building model airplanes and developed a habit of self-study in the science of aeronautics, while my peers played baseball or some other sport? Could I tell him that I never had the slightest interest in medicine? That I went into medical school because I wanted to please my family?

Curran's eyes narrowed and he looked at me shrewdly. "Who helped you? Who put you on to getting this grant?"

I answered innocently, "Well, you know I've been working with Dr. Reynolds and, at his encouragement and backing, I applied to the Josiah Macy Foundation."

With a knowing look, Curran snapped back, "Ah, I see. Reynolds is too aggressive, and he also breaks rules. But I must admit he has been a very successful investigator."

"Sir," I responded, "I also had the support of C. J. Wiggers and Walter Bradford Cannon." The last name was not quite true because I only met Cannon after I had already received the grant. But aware that Curran was a Harvard graduate, I knew the Cannon name would impress him.

Curran seemed to soften further. "You must have done some fine work to have such distinguished support. This time I am going to let you have the grant. But in the future, work through proper channels. Please keep me informed of every move you make with outside agencies. I may even be able to help you. It happens that I know Frank Fremont-Smith quite well."

With this, the interview was over. Curran actually shook hands with me. I expressed my thanks and made a graceful exit.

The next event in my young life is most memorable. I again owe this experience to good old Sam Reynolds who said to me one day, "How would you like to attend the federation meetings in Chicago and present a paper before the American Physiological Society? I was going to go myself, but I am so busy preparing for my fellowship that I would appreciate it if you would go in my stead. Besides, this reactive hyperemia work is more yours than mine. I have enough money in my grant to cover your airfare and hotel expenses." Of course, I jumped at this opportunity to present my work at a national meeting.

In the early days of these physiology meetings, all papers were presented in person, and there were no poster sessions. Researchers were allowed ten minutes to present and five minutes for discussion. My presentation was in the morning. About sixty people were in the audience, including C. J. Wiggers, G. B. Ray, A. J. Carlson, L. N. Katz, and other prominent physiologists. Katz, a bushy-haired aggressive individual, got up after each presenter to criticize the technology or the reasoning of each paper by quoting his own extensive work on the subject. An argument began among the distinguished physiologists in the front row, and the poor speaker usually staggered off the stage convinced that his career in science had just ended. This made me very nervous. When my turn came, my knees and voice were so weak that I could hardly walk to the podium, much less begin to speak. My previous dramatic and public speaking experience came to my rescue, however. I was surprised to hear my voice come out loud and clear, and I made my points in an assertive manner. I spoke directly to the audience rather than to my slides.

Sure enough, as soon as I finished L. N. Katz jumped up and, to my astonishment, said: "I congratulate these investigators for a piece of original work. They have put the observations of Sir Thomas Lewis on a measurable basis. This appears to be a practical method of assaying the peripheral circulation in man in both health and disease." After this laudatory remark, no one else was about to find error in my work. There were some questions on technology that I could easily answer. I walked off the stage elated, certain that I had now joined the brotherhood of scientists.

After the session George Ray told me that he knew L.N. Katz well, and this was the first time he had ever heard him actually congratulate someone on work well done. Ray was obviously pleased with me and invited me to have pre-dinner cocktails at the hotel bar that evening. When I arrived at the bar, Ray and Johnson had already had a couple of drinks and were obviously feeling good. When asked what I wanted to drink, I would have liked to answer a soft drink. But not to appear naïve, I said the first thing that came into my head: a dry martini with an olive. I never had one before. In fact, I had never had any hard liquor. The most alcohol I had experienced was a half glass of my father's homemade wine.

The first martini went down easily, and I felt a glow. Keeping pace with Ray and Johnson, who were experienced drinkers, I managed to down a total of five martinis in the space of 90 minutes. The conversation was animated with off color jokes. When I tried to stand, I discovered that I was very inebriated. When they invited me to dinner, I had the good sense to excuse myself on the basis of another engagement. I staggered to my room, weaving and almost falling several times along the way. I was terribly nauseous and probably would have vomited if I'd had anything in my stomach. I fell into bed in a stupor and woke the next morning with a terrible headache. I had planned to spend the next day attending meetings, but after forcing down some breakfast and two cups of black coffee, I decided to get some fresh air.

As I walked along Michigan Avenue, the breeze from the lake cleared my head, and I began to feel better. I discovered the Chicago Art Museum and spent the next few hours admiring the excellent collections, especially the more modern artists. My appetite returned. After a good lunch, I visited several camera shops for which Chicago was famous at that time. I was able to get several items of used equipment to complement my photographic paraphernalia. I'd acquired the habit of smoking a pipe, so it was a pleasure to find a fine tobacco shop. The purchase of the best briar and aromatic tobacco I could afford completed one of the finest afternoons I can remember. That evening I went to the conference dinner where I was able to hobnob with other young investigators from different laboratories.

The next day I attended meetings and visited both the scientific and commercial exhibits. On returning home, I felt quite satisfied with myself, but I also learned that I should never drink more than two cocktails. In subsequent years, I have attended scores of conventions and meetings in many different cities, but none had the flavor and impressions of this, my first one.

My final month as a medical student was hectic. Not only did I have to prepare to take the New York State Medical Licensing Examination, but I also had to prepare to start my research project. I was fortunately on an easy psychiatry rotation and had considerable free time to study. My main concern was finding a suitable assistant who could learn to do the reactive hyperemia test and work with patients. Miss Foster, who had worked with us on the initial project, didn't feel equal to working at Kings County Hospital where the bulk of patients with circulatory shock were to be found. After much searching and interviewing, I located Mrs. Blanche V. Richards, a registered nurse. Although she did not have a college degree, she was intelligent and had a fine appearance and personality. We worked very well together. Meanwhile, Ray got J. Hamilton Crawford, chief of medicine at Kings County Hospital, to secure a room that could be used as an office and laboratory. It was nothing more than a storage room, but it served as an indispensable base of operations. Phil Kendell promised to alert the residents to inform us of the admission of patients in circulatory shock. With these preparations in hand, I could concentrate on graduation and taking the licensing exam.

Graduation from medical school was a let down because I was not allowed to take my internship. Watching my classmates make plans for their graduate training, while I was committed to another year in nonclinical activities, was depressing. Unconsciously, serving the needs of others and saving lives grows on you and to be denied this opportunity when you have the training is deeply disturbing. I could comfort myself in the thought that the research I was going to do might save more lives in the end than all my classmates's clinical efforts. The truth is, however, that research is a lonely occupation with only intellectual rewards that are abstract and often not even realized. I nevertheless took consolation in my family's pride in my accomplishment. I took some pleasure in the fact that I graduated seventh in my class, which could never have been predicted from my college record.

The New York State Medical Licensing Exam was not easy. A full day of essay questions in all the basic sciences and clinical subjects, it was designed certainly to flunk foreign graduates. Most of us had writer's cramp at the end of the day and were convinced that we had messed up the exam. I definitely knew that I screwed up the pathology exam because I completely misinterpreted two of the five questions. But I must have done well on the rest of the exam because in a couple of weeks I received that precious document: The New York State Medical License. Now I could practice medicine legally because an internship was not required in New York State. As a passing fancy, I dreamed of giving up my academic position and research grant and opening up an office, simply plunging into medical practice.

I was twenty-five years old and felt fully mature and confident that I could do as well in practice as most generalist physicians. Phil Kendall advised me against this course of action by pointing out that I would later regret not having taken graduate training. He himself was going to take at least four years to round out his training for internal medicine. Besides, he said, "You're a natural for academic medicine, and you should round out your clinical training even if you end up doing basic science. I expect you to be a professor some day and perhaps a department chairman." I too felt instinctively that I would always enjoy research, even if I practiced medicine. And I had grown to like teaching and the academic atmosphere.

So on July 1, 1941, I plunged into a serious research and teaching effort with all the energy I could summon. Besides the scheduled work on circulatory shock, I planned four additional projects on reactive hyperemia. Mrs. Richards divided our time between Kings County Hospital and the Henry Street campus of the Long Island College of Medicine. Duplicate apparatus was constructed for both places so that there was no problem of transport. Gasoline was already rationed, but since licensed physicians could get more gasoline, my family let me have the old Dodge. I was able to get around quite handily even though the car had grown to be quite fickle. At the least it spared me the long subway train rides from my home in Queens through Manhattan to Brooklyn. The new connecting highway between Queens and Brooklyn had been recently completed, and driving enabled me to save an hour each day.

The work on circulatory shock went extremely well. By the end of the summer, we had already collected a variety of comparative cases. I lost no time in putting the data into shape and writing a full-length report. After submitting it to Sam Reynolds and Walter Bradford Cannon, both of whom made helpful changes, I decided to submit it to the *Journal of the American Medical Association* where, if accepted, it would get the widest attention. After many months of waiting, I finally received the paper back with a letter saying that it was acceptable, but I had to make some editorial changes. By this time, I had amassed more data that could enhance the paper, so some extensive rewriting ensued. More months passed, and finally the paper was published in 1943. It didn't create much of a sensation, but it did attract considerable attention in the way of reprint requests and invitations to give talks. To publish a paper in the *Journal of the American Medical Association* for one still in his internship year was a considerable feat, a very credible performance. But it brought an episode of embarrassment and unhappiness.

By the time the paper was published, I had obtained an internship in the teaching service of internal medicine at Kings County Hospital. As a result, I became quite friendly with J. Hamilton Crawford, the chief of service. He made morning rounds three times a week, after which Kendall and I would usually have lunch with him in the residents' dining room. Crawford was a Scotsman with a thick brogue and English mannerisms, of average height and slight structure, with a thin red face topped by jet-black hair. It was obvious from his conversation that he was very assertive and had a large ego. Almost every time we spoke, he let us know that he had been a fellow at the famous Rockefeller Institute. Then, as a sort of afterthought, he'd say, "You know I'm the only one of the faculty of the Long Island College of Medicine who knows how to do research." We listened with straight faces because we knew that his deep desire was to become chairman of the department of medicine, which would enhance his reputation as one of Brooklyn's foremost cardiologists. He had, in fact, done no significant research in years. His bibliography included but one or two papers written when he was a fellow.

Soon after my paper on circulatory shock was published, The Crawfish, as the residents called him, met me for lunch one day. His face was redder than usual, and the veins on his temples bulged. My immediate thought was that he was on the verge of a stroke. He was unusually quiet for a while, then he suddenly turned toward me and said in a sharp voice: "Why didn't you mention me in your *JAMA* paper? You acknowledged Reynolds and your assistant Blanche Richards, who doesn't even have a degree. Reynolds is an inconsequential person and yet you don't even refer to me, the only one qualified to do research. I am the chief of service and your direct supervisor! It is an insult to my reputation that a paper coming from my service has no mention of the head of the department!"

I was absolutely floored. Could I tell him that he'd had nothing to do with the work from the beginning to the end? But not wishing to aggravate the situation, I replied, "Sir, I have the most profound respect for your position and research accomplishments. May I point out that the work was done when I was an instructor in physiology and that the grant was under the auspices of that department? Because of the delay in publication, I put down my present position as an intern in medicine. If I have offended you in any way I apologize."

Crawford gave me a bitter look and said nothing else. Meanwhile, Kendall joined us and the conversation turned to lighter subjects. I sensed, however, that I had made a serious political blunder, that Crawford had deep resentment against me and would seek his revenge when the opportunity arose. He was pleasant enough on subsequent occasions, but there was always an uneasy feeling between us.

But now I've gotten ahead of my story and must return to earlier events that influenced my future. On the whole, the year spent as instructor in physiology was a success both intellectually and health-wise. I was able to do four other research papers and publish them in peer-reviewed journals, one of them the prestigious *American Journal of Medicine*, a Rockefeller Institute-sponsored journal. Then editor Peyton Rous, who latter won a Nobel Prize, was kind enough in his letter of acceptance to praise the novelty of the work.

I gained in strength and vigor. I had ample time to rest and enjoyed nourishing home cooked meals. I was able to do all the gardening and handyman jobs about the house, which my family greatly appreciated. My father, retired for nearly ten years, was not physically able to do much, while my brother Al refused to do anything that required exertion. Fortunately, he was still employed by the city that never fired anybody. Sister Catherine was a substitute French teacher and worked most of the time. Mary was again working for a Wall Street firm. With this combined income, including my salary (for we all still turned over our weekly earnings to Papa), the family was relatively well off despite the continuing national depression. It appeared that my sisters were going to be old maids. Al showed no interest in women. I was also backward in seeking the opposite sex, and my family definitely didn't encourage it. I felt that I was too young to consider marriage. Besides, that would have prevented me from securing an internship.

An amusing episode occurred about this time when a distant cousin on my father's side insisted on visiting our family. We had not seen them in years. I didn't even know who they were. They arrived from upper New York State: mother, father, and daughter, carrying a huge leather doctor's bag as a present for me. It soon became clear that they were intent on arranging a marriage between their daughter and myself. The daughter was rather stout, but not unattractive. She had only a high school education and was not an intellectual type. I was not interested and made myself scarce. My family, especially my mother, was not about to sell off their doctor son, no matter how good the dowry. The offer was politely turned down, but I kept the doctor's bag.

Another event had a more far reaching effect on my future, and everyone else's future, for that matter. On Sunday, December 7, 1941, I lay down in my bedroom for a nap after lunch. It was my habit to dose off listening to classical music on WQXR. Half asleep, the music suddenly stopped and an emergency message came on:

PEARL HARBOR IS BEING BOMBED BY THE JAPANESE!

The message went on to indicate that the loss of life and damage to our fleet was extensive. It was natural to anticipate that the United States would declare war on Japan, and Germany and Italy as well. A plan to draft all doctors of eligible age was already in effect, and I wondered if I would be excluded because of my tubercular history. Many thought that President Roosevelt had planned for this to happen so that he could drive the country into war. World War II had a great influence of the lives of all people. It had a great effect on mine, too, but one I could not anticipate on that Sunday afternoon.

The immediate effect on medicine was dramatic. A doctor shortage was declared. Medical schools were encouraged to accelerate medical education. Many schools shortened the curriculum to three years and doubled their student population by admitting classes both in July and December and by eliminating summer recesses. This put an enormous strain on medical school faculty, many of who were being drafted into service themselves. The military decided to allow recent graduates to complete their internships and residencies before being called to service. I was fortunate in this, for I was anxious to complete my graduate clinical training. Because of the shortage, I had no trouble in securing my training at Kings County Hospital, even though I suspected that The Crawfish would have preferred otherwise.

Many of my college friends were drafted, including Sol. This was truly ironic. Sol was denied a medical education despite excellent qualifications, yet he was good enough to serve his country. Sol paid a heavy price indeed. While riding in a motor pool jeep, he severely injured his shoulder and was left with a paralyzed arm. Phil Kendall was also drafted but allowed one more year of training. This was fortunate because I still had much to learn about the art and skills of medicine from him.

CHAPTER III

Internship and Residency

1942-1944

"After all the frills and conjectures of medical education are trimmed away, the most practical and useful education is apprenticeship to another physician(s)."

Rupert Black, M.D.

After ten eventful years from my first college day, I was finally able to consummate what I thought was my ultimate goal. I was doing clinical medicine at long last. I clearly remember the first patient I admitted as an intern at Kings County Hospital. Perhaps this was because I missed the diagnosis, but more likely because it was so dramatic and instructive a case. A very obese male was brought in a semistuporous state. He had been at the shore where he'd eaten large quantities of raw oysters. A few hours later, he had a gradual increase of abdominal pain located in the epigastrium. His family became alarmed as he sunk into an unconscious state and called an ambulance. On examination, it was obvious that he was in deep circulatory shock with very low blood pressure and cold clammy skin. His abdomen was rigid. There were no signs of hemorrhage, although his hemoglobin was low. Because it was the middle of the night, I could not persuade any attending physician to come in. I called in the chief surgical resident, who was unable to come any closer to an exact diagnosis than mine. Emergency surgery was ruled out because an exploratory laparotomy was not feasible in a man in such deep shock. A flat x-ray of the abdomen would have been of great help but could not be obtained at night. I did what I could for the patient by administering intravenous fluid and oxygen by mask. Blood cultures were taken in case the shock-like state was caused by bacteremia. The patient was put in a head-down, feet-up position to favor the circulation.

These efforts were futile, and the patient expired in a few hours. I was able to obtain permission from the family for an autopsy by convincing them that there might be a possibility of poisoning. The diagnosis was obvious as soon as the abdomen was opened. A large abdominal aortic aneurysm had ruptured and hemorrhaged into the retroperitoneal space. I had little consolation in the fact that the patient could not have been saved even if I had made the correct diagnosis. Only emergency surgery immediately after the rupture might have been successful.

With the vast amount of material on the wards, and admission duty every third day and night, even the dullest person would learn quickly. I soon had in hand a routine methodology of diagnosis and therapy that seemed to be satisfactory. Kendall was merciless and pointed out my errors with glee. From time to time, I tried to outfox him. Sometimes I succeeded. In the fall there was an epidemic of meningococcal meningitis. I had six cases lined up in the admissions ward one night. Fortunately, in 1942 sulfa drugs were effective in this infection, and I was able to save all but the most desperate cases. Before sulfa drugs, meningococcal meningitis was a uniformly fatal disease. It was gratifying to save lives.

Interns and residents were housed in a separate dormitory building at least two city blocks away from the hospital. This was not so bad in warm weather, but it was cruelty to be called in the middle of a winter night. The accommodations were not bad, but certainly on the Spartan side—two persons to a room with one dresser, one table between the beds, and one chair. There was a sink in the room, but the toilets and showers were centrally located. The intern who shared my room was a nice enough young chap, tall and thin, an athletic type. I no longer remember his name. We did not see too much of each other because he was on a different service, and we were on night duty at different times.

He suddenly vanished one day. Thinking that perhaps I had offended him, I made some discrete inquiries. It seems that after about one month of service, he came to the conclusion that he didn't like medicine, had never liked it, and just wasn't going to practice. He went back to a boat rental and fishing sideline on the north shore of Long Island. I was sorry that I didn't get to know him better for his case intrigued me. Like him, I was pretty much steered into medical school by family pressure; yet unlike him, I became enamored of the whole field. I wondered about medical school admissions committees and their ability to predict genuine motivation toward medicine. This fellow occupied the place of someone who was denied admission and might have made a fine physician.

Having the room to myself was enjoyable. I bought myself a small table radio and listened to classical music when I had some spare time. This might have disturbed the average roommate. But soon I became friendly with Julius Stolfi, who was about my age and on the open medical service. He asked if he could room with me.

"Sure," I said, "if you can stand my eccentric habits. I'm a night person who stays up till two and doesn't arise until at least nine. In addition, I snore and insist on listening to classical music."

"Fine," he replied, "I'm a day person who is asleep by eleven and up at seven-thirty no matter what else goes on. If my calisthenics on arising won't disturb you, then we will get along fine." The next day he moved in and we became close friends.

There were some 125 interns and residents at Kings County Hospital at that time. Social life on off-duty nights consisted of playing bridge, shooting craps, or playing handball. Those of a more amorous nature had girlfriends, mostly nurses who had apartments close by. Kendall, Stolfi, and Monty Cohen, another intern, plus I formed a foursome for playing bridge. Monty Cohen was a genuine expert and taught us many conventions and tricks that made the game much more interesting. We were occasionally joined by Bill Florio, a neurology resident, when he was not escorting an exotic female. Our sessions were not only for playing bridge, but also for medical discussions. The four of us formed close bonds, our friendship grew, and it has lasted a lifetime.

There were parties and escapades. Groups of five to ten fellows would go to the fourteen-ounce beer joint for a session of serious drinking. I would be roped in every once in a while because I didn't want to appear unsocial, but I really had no joy in drinking. The best I could manage was four glasses at the most. One fellow, O'Donald, the son of a policeman, was a big man in all dimensions. He held the record for the number of glasses of beer intake at one session—an astounding thirty-two glasses, or seven quarts! The beer joint got very boisterous. Everyone smoked, and the conversation was loud and disjointed. Our group would eventually stagger back to the dormitory in the early morning hours, singing loudly all the way. I often wondered what the neighbors thought of the Kings County Hospital house staff.

I was amazed at how little the house staff read. We had a small library room with a few of the major medical journals and a scattering of major textbooks. Occasionally a resident might be found reading there, but usually it was the daily newspaper. I determined that I would try to maintain an academic approach to medicine, so I read widely to keep myself abreast of recent research efforts, which I felt was necessary.

The syndrome of congestive heart failure (CHF), which was all too common and of current interest, fascinated me. I was determined to learn everything I could about CHF, and I decided that I would read the *Journal of Clinical Investigation* from its initial publication (about 1910) with special reference to CHF and related subjects. To do this, I had to go to the library of the Long Island College of Medicine. I enjoyed these weekly trips because I had the old Dodge, and this kept the battery from discharging. Besides, it was an opportunity to visit with Ray and Johnson and George Paff from anatomy. After some weeks of reading, I decided that I could conveniently do a nice bit of research using the ample clinical material available. I consulted with Kendall and naturally with

The Crawfish and both were agreeable. I still had access to a small room that I could convert to a laboratory. I used funds left over from my previous year's grant to buy the necessary apparatus and material supplies. With the large changes in fluid balance in the body brought about by the powerful mercurial diuretics, commonly the therapeutic modality used in congestive heart failure, I reasoned that there must be interesting changes in blood-specific gravity and blood volume.

Clinical research in 1942 was much simpler than it is today. One simply approached the patient, explained the procedure and its possible discomforts and risks, and usually gained approval—no signed consent form, no rigid protocol, no prior approval by an institutional review board. In that era, lawsuits for malpractice were practically unknown. This made clinical research more straightforward but increased the chance of a harmful outcome for the patient. From a moral and ethical viewpoint, my proposed research posed a minimum of discomfort and risk for the patient.

The main research procedure consisted of drawing blood samples. Evans blue, a dye used to determine blood volume, was not toxic and had been administered to humans many times before. The research progressed as I did all the work collecting samples and doing the determinations mainly in the evening and night hours. Two episodes of untoward events occurred that might seem amusing in retrospect, but at the time were serious maladventures. The first took place one night when I was pipetting serum for a blood volume determination. I accidentally sucked some serum into my mouth. Horrified, because I knew the patient had syphilis, I quickly spit it out and rinsed my mouth with 95% alcohol. In arrested syphilis, fortunately, organisms are not likely to be in the blood. Still, I was apprehensive for several weeks that signs and symptoms of that dreaded disease might appear. Research can be dangerous for the investigator as well as the subject! While I escaped infection, the second episode was more embarrassing.

Evans blue was a unique dye because it was not toxic and did not filter out of the capillaries because of its large molecular size. I made up the dye solutions and sterilized them myself. On one occasion, I must have made a serious error in calculation. I made a solution ten times more concentrated than required. To my horror, the patient who received this solution turned a bluish-ashen color. His cardiac failure had markedly improved and he was a grateful patient, but he wanted to know why his skin was so dark. I told him it was caused by his condition and that his normal skin color would return in a few weeks.

The next day The Crawfish was to make rounds and would surely ask about this strange case. Kendall and I moved the patient into the darkest corner of a side room where stabilized patients were kept and where often Crawford failed to see every patient. On rounds the next day, Crawford did not insist on making rounds in the side room, but he did glance in. He noticed the ashen color of our patient and, to show off his diagnostic prowess, he said, "I see you have a patient with argyria (silver poisoning)." We hastily agreed and ushered him to lunch.

The patient suffered no ill effects and his skin color gradually cleared, but I had to suffer the jibes of my colleagues for months thereafter. They referred to the incident as DiPalma's blue period— a parody on Picasso's similarly colored period of work. Despite these misadventures, the study turned out to quite interesting. I wrote it up and published in the *Journal of Laboratory and Clinical Medicine*. Kendall was a co-author, although he did little of the work, yet he was a very good critic and a great supporter of my efforts.

About this time, house staff physicians of Manhattan city hospitals had a confrontation with Mayor LaGuardia and demanded some salary support. They pointed out that porters got larger salaries than interns, even counting the room and board that the latter received. The "Little Flower" was sympathetic, but pointed out the deficit state of the city's finances. After much agitation and threats of a strike, the city decided to pay interns in city hospitals the starvation sum of $18 a month. Hardly even pocket money, but still better than nothing. Quite a few interns did some moonlighting even though it was strictly forbidden. This consisted of making house calls for attending physicians, especially at night, or working in the emergency clinic of private hospitals that didn't have a house staff. I did not moonlight, as it would have precluded doing any research or even any serious reading of the medical literature. Consequently, the miniscule salary was much appreciated for sundry items like pipe tobacco, an occasional movie, and a tasty sandwich at the corner Greek restaurant.

It surely did not allow for any fancy courting of the opposite sex. Nurses, who were the most frequently dated, knew this and did not expect fancy dinners and shows. A movie and maybe a soda or hamburger was the usual date. Nurses were much better off financially and could share apartments in the vicinity. If a nurse thought that an intern was a serious potential catch, she would invite him to the apartment for dinner. More romances developed as a result of the intern's poverty than if he had been well off. Some interns played the game purely for sexual gratification, and some accommodating nurses satisfied this demand. There was not the degree of promiscuity evident today, however, and where there was, it was kept "under the covers."

Kendall revealed to me one day that he'd been married since his junior year in medical school. In fact, he already had two young daughters. His wife worked as a secretary and his mother-in-law took care of the children. He had managed to keep this secret from the authorities and pledged me to silence. I spent some pleasant afternoons at his apartment. Kendall was quite a drinker and educated me in this art, to which I fortuitously never gained real addiction.

We had clinical material available that was the equal of any hospital in the United States. We had some very fine, dedicated attending physicians whom we greatly respected. There were also some brilliant residents. One was Jacob Halperin, whom we called "Jake the Rake" because of his many love affairs. He was academically the top man in our class. Whenever he had an interesting case on the open service, he would let me know so I could examine and study it. He was greatly interested in Addison's disease. We once had a sixteen-year-old girl with this disorder that we let Jake study. When I was on admitting duty one night, I made a diagnosis of

Addison's disease in a fifty-year-old black woman. Since one of the hallmark features of the disease is an increase of skin pigmentation, everyone wanted to know how I could tell that her skin was darkening beyond its normal hue.

"Easy," I replied. "She told me her skin had been getting darker."

I explained that black people are just as observant about the shade of their skin as are white people. When the blood chemistries came in the next day, they showed the characteristic pattern of Addison's disease dominated by a very low sodium level. Meanwhile, I had started to treat her with saline infusion, and she showed marked improvement that clinched the diagnosis. I probably saved her life by this prompt diagnosis and treatment. That case brought me some modicum of fame as a clinician, which pleased me because I had always been considered more of a researcher than a clinician. I noticed that the medical students now began to seek me out and follow me on my rounds.

The salt and fluid therapy of Addison's disease could save lives, but not prolong them. The disorder was caused by the failure of the adrenal gland to produce its cortical hormone, cortisone. In 1942 cortisone had not been synthesized and only a crude extract was available which was weak, expensive, and in short supply. To have Addison's disease then was a virtual death sentence. Jake was able to get a supply from Ciba of desoxycorticosterone (DOCA), which was a synthetic cortical hormone. It was able to control salt metabolism, but not the hormone effects on glucose, fat, and other actions of the true hormone. Nevertheless, DOCA could greatly improve the quality of life and longevity in this disease.

Jake and I devised a special instrument to implant pellets of DOCA underneath the skin. This implant provided the patient with a constant drug supply for six months. Eventually, Jake had about a dozen patients with Addison's disease, a large number for this extremely rare disease, and he treated them expertly. I implored Jake to publish his results, but he was not the publishing kind. He never had the confidence that his findings were meritorious enough to commit to print. This was most deplorable because Jake had as much knowledge and expertise as George Thorn, then professor of medicine at Harvard's Brigham Hospital and considered the world's expert on Addison's disease.

It has always been a mystery to me why some people with little ability and experience publish profusely, while real experts sometimes hesitate to let the public see their results. The medical world never got to learn of Jake's fascinating series of patients. In a few years it didn't make any difference because cortisone, the true hormone of the adrenal, was synthesized in 1950 and made widely available. Addison's disease could now be completely cured and normal quality and expectancy of life restored. Jack Kennedy, who had the disease, would never have been able to run a vigorous campaign and become president had cortisone not come along in time to cure his disease.

My first year of internship came to an end all too soon in June, 1943. The war had greatly intensified. A great many doctors were needed, and many were drafted even though they had not finished their training. Among them, my roommate Stolfi rushed to get married before going overseas. Kendall had finished his training and had no excuse. He made the unfortunate choice of joining the Army Air Force and was sent to a godforsaken base in the middle of Oklahoma where there was nothing for a physician, especially one of Kendall's abilities, to do but drink at the officers' club. Many became alcoholics. I was declared 4F because of my tubercular history and thus ended up as chief resident of the internal medicine service, although I am sure The Crawfish would have preferred otherwise. The house staff was reduced to about half its former size, and everyone left behind had to do double duty.

We had to work every other day for twenty-four hours, which meant that we got practically no sleep. And the work itself was exhausting. I was in charge of 140 patients and had to make rounds twice a day. Just passing by each patient briefly and glancing at their charts took hours. We spent more time, of course, on new admissions and the acutely ill. Many attending physicians were also drafted. Those who weren't were busier and consequently tended to come less often to the city hospital to do free work.

Opportunities for moonlighting also increased, and this put an additional strain on the work effort of the house staff. Despite all the shortages we carried on, but many thought the lucky ones were those who were drafted.

I soon found out that my job as chief resident was largely administrative and custodial. The main problem was keeping the census down. People at the poverty level use a city hospital as a hotel, even a vacation resort. This was still the age when bed rest was the main cure for every ailment. A diagnosis of suspected myocardial infarction was welcome because it meant at least six weeks of absolute bed rest. Malingering was fairly common. Case in point: a sixteen-year-old girl with a history of spitting up blood. Surely this meant tuberculosis and required a complete and exhaustive work-up. We learned later that she wanted to get away from her parents who were disciplining her for an escapade with a fifty-year-old lover. She cleverly sucked blood from a loose tooth socket, scared her parents and fooled the doctors. She did have beautiful breasts, and all the interns wanted to examine this interesting case.

Another malingering trick was to fake fever by rubbing the thermometer briskly on a bedsheet when the nurse wasn't looking. It didn't work too well because it was tried so often that the nurses were on to it. Most of the custodial patients did have some chronic disease that could be used as an excuse for hospital admission. Arthritis, hypertension, diabetes, and heart disease were the most common. Most could easily be treated on an ambulatory basis, but the rule was that no one could be refused admission so all had to be admitted and receive an expensive work up and hospital stay. Then there was the all-too-frequent syndrome of old age—weakness and disability. Children and relatives tired of taking care of aged parents dumped them in the receiving ward and left without leaving a history or even a name or address. Sometimes this backfired. An elderly, demented man, who hadn't had a bath in years and was crawling with lice, was so dumped. When cleaning him up, the nurses found a packet containing $10,000 sewn to his underwear. The story got into the newspapers. Relatives and lawyers soon appeared with papers for the old man to sign. Because he was demented and in no position to sign anything, he was put in isolation to prevent the thieving relatives from sneaking in unobserved.

Despite my administrative duties, I managed to dabble in some research. With Stolfi in the army, I acquired a new roommate, Jeremiah Stammler. He wanted to associate with me because he was interested in research. His main interests were in cholesterol and arteriosclerosis. I had no facilities for this type of research. After much discussion, we settled on trying to measure the osmotic pressure of blood under various circumstances. I volunteered to construct certain suitable chambers out of plastic that enclosed a cellophane barrier and connection to a manometer. We had to give up after many trials and modifications of the apparatus because our results were too inconsistent to be reliable. Jerry was a very interesting and most persistent character. After he finished his clinical training, he took a fellowship with L.N. Katz in Chicago where he worked on arteriosclerosis in chickens. Among my younger colleagues, Jerry achieved the greatest success in research and medicine. He eventually became a professor and chairman of the Department of Preventative Medicine at Northwestern University School of Medicine. His greatest contributions were conducting one of the first Coronary Drug Trials and later a model for large-scale prospective clinical trials.

My clinical training progressed satisfactorily. I developed suitable personal algorithms for most clinical problems. I became convinced that the practice of medicine was actually quite simple. My overconfidence was unjustified, but one which afflicts most senior residents. As the year began to draw to a close, I decided that I had gained all I could from Kings County Hospital. Ordinarily, I should have spent another year as a resident. I knew that Crawford expected this, but I felt that I should take training in another medical center, preferably a fellowship that would allow me to exploit both my research and clinical experience. I arranged an appointment with Jean Alonzo Curran, who was still dean at the Long Island College of Medicine. He reacted favorably to my ambition and volunteered to explore the possibility of a fellowship at the famous Thorndike Laboratory at Boston City Hospital, connected to the Harvard Medical School service.

To my surprise and great pleasure, Boston City Hospital responded favorably—undoubtedly because the draft still caused a physician shortage—and I was granted an interview with George Minot of pernicious anemia and Nobel Prize fame. The interview went well, but Minot was noncommittal. After a couple of anxious weeks, I received a nice letter confirming my appointment to start on July 1. I was floating on air! At last I was in the right groove for an academic career. With credentials from the Thorndike laboratory, I was sure to be able to secure an academic position, even in the most prestigious medical school or clinic.

But my good fortune was short-lived. Against all odds, I was drafted and passed the physical exam. I was told that my history of tuberculosis did not exclude me from service. I made preparations to enter the army, and was forced to call Dr. Minot and tell him that I couldn't take the fellowship. Just three weeks later, diabolical fate dealt me another blow. The army changed its mind and declared me 4F again. I immediately called Boston to see if the fellowship was still open. Unfortunately, they had hired a female physician not subject to the draft. I was left without a position. I probably could have stayed on at Kings County Hospital or secured another residency, but I was so disgusted and frustrated that I decided I would simply go into private practice.

During this last year of residency, I had grown thin and was often exhausted. I badly needed a vacation. An opportunity presented itself to be the camp physician at the Vermont camp where I'd been the arts and crafts counselor a few years earlier. It was a good deal. The $500 I'd earn for two summer months would serve as a financial nest egg to open an office. And as the camp physician, my duties would actually be lighter than those of a counselor, and I would spend less time with the children.

With a light heart, I got into the old Dodge and set off for Lunenburg, Vermont. I was looking forward to a triumphal reunion with my former fellow counselors. I didn't expect any calamities of a medical nature because most of the campers were healthy kids who were cleared by their physicians before coming to camp. There might be a few asthmatics and perhaps one or two well-controlled diabetics, but other than minor injuries or upper respiratory infections, I anticipated little action. I looked forward to getting plenty of sun, swimming, canoeing, and perhaps some horseback riding. The camp nurse fortuitously turned out to be a very pleasant woman in her late thirties who was more than capable of taking most minor sick calls. Marion Bruno was a registered nurse who took on duties as a private nurse when her husband died of an apparent heart attack. The camp owners knew her well because she'd taken care of Cy, their chronically ill son. She was almost a member of their family. Hungarian by birth, she immigrated with her parents when she was about 15 and retained a continental flavor that I found attractive.

The first week of camp went by smoothly, and I was congratulating myself on the decision to spend the summer in Vermont. Then my luck ran out. The camp owner's wife an elderly hypertensive, excitable woman, was standing on the porch of the main house yelling directions to some young campers when she suddenly fell to the ground unconscious. I was called to the scene and immediately saw that she was gravely ill, the victim of either a stroke or heart attack. With the aid of several husky counselors, we brought her to the infirmary where she stabilized somewhat, but did not regain consciousness. Examination demonstrated a very low blood pressure with a weak, rapid pulse. She was extremely pale with cold clammy skin. Her reflexes were equal on both sides of the body, and she responded to painful stimuli. I was sure that it was an acute myocardial infarction with cardiac shock, but I had no electrocardiograph to confirm the diagnosis. Her husband was a dentist and very intelligent. Conferring with him and their daughter Rose, we came to the conclusion that she could not be moved to the hospital in a nearby town. I advised them to call in a local doctor to confirm the diagnosis and expedite getting a tank of oxygen and a suitable mask. I also wanted an intravenous infusion setup, which was only available from the local hospital.

The local medical doctor showed up shortly. He was a tall, sparse man of middle age who might well represent a typical New Englander. His conversation consisted of short bursts of grunts that presumably confirmed what I had just explained. After a brief examination, and some questions from the family, he appeared to agree with my diagnosis and proposed therapy. He then opened his bag, pulled out a syringe and a vial of digitalis, and proceeded to administer it intramuscularly. He watched Mrs. Jaffe for a while as if he expected a sudden change for the better. As I expected, there was no change because digitalis, although a wonderful drug for congestive heart failure, was of no value in this type of heart failure. Whether he knew this or not, or just gave an injection to impress the family, remained a mystery to me. He grunted a promise to speed the delivery of an oxygen tank, mask, intravenous apparatus, and sterile saline glucose solution before he abruptly departed.

I was disappointed because he left to me the unpleasant duty of telling the family that the prognosis was very grave and that, unless a miracle happened, Mrs. Jaffe was going to die in a matter of hours. I had this onerous duty many times as a resident, but this was different. Here was a private patient, my employer's wife whom I had known for years, and I was on my own without the blanket coverage of the hospital and all its impressive facilities. The family, however, seemed to take the news very calmly and bravely. They appeared to be more worried about keeping the whole episode secret from the campers so as not to disturb the camp routine.

Nurse Marion and I decided to treat our patient jointly and do what we could to ease any pain and suffering. The oxygen and intravenous solution improved her skin color and circulation somewhat, but she never regained consciousness. She passed away quietly the following morning. None of the family had come to visit or even inquire about her during this long deathwatch. The mortician came promptly; the body was spirited away, and shipped to New York City for burial. Camp life went on as usual. Mrs. Jaffe was not even missed.

There is an aura about watching a person hover between life and death. It is not only a solemn occasion, but also one that inspires introspective thoughts. As the minutes and hours tick away, you wonder when a similar fate will affect you. Events of your life flick by, and you reflect on past misadventures. Marion and I, watching the dying woman in the dimly lit room, were drawn together by parallel thoughts. We confided in each other intimate episodes in our past lives that ordinarily were kept private. We took turns sleeping on a couch in the same room. In her turn, Marion leaned against my chest and, when it came to my turn, my head was on her lap. We might have been husband and wife or brother and sister. I doubt that either of us had any amorous thoughts at the time.

Over the next few days, it became obvious that we had developed affection for each other that went beyond the bounds of friendship. During the next week, we met each night and sat on the back porch of the infirmary. We chatted and enjoyed the night air and the brilliant Vermont night stars. Marion was friendly with the cook, and she would whip up delicious late night snacks. There were no endearing words between us, but I accompanied her inside the infirmary one night to examine a patient. On the way out I suddenly felt compelled to embrace her and kiss her full on the lips. She responded passionately, as if she expected it. I began to fondle her breasts, and she responded by massaging my male member. She bit my ear lightly and whispered, "Do you want it?" I replied simply, "I do." We hurriedly undressed in her bedroom and joined in a very satisfactory sex session.

I was twenty-eight years old, and with the exception of one or two unfulfilled experiences, was a virgin. This experience was a revelation to me. This was the start of many such amorous adventures in succeeding weeks. Yet I knew that I was not really in love with Marion. I believe that she sensed this. We kept our affair secret from the rest of the camp.

CHAPTER IV

Private Practice

1944-1950

"Many a good mind is wasted in the rigors and rewards of medical practice. Combining creativeness and innovation with practical service to fellow man is seldom satisfactorily achieved let alone also having an ideal family life."

Rupert Black, M.D.

Medically, the rest of the summer was uneventful. I managed to get in plenty of swimming and canoeing and even some tennis and horseback riding. All too soon the summer ended, and I was back in the city ready to start up a practice. Armed with the $500 I received as camp physician, I rented a one-room office with a spacious bathroom and tiny waiting room on the ground floor of an apartment building at 38 Livingston Street in Brooklyn. The medical school and hospital were only a few blocks away, and the subway was convenient. I purchased a second-hand desk, examining table, instrument cabinet, instruments, sterilizing equipment, and a screen. The screen divided the room into a consulting section and an examination section and provided privacy while undressing. A day bed that served as a couch, two chairs, and an end table furnished the waiting room.

I had stationary printed to send announcements to all my physician contacts, friends, and selected relatives. Despite handsome drapes that my sisters contributed, the office wasn't much, but it was all I could afford. As luck would have it, Luigi Minetto, a classmate, opened a handsome, well-furnished office on the corner of Livingston Street. He was a shrewd businessman and put me to shame in the art of building a practice.

Waiting in the office for the phone to ring those first few weeks was a dismal and depressing experience. George B. Ray came to my rescue and offered me a part-time position as assistant professor of physiology and pharmacology at a salary of $1,800 dollars a year. I gratefully accepted this opportunity because it enabled me to keep body and soul together if no patients crossed my door. Gradually, doctors I knew from Kings County Hospital and the Long Island College Hospital began to let me make some of their house calls when they were busy or simply didn't feel like making them. Milton Plotz had a huge practice and often referred house calls to me. I couldn't charge more than he did, which was $3. Since the patients usually lived in the far reaches of Flatbush or East New York, I had to drive an average of ten miles to and from their homes. I made less than a taxi driver on a single call. It wasn't too bad if I could stack three or four calls together. I must admit that Plotz occasionally let me make house calls on his more affluent patients, allowing me to charge five or even ten dollars.

My teaching job and attendance at free clinics at both Kings County and the Long Island College hospitals limited my office hours to evenings from seven to nine, five days a week, and one to three on Saturdays. Since I still lived at home and had to travel to Queens at night and back to Brooklyn in the morning, my day ran from 7 a.m. to 10 p.m., as long as I didn't have any night calls. I slowly built up a small office practice.

Although I was qualified as an internist, I really did general practice. I had a small reputation as an expert in peripheral vascular disease because of my recent published research on circulation, and from time to time some friendly doctor would send me a patient for consultation. This would bring me a fee of ten dollars. These consults required a written report, which I laboriously typed out myself because I had no secretary.

We were still in the middle of the Great Depression, and people didn't spend money on doctors unless it was absolutely necessary. Walking down Henry Street looking quite dejected one day, I met an old time doc who stopped me and said, "Joe, why are you looking so glum?" I replied that I hadn't seen a private patient in the past two days. He smiled and said, "Don't worry, God will provide"—a prophetic statement because the next day a small pox epidemic was predicted by the N.Y. City Health Department. Everyone had to be vaccinated who hadn't been in the last ten years. Two local restaurants called me in to vaccinate all their workers. This netted me several hundred dollars for a couple hours of work. Although my competitor, Luigi Minetto, acquired a bigger, more affluent practice, I was too busy to be jealous. His business methods were, if not illegal, almost unethical. He definitely overcharged and ordered excessive laboratory tests. Disenchanted with Mineto, one young patient came to me after Minetto had charged him $95 for treating the common cold.

My first six months in private practice ground along their weary way. It was exhausting work. My patients were mostly routine cases, which was a let down from my resident days when I had a wealth of fascinating cases. I was a slave to the telephone and had no time for intellectual pursuits. Yet I did not dislike practice, and I adjusted to the routine after a time. Grateful patients proved to be a great source of satisfaction and made me feel that I was achieving my true potential. On the difficult days, I wondered if I could continue for long at this pace. In contrast, this thinking alternated with a great feeling of elation when things went well.

About this time, William Dock was appointed the new chairman of the Department of Medicine at the Long Island College of Medicine. About forty-five years old and controversial, he was considered to be one of the most brilliant contemporary physicians. He had trained under Henry Christian at Brigham and had gone from there to Stanford Medical School where he was assistant professor of pharmacology and medicine and in private practice. His fame stemmed in part from his heritage as the son of George Dock who, next to Sir William Osler, was perhaps one of the most respected physicians in America. Bill Dock had published extensively and was a member of the American Society for Clinical Investigation and the American Association of Physicians. His most recent position before coming to Brooklyn was professor and chairman of the Department of Pathology at Cornell University School of Medicine.

With a quick, witty mind and a "triple threat" background in internal medicine, pharmacology, and pathology, Dock could not be outdone in any conference or discussion group. His approaches were always unique and contrary to the general view. Adoring students and residents followed him on rounds hoping to gather every pearl that dropped from his lips. Fellow clinicians didn't like him because he was openly critical of their methods. The Crawfish especially hated him in part because he had expected to receive the chair of medicine himself. Despite Crawford's feelings, there was little doubt that Bill Dock was one of the best additions to the school's faculty. He stimulated and changed the academic careers of many people, including my own.

Dock showed up in my laboratory one day with what appeared to be a box of Fanny Farmer's candy in his hand.

"Joe, I've just spent the weekend with my old colleague in pharmacology at Stanford, Maurice Tainter, who has an interesting project that you might be curious about," he said. "He is now medical and research director at the Sterling Winthrop drug company in upstate New York. Have you ever heard of alpha fagarine?"

I admitted that I hadn't. Dock explained, "It's an alkaloid extracted from a plant in South America that has been reported to have unusual antiarrhythmic properties on the heart exceeding those of quinidine. The exact chemical structure is not known, but Sterling Winthrop chemists have made a number of close chemical compounds which they wish to have screened in animals and compared to alpha fagarine and quinidine for antiarrhythmic activity."

Dock removed the cover of the candy box and showed me about twenty vials, each containing white powder identified by a number. There was also a stack of cards identifying the chemical structure of each compound. I saw immediately that they were a series of homologous compounds, which would allow comparison of the relationship of chemical structure to antiarrhythmic activity.

"Why don't they do the screening themselves?" I asked.

"They are just getting reorganized and have neither the personnel nor the laboratory and animal facilities to do the work," Dock replied. "They want to farm this one out."

"Are these compounds patented and can I publish the results even if they come out negative, without interference from the drug company?" I inquired.

"Yes, on both counts. I have Tainter's word on this," said Dock with a smile. "Anticipating your next question I arranged that you should have a $3,000 annual grant from the company. It's not much money, but it will at least allow you to hire an assistant and pay for animals, supplies, and some equipment."

This seemed fair enough, and I indicated my interest in doing the project. Dock seemed pleased and left me with the candy box, its vials, and Tainter's phone number. I was once again plunged into research, despite the fact that I was in private practice, had a part-time teaching job, and was doing much free work in clinics and wards of two hospitals.

It was late spring. My plan was to start the work in July so that I might have a full academic year to do the work. I first had to devise a screening method that would be cheap, scientifically valid, and simple. Not an easy order because, up to this time, there'd been relatively little work on this subject. I began by doing experiments on frogs. Although partly successful, I abandoned them because work done on a lower animal order might have less clinical significance in humans. Cats proved to be the best choice. The cat's heart is in some ways closer to the human's than a dog's or pig's heart. Using an open chest preparation with artificial respiration, it was possible to measure the threshold amount of current needed for an electrical pulse of 600 cycles per minute just to fibrillate the atrium of the heart. Better methods have since been devised, but this original method of screening antiarrhythmic drugs still remains valid today.

My plans turned next to securing assistance. I could hire a technician, but I felt that the work required someone more mature and more capable of making clinical correlations. Meanwhile, the war had ended, and my good friend Julius Stolfi had returned to the Kings County Hospital to complete his residency training. I asked him to find me a bright resident who would be willing to spend a year as my research fellow. I could only offer a stipend of $1,500 a year, but the work would be rewarding and would count as educational credit toward the boards of internal medicine. An enthusiastic and convincing character, Stolfi talked Richard Reiss into accepting the job. Dick was a young resident who turned out to be a great find by not only doing what was expected of him, but also contributing original ideas.

We began to collect significant data. The work was going well when fate again twisted my plans. My kind benefactor, George B. Ray, suddenly died. Meanwhile Raymond Johnson had found himself a better job in Nebraska, so the Department of Physiology and Pharmacology was left with no one to teach the courses except a part-time person—notably myself.

Dean Curran asked if I felt capable of running both courses for the year until they could find another chairman. Against my better judgment I replied that I could, but in order to run the department I would have to hire at least one more person and retain the present secretary and diener (the person who builds lab equipment and handles electronics). I would also require an additional stipend because this teaching load was full-time and would cut into my practice and research efforts. Curran was agreeable to this, but the stipend he offered was not overly generous considering that he was saving the salaries of a chairman and two professors. I accepted the challenge, nevertheless, because any money looked like big money to me at that time.

Dick Reiss, my research fellow, was bright, vocal, and made an excellent instructor. Of course, I made sure to provide him an additional stipend. He had just been married and could use the extra cash. Youthful energy is wonderful. I rapidly made plans and organized a course of instruction based on the previous course, but with some ingenious innovations of my own. The laboratory work was increased somewhat. When I look back now, I cannot believe that I gave practically all the lectures, attended all the labs, made out exams, and did all the paper work required.

I also kept my office hours and attended to all my clinical duties, but I made very few house calls. This was no way to build a large practice, but I managed at least to maintain what I had and even make a small profit. I received invaluable help from the department secretary, Mrs. Danziger, a lovely and capable woman, and Carl, the diener. Dick Reiss proved to be most capable and efficient at running all the laboratories while carrying on the research work with ease. From a critical viewpoint, the course we ran was undoubtedly mediocre, yet the students did exceedingly well in the national boards in physiology and especially in pharmacology where they received the highest score in the country. Credit for this must be attributed to the fact that we had some of the brightest students in the country at that time. A good many came from City College and many had advanced degrees.

Despite these successes, the academic year came to a tragic end. With the extra stipend Dick had received, he bought a used car and planned a vacation trip to Chicago with his wife and young daughter. Just outside Chicago the car hit an oil slick, went into a spin, and overturned in a ditch. Dick's chest was crushed by the steering wheel, and he died within minutes. His wife and daughter were badly shaken but not seriously hurt. Thus ended a brilliant career of a young physician. I was particularly depressed by this tragic loss because I'd grown to respect and admire Dick for his many fine qualities. I also felt a sense of guilt because I was responsible for his opportunity to make extra cash available to buy the fatal automobile. I did what I could for the wife and daughter. She eventually remarried after a period of severe depression and went on to lead a useful life.

The work on the alpha fagarine compounds, although promising, was far from being completed so I asked Maurice Tainter for a year's extension of the grant. He was agreeable. I sought another research fellow, Joseph Lambert, a pleasant, happy go-lucky type, who was not as bright as Dick but capable enough. He had been married for three years and already had three offspring. He worked out very well, and together we published several papers. Lambert was inherently not a research type, but he ended up as a very successful internist with a large practice in Bayshore, Long Island.

Dean Curran meanwhile had secured a large grant from the Rockefeller Institute to rebuild the Physiology Department. He was able to secure Chandler Brooks as the new chairman. Chandler was a rather stiff person. Although the students called him the "The Mortician," he was actually a very fine, generous person. His main work had been in neurophysiology and merited eminent recognition. He had worked and published with Eccles, who was considered one of the world's most distinguished neurophysiologists and resided in New Zealand. There was no doubt that Chandler was a great addition to the faculty of the Long Island College of Medicine. He wisely recommended that the subjects of physiology and pharmacology be separated into individual departments. As a result of this decision, Guilio Cantoni was recruited to run the pharmacology course. Guilio was really a biochemist, and a good one at that, and a very keen researcher. He hired a young biology major named Elizabeth Moore, the daughter of the chairman of the newly established Department of Preventative Medicine, and someone who would soon become more involved in my life. I was kept on as a part-time assistant professor to teach both physiology and pharmacology. This allowed me to maintain a research laboratory and continue my own work. I also had more time now to devote to my practice and to the Department of Medicine.

Such is the contrariness of life that during this period of my life, when I was so busy and involved in my work, I was more in tune with the opposite sex than ever before. As I approached the age of thirty, perhaps I felt that there was a danger of becoming a confirmed bachelor. I had dates with Marion from time to time, but I knew that she would never be a permanent mate. I tried to turn the affair into one of friendship alone, but such arrangements never work out.

I meanwhile became attached to Elizabeth Moore who was a

more suitable age. Tall and attractive, with dark eyes and hair, she had a wonderful smile. Her prominent cheekbones suggested an Asian influence that she inherited from her father who was part American Indian. Her mother was decidedly English. I managed to see Elizabeth nearly every day at the laboratory, and we went out to dinner and sometimes a movie once a week. I often had dinner with her family in Queens. I even had her over to my house for dinner. As I expected, my family reacted rather coolly toward her. They did admit, however, that she was a step above other dates I had managed to drag home for their inspection. Since my siblings were all unmarried themselves and had little prospects, I suppose they were in a position to be hypercritical. My mother naturally felt that no woman was good enough for her son. It so happened that my cousin, made a seemingly fabulous marriage to a lovely Italian girl who came from wealthy, well-connected parents, which my family made sure to point out to me. Elizabeth and I got along with each other, and had not other events conspired, we may well have eventually married.

Our research indicated that some of the alpha fagarine-like compounds had superior antiarrhythmic activity to quinidine and appeared to be less toxic. We settled on one compound, numbered 1227, as the best of the lot according to the data we had collected. I asked Maurice Tainter if Sterling Winthrop was agreeable to testing this drug in humans to learn if it was effective. I also consulted with my medicine chief, Bill Dock. All gave their sanction so I proceeded to do toxicity studies in mice, rats, and dogs.

I had a medical student who'd worked at New York University with Bernard Brodie who first developed a methods of measuring the blood level of drugs. The student knew how to do a chemical procedure that Brodie had devised to measure the blood level of alkaloids. I took Number 1227 orally myself, and then gave some to healthy volunteers, measuring the blood levels obtained. The study indicated that the drug was well tolerated with a minimum of side effects. Absorption by the oral route was poor, but sufficient, as shown by the blood level studies. This suggested, however, that intramuscular administration might be advisable. Indeed, this was one of the first pharmacokinetic studies done on any drug prior to clinical use.

At the time there was no controlling Food and Drug Administration (FDA) legislation that required special approval for new drugs to be administered to humans. It was not mandatory to obtain written informed consent from patients as it is today. It was considered good medical practice to let patients know what drugs were being prescribed and what risks were to be expected. I always explained to each patient what drugs I was recommending and the possible benefits and dangers of each agent. My experimental data indicated that in every respect Number 1227 was as safe as quinidine, the drug most often used as an antiarrhythmic. Having taken some of the drug myself and tested it on other human volunteers, I considered it ready for a cautious clinical trial.

I had a male patient with diabetes and hyperthyroidism in my practice who was satisfactorily treated with insulin and antithyroid drugs. He also had atrial fibrillation that did not respond to quinidine. He was not an ideal patient because of his co-morbidities, but I decided to try 1227. After informing him of the experimental nature of the drug and its possible dangers, I prescribed the lowest calculated dose. His arrhythmia did not respond, but after doubling the dose, I was pleased to observe that he had converted to a normal sinus rhythm. The patient felt much better and thought I was a magician, while I was much encouraged to carry on the investigation.

Administration of 1227 to the next nineteen patients by the oral route showed that about 30 percent who had not responded to quinidine could have their arrhythmia corrected by 1227. This was very encouraging, but there was the problem of inconsistent oral absorption. I was therefore moved to study intramuscular administration. I now had a third research assistant, John Shults, whom I encouraged to find inpatients at Kings County Hospital with a recent onset of atrial fibrillation but had not responded to quinidine. His first patient was a seventy-eight-year-old man with a long history of heart disease. After obtaining consent, he administered the calculated therapeutic dose of 1227 intramuscularly. The continuous recording of the electrocardiogram showed a conversion of the atrial fibrillation to a regular rhythm in ten minutes. In a few more minutes, the patient unfortunately, developed ventricular tachycardia, which soon degenerated into ventricular fibrillation—a uniformly fatal arrhythmia. Attempts to revive the patient proved useless and he expired.

Needless to say, Shults and I were devastated. I even seriously considered giving up the practice of medicine. Bill Dock, my medical chief, was very kind and pointed out that such medical misadventures occur to every physician, especially those who are courageous enough to conduct investigations. Dock took me to his office and pulled out a file of patients who in his experience had died as a result of misdiagnosis or physician error. The important thing, he pointed out, is to learn from the episode and avoid the error in the future. The case should be published so that other physicians may avoid the same error. I resolved to follow his advice.

As I studied the case in retrospect, I observed that the patient had an intraventricular block besides his atrial fibrillation. Search of the medical literature uncovered a few cases reported by other physicians of the fatal consequences of quinidine administration in patients with intraventricular block. Oddly, this was not mentioned in the two foremost texts of cardiology authored by Sam Levine and Paul D. White. I searched the medical records of Kings County Hospital and found that a similar sudden death had occurred in three other cases receiving quinidine when intraventricular block existed. At the time the significance of the long Q-T Syndrome was not known which this patient may have had making him susceptible to a fatal cardiac arrhythmia.

I resolved to write an authoritative article on antiarrhythmic drugs pointing out this danger. With John Shults' help and the critical advice of Bill Dock, the article was eventually written and published in the journal *Medicine* in 1950. In my rounds at Kings County Hospital, I spotted many such cases before the quinidine had a chance to do its deadly work. So in an indirect way, my medical misfortune ended up saving countless lives. This phenomenon has been rediscovered and studied in great detail in recent years. As many new, more potent antiarrhythmic drugs have been developed and used, the "sudden death syndrome" has become an epidemic. A large clinical study sponsored by the National Institutes of Health has demonstrated that chronic use of antiarrhythmic drugs under inappropriate conditions increases mortality. As a result the FDA has caused some of the more culpable drugs to be withdrawn and certain others to be restricted in use. The ideal antiarrhythmic drug has yet to be discovered.

As to 1227, Sterling Winthrop lost interest in it following my report, but especially when it was learned from South America that alpha fagarine was causing fatal ventricular fibrillation. The company was generous enough to let me publish several papers on the relationship of chemical structure to antifibrillatory activity of the compounds they had supplied to me. The work was of scientific merit and could help other scientists in the study of drug action on the sensitive membranes of the heart.

Another spin off was the stimulation of my interest in the physiology of the sensitive and excitable membranes of the heart, notably the sinus and atrio-ventricular nodes, but especially the purkinje fibres. An isolated papillary muscle of the cat's heart, which had recently been devised, proved to be ideal for the experiments I contemplated. NIH had started to provide grants to young investigators, and I made haste to get one. This enabled me to take on another research fellow, Antonio Mascatello, and continue in research even though I was still in active practice.

To continue my research, I needed a square wave dual pulse electronic generator in which the second pulse could be separated from the first by incremental amounts. This apparatus was not available commercially. I explained my problem to department chairman Chandler Brooks, who was sympathetic to my research ideas. He had imported from New Zealand an electronics wizard, Peter Suckling, who could help me. With Peter's know-how, I was able to build myself this complicated stimulator. This enabled Mascatello and me to conduct some classical experiments on the excitability of the isolated papillary muscle of the cat and the effects drugs had on it.

As an aside, my theories about the excitability and refractory period of heart muscle did more for Brooks than they eventually did for me. He saw the potential value of my ideas and decided to exploit them himself. He took on a research fellow, Brian Hoffman, who had been a former student and had just finished his tour of army duty. Brooks asked me about Brian's aptitude for research, and I gave a lukewarm answer because I had never observed any research interest in Brian. How wrong I was! Chandler Brooks and Brian Hoffman went on to establish the field of cardiac electrophysiology that has had tremendous impact in the diagnosis and therapy of heart disease. Brian became chairman of the Department of Pharmacology at Columbia's College of Physicians and Surgeons, and has had a truly distinguished career. In science, who first has an idea is less important than who exploits and develops it to the point where other scientists can use it. It has always been a source of pleasure to me that I have been a small, but perhaps significant, instigator of cardiac electrophysiology.

I did not neglect my practice even though my research work continued to blossom. I had a waiting line of loyal patients spilling out into the hallway from my small waiting room. My medical chief at Kings County Hospital was now Bill Dock, who had gotten into some altercation at the Long Island College Hospital and, as a solution, changed places with Crawford. Kings County suited him much better and Crawford was also happier at Long Island. I often made rounds with Dock and learned many clinical pearls from him. I was pretty much second-in-command in the academic medical department. The course in physical diagnosis was put in my charge. This was quite an assignment because it consists of one-on-one instruction. Luckily I was able to recruit many young doctors to assist me for a small stipend. When Dock was on a trip, which was often because he was a very popular speaker, I would substitute for him on rounds. Residents who must accompany the chief on rounds have an appropriate name for the exercise: "shifting dullness," a parody on a famous physical sign of fluid in the chest. Contrary to most clinicians, Dock made rounds interesting and instructive. He had an endless fund of anecdotes and practical wisdom that offset the boredom of seeing the same disease or symptom repeatedly. I tried to emulate Dock when I made rounds, but I could never equal his skill and fund of knowledge. My years of teaching physiology and pharmacology, however, gave me enough background so that I had insight and information that many physicians lacked and could make my comments reasonably interesting and informative. I was gradually getting a considerable reputation as a clinician, sought after by residents and students.

Meanwhile, I was getting more attached to Elizabeth. We dated at least once a week and saw each other daily. We seemed to enjoy the same things. Her family was cordial toward me. Papa was a great golfer and a heavy drinker. I had the impression that he would have liked me better if I too was a golfer, which I definitely wasn't, but I did bend the elbow with him once or twice. The desire to find a permanent mate was slowly infecting me, and Elizabeth appeared to be an ideal candidate. Although we got to the stage of some heavy petting, we never made sexual contact. Perhaps this was because I was still seeing Marion on occasion and my sexual appetite was appeased. And although I was now making a decent income, I still had not built up enough of a nest egg to consider setting up a domicile. As I still lived at home, I felt it only fair to pay board as well as pay back on the monies my family had spent on tuition.

Although I was successful in practice, the physical work was exhausting and there was not much time for intellectual development. The hankering to become an academic physician was always in the back of my mind. Such positions were difficult to acquire and did not, as a rule, pay wages comparable to what could be earned in even a modest practice. I bitterly missed the opportunity that I'd nearly had to spend a year or two at the Thorndike Laboratory in Boston. That would have undoubtedly set me on the right track for an academic appointment. When I consulted with Dock and Dean Curran, both advised me to take six months off and spend it in a first-class research lab. Curran was particularly helpful and offered to continue my modest part-time salary while I was away. I would have to continue paying my office expenses, of course, and secure someone to take care of my patients.

Despite these anticipated hardships, I determined to find an opportunity before I became too old and burdened with family obligations. Gene Landis had recently replaced Bradford Cannon as chairman of Physiology at Harvard. He had done outstanding work on the capillary and peripheral circulation and might well be agreeable to have a guest research fellow who had done work on the small blood vessels of the skin. In fact, he had himself spent a year with Sir Thomas Lewis in England. I asked Dean Curran to contact Gene Landis about the possibility of my spending time in his laboratory. To my great pleasure, Landis agreed to have me as a teaching fellow in the Department of Physiology at Harvard from February to June 1946.

I set off for Boston early in the morning one fine day in the middle of winter. The old Dodge had new tires and brakes and purred along the old Post Road until just outside of Hartford, Connecticut. As the skies darkened, it began to snow lightly. I managed to get through Hartford, but then the snow really began to fall. It soon became impossible to make any headway. Fog and swirling snow made visibility poor. As I crept along, I must have deviated into an off-road because I was suddenly stuck in deep snow in the middle of an open field. No one was in sight. I had the eerie feeling that I was completely lost without hope of rescue. I did have the foresight to pack a pair of chains with the rest of the junk I carried. Putting a pair of chains on the rear wheels is never an easy job. In the midst of deep snow, it is even more difficult because the car must be jacked up on a slippery surface. I managed to get them on and was able to back up the car in its own tracks to the main road. With the chains still on, I proceeded slowly and tediously to Boston.

I arrived late in the evening. The snow had stopped but at least 12 inches were on the ground. The main thoroughfares had been plowed, and I was able to find my way to Harvard Medical School. The ancient Peter Bent Hotel was across the street on

Commonwealth Avenue. I parked in front, entered the hotel, and was greeted by a sleepy clerk who seemed surprised to see me. After I registered, he led me to an old elevator and a third floor room that could not have been bigger than six by eight feet. It was sparsely furnished with a single iron post bed, a wooden chair, and a nightstand. A big cast iron radiator sat underneath a large window. It might have been a prison cell except for the window. But the price was right—only $3 a night—and it was only a block away from my place of work.

Early the next morning, I made my to the Harvard Medical School campus, the most impressive campus I had ever seen. Built on the Greco-Roman style of architecture of massive stone and marble with colonnades, it occupied an enormous rectangle bigger than a football field. An administration building was at the head with separate but matching buildings at the sides of a large central courtyard. The Roman forum must have inspired the architect. I inquired at the administration building where I might find Dr. Landis and the Department of Physiology. Directed to a corner building at the right of the campus, I made my way to the second floor to a large office laboratory suite. A nice Irish secretary pointed to a chair and said that Landis would see me soon. Presently, a very professional looking man of average size came out and shook my hand. He wore an immaculate white starched laboratory coat and appeared too neat to be a professor or a scientist. He was most cordial and said he had read my work on reactive hyperemia of the skin blood vessels and was impressed by it. He felt my work would make a good fit with the research of Clifford Barger, a young instructor who had been collaborating with Landis for about a year. Landis hoped that we could work together on the mechanism of heart failure. Without further fanfare, he led me down to the large first floor laboratory that contained an enormous machine built into the floor. I later learned it was the first treadmill built in the United States. Landis introduced me to Cliff Barger who sat at an old desk in the corner. Then Landis left abruptly.

Cliff was a thin, rather tall young fellow with a square decisive face, deep-set piercing black eyes under thick black eyebrows, and a broad high forehead. His hair was jet-black and combed back. He smiled and said, "Let's start by you calling me Cliff. I'll call you Yousel. Welcome to Harvard."

By calling me "Yousel," I felt he was telling me that he was Jewish and that he accepted me although I was Christian. That was fine with me, as my best friends were Jewish. Indeed, with my Brooklynese accent and large nose, I certainly looked and sounded more Jewish than he did. I soon learned that he knew my former research fellow, Dick Reese, and his wife so we immediately formed a common bond. I didn't know it then, but Cliff and I were to become lifelong friends in many ways, with a bond even stronger than that between brothers.

That first day we spent an hour or more discussing our research interests. Cliff studied venous pressure as it related to exhausting exercise and heart failure. His plan was to measure venous pressure of both humans and dogs in progressively severe exercise, along with other modalities. I felt that we could measure the responses of the small blood vessels of the skin with my reactive hyperemia device and that it would add significant data. This could only be done in the human subjects. By using dogs, we could measure central venous pressure directly in the right atrium by means of a catheter passed through the jugular vein. Cliff then showed me how to operate the treadmill. I tried it out myself and found to my chagrin that I could only run five miles an hour at a ten-degree slope for four minutes. After catching my breath and assured by Cliff that my run was not too bad, I followed him on a tour of the department.

First we visited the former laboratory of Walter Bradford Cannon. The room was bare, but just standing in the laboratory where this great man had conducted his most famous experiments was an impressive feeling. A notable feature was a working fireplace, suggestive of an ancient alchemist's laboratory. The department also boasted of its own extensive physiology library, separate from the main medical library, with its own librarian and indexing system. I was much impressed by this but more so by the large, well-stocked storeroom. Next to the storeroom was a workshop, which to my delight held a South Bend Lathe complete with accessories. Another room contained an electronics workshop, also well equipped. Dr. Grass, the famous electronics instrument inventor who had recently left to establish his own factory and business, had occupied it. An animal facility with its own caretaker was on the top floor. There were student laboratories and laboratories of the various faculty members. I thought this facility was probably one of the best facilities for study and research in physiology in the entire country.

During the tour of the department, I had a chance to meet with other faculty members. John Papenheimer, an assistant professor, was a tall, slightly stooped, very intellectual looking young man. His father was A.M. Papenheimer, an eminent pathologist in New York City. John was cordial but had a reserved manner. He took pains to explain his method of using electrical conductance to measure the caliber of small vessels. There was little doubt that he had skill and a first-class research mind. Assistant professor John Perkins, a thin man with the look of an aesthetic, was most pleasant and deeply dedicated to the science of physiology. I never did find out exactly what his strength in research was. Cliff whispered to me that he was independently wealthy and probably worked for a nominal salary. It was impossible not to like Perkins. He was so sterling a character, concerned with everybody's welfare, and so deeply interested in the science of physiology.

Several other young scientist fellows seemed to be more detached from the mainstream. One was a young woman, Ellen Allen, who related directly to Landis and barely to the rest of us. All these people were intensely competitive and worked as if their life depended on it. I soon found out that Landis made rounds every morning starting at eight o'clock, visited each laboratory and inspected the data collected from the previous day. He made pertinent comments, often very kindly intended, but certainly designed to exert some pressure to produce. He also had a curious system of colored cards—green, yellow, and pink—on which he scribbled assignments. I never did figure out what the colors meant. All this produced an atmosphere of intense competition and raised the level of performance. This was Harvard, and we were expected to do the best work or get out. In some ways, I was amused by this because I was already an accomplished scientist and, to tell the truth, although much younger than Landis, I had almost as many publications as he did and in as many good journals as he had. I adapted to the system nevertheless and became an eager beaver just for the joy of the game. After all, I didn't need any more publications. All I wanted was a good mailing address and fine recommendations to put my curriculum vitae in the right groove. I certainly had no intentions of remaining at Harvard. I was there to learn, and I was determined to accomplish as much as I could in the allotted time.

On Cliff's advice, I soon found myself a furnished room in a boarding house on Beacon Street in Brookline. It had a much better atmosphere than the hotel and provided a continental breakfast as part of the modest rent. Parking was available in a middle strip on Beacon Street, and it was no more than a ten minute ride to the school. Meals were a problem because restaurant food and my stomach did not agree. I began to lose weight. Cliff and his wife invited me to their apartment about once a week for a great home cooked meal.

I had much in common with the Bargers. Cliff had a history of tuberculosis similar to mine. His diagnosis was the main reason he had gone into physiology instead of medical practice. Claire, his young bride, was a lovely girl, spirited, full of fun. Her father was in the wholesale grocery business in Connecticut, so we had a common thread since I was a retail grocer's son. Between the fruit her father sent her and the cuts of beef Cliff's father sent from the family farm and butcher business, they had an ample supply that they generously shared with me. They also provided what recreation I had time to indulge in. Once we went bicycling; another time horseback riding; several times to musicals and shows. Cliff had a former patient, a South American diabetic who came to Boston to the Joslin Clinic to get his diabetes straightened out from time to time. He provided the Bargers with tickets to shows. I remember seeing Carmen Jones with the Bargers. Thus, with our research and teaching interests, Cliff and I became close friends, closer than I'd been to anyone else. The Bargers made my stay in Boston worthwhile, even beyond the academic benefits of working at a great university.

Teaching students at Harvard was no different from my experience in Brooklyn. On the whole they were quite bright but not as capable as my best New York City College students. I had the distinction of teaching the first Harvard Medical School class that had females. This was nothing new to me because we had women in the class long before Harvard succumbed to the opposite sex. I was assigned mostly to laboratory teaching, which suited me fine because it allowed me to get to know students personally. The students were more genteel and seemed to have more versatile backgrounds than my Brooklyn students. One group appeared somewhat less able than the rest. I found out later that they were dental students; the course was being given simultaneously to both medical and dental candidates.

Among the eleven female students, one was older than the rest. Rumor had it that she was a Hollywood movie actress who had been married but was now divorced. She decided to go into medicine for unknown reasons and was bright enough and financially able to do it. Cliff warned me that she had her eye on me, which I didn't believe. We had an experiment one week that required sacrificing rabbits. Our actress student took two of them home and prepared a Hassenfeffer stew. She invited me to her apartment to share in this feast. It was a delicious meal complete with trimmings and wine. I left as soon as possible, claiming important work had to be urgently done. I will never know whether she had amorous intentions or was merely trying to earn brownie points to pass the course. Not wishing to engage in any more entangling affairs, I stayed clear of her.

Landis had designed a very complete, well-organized laboratory course. A detailed manual made the experiments clear. Students could volunteer to do additional experiments to gain extra knowledge and some honor points. At Landis's suggestion, I devised an endocrine experiment using some experience I had gained from working with Sam Reynolds. It involved doing vaginal epithelial stains in female rats. The estrus cycle of individual rats could be studied by making daily observations for a week or two. The effects of estrogens could also be observed. An amusing sidelight of this experiment was the requirement for students to insert their arms into a large cage of rats to pick out their particular specimens. If they didn't insert their arms determinably or their hands trembled, their clumsy handling of the rat would usually result in a nasty bite. I got the reputation of teaching Harvard students how to handle rats!

As a gadgeteer, I had a lot of fun with our experimental work. My experience with the South Bend Lathe came in handy to turn out special cannulas for catheterizing the dogs. In the human experiments, we had to measure respiratory rate as the subjects exercised along with many other observations that kept us very busy. I was able to devise a gadget that digitized the rate with a counter. Then I arranged a movie camera to photograph the counter as well as a clock so that we had a permanent automated record of this data. I bought a surplus Army Radar Scope and converted it into a useful laboratory oscilloscope. I spent many nights working on this project until two in the morning. The electronics shop, which contained meters, resisters, condensers and tubes, came in very handy.

A large, prestigious university is a mecca for scientists, both local and international. In my brief stay I met personally more prominent scientists and Nobel Prize winners than I have met since. One of these was August Krogh, a most impressive elderly gentleman. I also had opportunities to talk with Hallowell Davis, the famous neurophysiologist. He was in the process of leaving the department to head a large new laboratory on hearing defects in St. Louis. He and Authuro Rosenbleuth, who had been prominent members of the department under Cannon, were apparently not too happy with Landis and decided to leave for greener pastures. Rosenblueth went on to establish the Cardiovascular Institute of Mexico, which achieved considerable prominence and fame. The famous physiologist Alexander Forbes, a retired member of the department, maintained a small office. Younger men like myself gained much from friendly conversations with Forbes, who had done so much useful work for the Navy in World War I.

I missed my family. I especially felt the lack of female companionship. Elizabeth came up to Boston one weekend to visit her aunt. We made a day of it, spending some time with the Bargers but much of it with each other. She was very affectionate on this occasion. I had the feeling that if I had asked her to marry me that weekend, which I was considering doing, she would have accepted. Some instinct made me hesitate. I decided to delay asking her until I returned to Brooklyn. As events later developed, this was a wise decision.

Landis invited us all over to his house in the suburbs one Sunday afternoon. Although it was already spring, snow and ice were still on the ground. Landis's afternoon tea was a bit formal and stiff, as everyone was trying to be on their best behavior. Landis had a charming wife who did her best to soften and lighten the atmosphere. The intellectual talk of professors and scientists is at best boring, except to the people expressing it. The affair was a nice gesture, but did little to allay the fears and ambitions of the young fellows who were so competitive.

I was flattered when John Papenheimer asked me out to dinner one evening. The son of a prominent pathologist, he had a brilliant mind with an IQ far above my own and an upbringing far different from mine. I wondered what interest he could have in me. Our dinner conversation explained it. We had extended discussion about the virtues of a career in pure science as contrasted to one devoted to medical practice. He spent considerable effort trying to convince me to give up my practice and devote my time entirely to teaching and research. I suspected that he was, in effect, convincing himself that he had made the right decision to devote himself entirely to science.

I actually believe this is mainly a question of personality. He was of a reticent nature and uncomfortable with people, particularly those of lesser mentality than his own. I was much more outgoing, liked being with people, and had a stronger need to earn money, which was not available in a pure science career. Our conversation of that evening stuck in my mind because it is difficult to divide your attention between the requirements of research and those of practice. Each is a severe taskmaster and wants to consume all your energies. Indeed, few manage to combine the two successfully. Sooner or later, you must yield to one side or the other.

Cliff and I enjoyed each other's company and worked very well together on our research. We were beginning to get results and made efforts to write them up for publication. Landis, however, was far from satisfied with either the data or the writing. This was probably justified. It took one more year and several more research fellows to complete the work to Landis's satisfaction.

Working with the dogs proved to be difficult. It was virtually impossible to run them to the point of exhaustion. They would willingly run until their feet would bleed at any speed or incline of the treadmill. It was a lesson in the superior efficiency of the horizontal posture in contrast to the upright, and that of four legs to that of two legs. One dog subject was especially able. He was undoubtedly a mongrel, but resembled a gray colored German Shepard. We called him "Speed" and became as fond of him as if he were our personal pet. We took turns walking him about the courtyard and brought him special food snacks. After our daily experiments, the dogs had to be returned to the general pool of animals. Afraid that Speed would be used in a lethal experiment, Cliff managed to keep him free of harm for many years. Contrary to the interdictions of antivivasectionists, most scientists I have known grow fond of the animals they work with. One female biologist worked with bats and had an uncanny ability to grow and handle them. She was appropriately known as the "Bat Lady." George Koelle, a famous pharmacologist, worked with cats. He adopted several crippled ones and kept them as pets. When he sat for a portrait to be hung in his honor at the University of Pennsylvania, he insisted that it be done with him holding a cat.

The end of my sojourn at Harvard came all too soon. After a final dinner with the Bargers and promises to visit soon, I packed my old Dodge and returned to Brooklyn to take up where I had left off. My practice was much reduced, not surprisingly from my long absence, but many patients were overjoyed to see me return. I was soon busier than I wanted to be. Academically, Dock offered me a position as assistant professor of medicine, full-time and at an agreeable salary. I accepted, provided I could keep my private practice and my affiliation with physiology and pharmacology. The administration agreed to my request. There was no provision for a practice plan for full-time physicians as there is today. This meant that I must concentrate my time at Kings County Hospital.

With all good intentions, I set up a laboratory to study peripheral vascular disease. Kings County provided an ample supply of human clinical material for these studies. It was a good fit with my research background. Dock provided me with a fellow, so I had some help. Together we provided a valuable consultative service, but the research aspects did not seem to gel. My teaching and clinical duties were heavy. I didn't have time to devote to original ideas in research. One of my old professors told me that leisure time was important to think. Now I realized that this was only too true. Unfortunately, leisure time was the one thing I did not have.

Elizabeth and I began to see each other again on a regular basis, but she was somehow a little distant and less affectionate. I suspected that perhaps my sisters, who had her over to dinner in my absence, had somehow adversely affected her. Guilio Cantoni, for whom Elizabeth worked, called me over one day for a private conversation. In a paternal manner—which I considered strange for we were the same age—he advised me that Elizabeth would not make a good wife for me. She is dating other fellows, he said, and "is just stringing you along." I had half suspected this but didn't want to believe it. I resented Guilio's well-intended advice and was disturbed that he took the trouble to advise me since we were by no means close friends. Yet, as I reflected on this later in life, I realized that he must have thought highly of me to make what must have been an embarrassing effort for him.

As fate would have it, Guilio did not last much longer at Long Island. His laboratory just above the library had a severe water leak and flooded the floor below, causing serious water damage to valuable and irreplaceable books. The cause was a glass water still that was let run over night. As the water pressure rose, the rubber hoses slipped off the condenser and caused the flood. When the Dean called Guilio in to chastise him, Guilio instead gave the Dean a piece of his mind. He faulted the institution for being too cheap to have security guards to make rounds at night to prevent such accidents. This didn't sit well with the Dean, and Guilio soon left for greener pastures. This was a great loss because Guilio was one of the most brilliant researchers I had ever met. His subsequent work on biochemical aspects of cancer was seminal, and he received much acclaim for it.

Guilio's replacement was Nicholas Dreyer, a tall gangling Africaner. He came from Nova Scotia and was a friend of Professor Moore, Elizabeth's father. Nick was a most interesting character who had his training in England with the famous group of physiologists and pharmacologists at the University of London and at Edinburgh. He told vivid tales of these great men and their idiosyncrasies, including even Sir Charles Sherrington, the very famous neurophysiologist. Nick and I became close friends and collaborated on several research projects. Elizabeth served as his technician. My association with Nick made me feel that I was experiencing some aura from the fathers of physiology and pharmacology.

While I maintained an active connection with both basic science and academic clinical medicine, my growing private practice prevented me from engaging in major research projects. I soon discovered that one really sick patient can keep you occupied all day, not only with visits with the patient, but with conversations with relatives, and residents anxious to try every new treatment. I was working seven days a week, usually fourteen to sixteen hours long. Yet, I managed to do a few arbeits, or potboilers, in research.

One of these was with Dick Gubner, a fellow physician maybe a year or two older than I. Compared to me, he was born with the proverbial silver spoon in his mouth. His father was a very successful otolaryngologist who indulged his only son. Dick didn't have to scrounge for a living, as I did, and had some leisure time. He had a nose for money and managed a number of jobs with the Pennsylvania Railroad, as well as insurance and drug companies that allowed a very comfortable living without the necessity of seeing endless private patients. He also had an uncanny ability to ferret out interesting research projects, mostly with immediate clinical significance, but he had little ability or facilities to carry them out, especially if they required actual experimental work. Versed as I was in peripheral vascular disease, he succeeded in persuading me to explore the potential of using glycine—an amino acid that in most people has a specific dynamic action (increases the basal metabolism)—to improve the blood flow in the limbs of arteriosclerotic patients.

Rescuing an old but still useful plethysemograph from the pile of junk that collects over time in every laboratory, we measured the blood flow in the legs of every subject we could convince to sit imprisoned in the device for several hours. Sure enough, glycine administered as ordinary gelatin did significantly increase the blood flow in the lower limbs. The disadvantage was that glycine in the amounts required to achieve this improvement was nauseating to most subjects. Nevertheless, we proved the point that the specific dynamic action of foodstuffs might be used to therapeutic advantage in patients with peripheral vascular disease. We published a paper covering this work in the *American Journal of Medicine*.

I passed my time doing some research but hardly in the mainstream that I had been used to when my practice was less demanding. I had many occasions to rue the statement of Meltzher, a famous clinician and researcher, who said: "The practice of medicine is the graveyard of many fine medical minds."

Although I saw Elizabeth every day, we somehow became more distant and dated less often. She confronted me one day with the statement that we probably should stop seeing each other. She suspected that I intended to ask for her hand in marriage. It would not work out, she said, because we had conflicting characters. She hoped we could remain friends, but our relationship could not go beyond that. I was devastated and depressed, but no amount of arguing would change her mind. She knew herself better than I did. She tended to be a carefree person little interested in science and intellectual pursuits. My own dedication to science and medicine would lead to inevitable conflicts. I later discovered that she had found someone who suited her much better. Within six months she was married and moved to Chicago. I never saw her again.

It has been said that those disappointed in love soon fall into another relationship. Jim Hamilton, the chairman of Anatomy, had a technician who was also a graduate student working toward a Ph.D. in anatomy. I didn't know she existed, but she knew something about me because George Paff had gotten her to use some spring clamps I'd devised to expedite the adrenolectomies she was doing in rats. Chances were that I would probably never have met Mary Solowey except for a coincidence involving her sister, Elsie.

A few years older than Mary, Elsie was working toward a degree in physics at New York University. After having received a required immunization, Elsie became intensely jaundiced and feverish. Alarmed, Mary asked about for a good internist. Paff and Hamilton recommended me. Mary promptly called and asked me to see her sister who was at home in the Bronx. I explained that I didn't make house calls in the Bronx. Besides, it sounded like a hospital case to me, so I advised her to put her sister in a taxi and take her to the Long Island College Hospital where I would arrange to admit her immediately. As soon as I saw her, it was obvious that Elsie either had obstructive jaundice or hepatitis. I leaned toward the latter diagnosis. I ordered the appropriate liver function tests and reassured her that she would recover. Our knowledge of hepatitis in 1947 was primitive compared to today. We didn't have types A, B, and C, nor did we have vaccines. There was only one kind of infectious hepatitis, and there was no specific therapy. Fortunately, like most patients Elsie got better. It was a case of "I treated her, but God cured her." In five days, the fever and jaundice disappeared, and I sent her home with the usual instructions to take it real easy for a month and to eat a light diet. The interesting thing was that I only saw Mary once during Elsie's admission. Apparently, Mary would sneak in to see her sister only when she was sure I wouldn't be there. I thought nothing of this at the time, but I did think she was an attractive girl, someone I would like to know better.

A few months passed. I had pretty much forgotten the whole episode when I received a wedding invitation to Elsie's wedding. I would ordinarily turn down such an invitation politely, but a lingering desire to see more of Mary gave me impetus to accept. When I got to the reception, I surmised that the only reason the sisters had invited me was to match me up as an eligible bachelor with one of the bridesmaids who didn't have an escort. Her name was Ethyl, a big freckled, redheaded Irish girl with a raucous voice who was as little attracted to me as I was to her. Mary didn't seem to have a particular escort, and I found it easy to spend my time with her. We danced together and made light conversation, which came naturally because of mutual acquaintances at the Long Island Medical College. I found her to an extremely forthright, a dedicated person who had had a strict upbringing. She was fairly tall with a husky but not unattractive body, a round face, clear blue eyes, and blond hair. Her voice was pleasant, and I learned later that she was a very good singer who had been featured on several radio shows. She was of Russian extraction; both her parents were born in Kiev. It was no exaggeration to admit that I was smitten with her. I made her promise to consider having a date with me soon, but she was going on vacation and would not be back until the fall. I was left wondering if she would ever have a date with me. I wrote her a nice note telling her that I would contact her when she got back.

Weeks later and quite unexpectedly, I met her head-on in the street. She blushed intensely, so I knew that she had been thinking about me. She agreed to a date the next Saturday after my office hours, which ended about two o'clock. She arrived promptly, bringing sandwiches so that we would not lose time going out for lunch. It was a fair day and we walked hand in hand toward lower Borough Hall, the foot of Brooklyn that affords a fine view of Manhattan across the bay. Then we walked back to my car and drove to the vicinity of 42nd Street and Broadway. On a Saturday afternoon it was possible to find parking space. We hunted for a good movie and held hands during the entire show. I doubt that each of us remembered much else. After the show I took her to the Brass Rail for dinner. I offered to drive her home, which gave her an opportunity to chide me.

"You wouldn't make a house call in the Bronx to see my sister, but you're willing to drive me home?" she asked.

I told her that this was my free time and I could spend it as I wished, but it was impractical to make long distance house calls during business hours. I didn't tell her that I also wished to see where she lived. After an uneventful ride to the Bronx—she lived on Lurting Avenue not far from Pelham Parkway—I escorted her to the door of a private, three-story brick house. She didn't invite me in, so I made a motion to kiss her just as she turned her face to the side. I only made contact with her cheek. I didn't press the matter any further, said good-bye, and promised to call on her again.

We had regular dates after that. I called her every day at a set time in the afternoon. My friends in her lab told me that she would anticipate the call and get nervous when it was a little late. She invited me to meet her parents who were simple, honest folk. Her father was a tailor who had owned his own business but now worked for various jobbers in season. I liked him because he had a good sense of humor and was very handy with his hands.

One weekend Mary invited me to go sailing with Elsie and her husband, Kenneth. Elsie had bought a sailboat the year before, and it had become the family's main recreation. I could only go on Sunday and had to get back to the dock by six p.m. to make house calls. They assured me that this was feasible. The day turned out fair with a nice breeze. We sailed to the opposite shore of the Long Island Sound with ease. After a nice lunch, we lazed around until about five o'clock when I insisted that we start back. When we raised the sail, it hung like an old rag. The water was smooth as glass. It was obvious that we were in a dead calm. They all smiled, admitted that this usually happened at this time of day, and told me not to worry—the wind would soon pick up. But it didn't, and I was furious. The boat had no auxiliary motor. I insisted on paddling back across the sound. This did not ruin my relationship with Mary fortunately, but I never went sailing again.

Beyond the joy and satisfaction of a successful relationship with a woman, my practice and the little research I was doing perked along quite well. The only dark cloud was the perennial trouble my medical chief, Bill Dock, was having with the administration both of Kings County Hospital and The Long Island College of Medicine. He was dissatisfied with the policies regarding internships and residencies and was also concerned by the lack of financial support to staff the department adequately. When Dock was not pleased, he wrote letters that were embarrassing to the administration. This caused great irritation among the powers in charge who would have liked to get rid of Dock on the spot. He was much loved by the faculty and students, however, and a kind of truce developed that allowed the situation to simmer along.

We all knew that sooner or later Dock would offer to resign, and the offer would certainly be accepted. I was kind of second in command in the small department so I had to settle diplomatically what situations I could. Meanwhile the medical school, which had been in a precarious financial situation, was making a bid to become a state-supported school as part of the University of the State of New York. Delicate negotiations were going on. Because Kings County Hospital was to become the main teaching hospital and the school campus was to move adjacent to Kings County, Dock's letters were of particular concern. The faculty and staff all favored the move because it promised an influx of stable financial support and vastly improved facilities. The Long Island College Hospital, which had been closely affiliated with the medical school since it's beginning, was unhappy with this move. The hospital people wanted the campus to remain at the Henry Street location. There was not much that could be done about it, however, because the hospital and the school had separate boards and reached decisions independent of each other. About twenty years earlier, some very wise fathers of the institution had brought about the separation of the hospital and medical school. The affairs of academics and those of healthcare delivery must work together for the benefit of both, but their different aspirations inevitably lead to conflict. Most hospital-medical school organizations have found this out to their disadvantage.

As a faculty member and an alumnus, I was strongly in favor of a state takeover of the school. It deserved much greater financial and community support as the only medical educational institution in Brooklyn, a borough of over three million people. Older alumni opposed the move because they felt that the school's name and atmosphere would change from what they had known and considered an ideal. This created some schism in the faculty and staff, but not serious enough to impair the movement.

At this period in my life, I was mainly consumed with my romance with Mary. I had her over for dinner so my family could inspect her. As expected, they had all kinds of subtle and not-so-subtle objections: She was of a different faith (Russian Orthodox). She was Russian (and that was considered inferior). Her legs were too fat. She was too strong and too heavy for me (and would crush me). They didn't like the fact that Mary came from a humble background and pointed out that my cousin Charlie had married near nobility. When pushed to the wall, however, they had to admit that essentially there was nothing wrong with Mary. She was a bright, well-educated girl who would make anyone an excellent wife. Mary nevertheless picked up on these innuendoes, perhaps by body language, and they were a great source of unhappiness between us. On this basis, I hesitated to ask for her hand in marriage because I feared a turndown.

An event on December 27, 1947, sealed our fate. It began to snow heavily about 10 a.m., and in a few hours over a foot of snow was on the ground. I had patients in the office and hurried them on their way. Then I set out in my car to make house calls. Within minutes I got stuck two blocks from my office. I left the vehicle and returned to the office. Then I remembered that Mary and I had tickets to a major Broadway show that evening. Mary was to come to my office, and we were to go to dinner and the show. I tried to get in touch with her to tell her not to come because of the snow. She had no phone at home so I was unable to reach her. I waited for her, fully expecting her not to show, but sure enough she did come. By this time the snow was at least a foot and a half deep. We decided to go anyway. The good old New York subways were running on schedule although the streets were deserted. Broadway looked like a scene on the moon—completely deserted and strangely silent. We had a wonderful evening together and enjoyed the show immensely in the dramatic setting of a city completely paralyzed by the heavy snowfall.

Getting home after midnight was another matter. I could get home easily by subway without much walking. Mary, however, would have to walk about a mile in deep snow because the surface train that completed the last part of her journey was not running. We decided to go back to my office where Mary could sleep on the day bed that served as a couch in the waiting room. I made her as comfortable as possible, left, and promised to return in the morning. I believe that she fully expected me to make a sexual advance. She told me later that she didn't sleep all night and expected me to return with amorous intentions.

My failure to take advantage of her sealed our relationship. I suppose that today the opposite might be true—that failure to take advantage of such a situation might mean a lack of sexuality. In our case, Victorian ideals still held sway, and most girls protected their virginity until they were married. After our adventure in the blizzard, I noticed that Mary was more affectionate than ever. She wore the gold locket I had given her containing my picture every day. This encouraged me to make a marriage proposal, which she accepted after appropriate hesitations and exceptions. She knew my family did not completely approve of her. She mentioned our differences in religion and said she wished to complete her degree requirements. I assured her that if we loved each other enough, we could surmount all difficulties. I had fortunately saved enough money for us to live independently of our relatives. Religion did not matter, as I was an agnostic, and I didn't care if she did or did not practice her religion. I encouraged her to pursue her degree.

Yet all these small details can add up to be major annoyances, if not immense problems. My family wanted us to be married in a Catholic Church; hers in a Russian Orthodox one. Well, one has to give in to the other, and somehow the Catholic Church won out. Through one of Mary's friends, a Catholic priest was found who happened to belong to the parish of St. Patrick's Cathedral in Manhattan. He could give the necessary indoctrination and marry us. We soon found out that Mary had to have some fundamental indoctrination in Catholicism, and that she had to pledge to raise any children from the marriage in the Catholic faith. Mary was quite good about going through this tiresome ordeal. Even with this, we learned that we could not get married in the main church but were relegated to a side chapel.

Our faith in each other must have been very great for these events not to spoil our determination to join in matrimony. Other irritating details added to controversy, of course, such as what relatives rode in which limousine, who wore what flowers, and what was the order of procession. Before the event I was very busy with my practice and teaching duties and pretty much in a daze most of the time. The date for the great event was set for Saturday, June 26, 1948. The best man was Julie Stolfi; the maid of honor, Mary's sister Elsie.

We planned on a month-long honeymoon, and I arranged to have my practice cared for in my absence. When the time finally came to walk down the aisle, I did so in rented, ill-fitting tails. I think I performed reasonably well. Mary's mother somehow got lost, and the wedding was delayed with all of us biting our fingernails until she finally showed up.

The reception is a blur in my memory, but I have spotty visions of my friends George Paff, Julie Stolfi and Cliff Barger, who came all the way from Boston for the event. I had three or four drinks. With my poor tolerance for alcohol, this was enough to anesthetize the occasion. Mary looked beautiful, and I was reassured that I had made a good decision. After we cut the wedding cake, we made our exit and went to my office, where I had set up photographic equipment so that we could take additional photos. These proved to be in some ways better than the professional photos. I still have one of these on my desk some fifty years later. We spent the first night in each other's arms on the day bed in the waiting room. Young love is so endearing and puts up with discomforts that would not be tolerated in later life.

The next morning we went to Child's restaurant for a hearty breakfast. We packed our sparse belongings into the 1942 Dodge that I'd bought from my brother Al for $700 and returned the 1933 Dodge to him, which could not make the trip we planned. Our itinerary was to cross the country by car and stop at as many national parks and places of interest as a month's time allowed. With great anticipation, we started off on one of the great adventures of our lives.

The first day we got as far as Harrisburg, Pennsylvania, where the then-under construction Pennsylvania Turnpike ended in a dirt road. We found a small motel and a hamburger joint and made a night of it. Early next morning we made our way west along primitive roads, bypassing Pittsburgh, and into Ohio and then Indiana. There were no turnpikes. Most of the roads were just two lanes. Many stretches of highway were under construction, and the roads were often gravel. We were lucky to average 35 miles an hour.

We finally got to South Dakota where we saw the Badlands and the partially finished Mount Rushmore. We were much impressed by the change in scenery and terrain west of the Mississippi River. In contrast to the east, there were far fewer cities. A town was little more than a gas station and a general store with a cluster of a few houses. We were impressed that, despite the wide open spaces, all the land was fenced off and apparently claimed by someone. I found it interesting that we could always spot a town of any size in the distance by the ever-present church spire.

My previous camping experience came in handy, especially being able to cook outdoors. I had the presence of mind to bring along a gas-fired stove and an insulated box that served as an icebox. We made our food purchases in town and then set up at a convenient scenic spot to eat. Mary was an excellent cook. We had many delicious meals under the most pleasant circumstances. At night we usually found roadside cabins for rent for as little as three to five dollars. On the whole, they were very comfortable and afforded clean beds and toilet facilities. I'd brought along a sleeping bag that I borrowed from Bill Dock. We only used it once at a very scenic spot in the mountains of Wyoming. The stars were awesome, and it was very romantic to sleep with my wife all alone in the wilderness. But soon the mosquitoes attacked our faces and we had to keep them covered. Then Mary was sure a bear or other creature was about to attack us. Although we survived the night without incident and were able to watch the sun rise over the mountain, we never used the sleeping bag again.

The next morning was a beautiful summer day as we continued on western journey. We could see the Rocky Mountains, or Continental Divide, in the distance several hundred miles away. Vast fields of wild flowers were in the foreground, and it made for a most picturesque scene. I wondered whether the early pioneers had the same exciting view. By July 3rd, we reached the outskirts of Yellowstone National Park. We stayed at a cabin settlement called Pasha Teepee. After a good night's rest, we decided on a day of relaxation before entering the park itself. The terrain and surroundings were beautiful, and we thought a leisurely hike up the mountain would be fun. Though there was no trail, we were confident that we could find our way. After all, we only had to climb uphill to reach the top. It turned out to be much steeper and harder going than we expected. About halfway up, Mary was ready to turn back, but I insisted on going ahead with Mary trailing behind. We finally got to within fifty yards of the peak, which was very steep and just plain rock. Mary sat down and said that she had reached the end of her determination to climb and that we should rest and turn back. I foolishly decided to climb the remaining distance and bravely set off. Halfway up, clinging to the steep rock face, I discovered that there was an eagle's nest on top. Disturbed by this rash intruder, the eagles began to shriek, flap their wings, and scratch their claws—which loosened rocks and caused a small avalanche aimed at my head. I strained to hold on to the steep rock face and felt a sharp pain as if something ripped in my right groin. In my anxiety to get down safely, I didn't think much of it at the time, but it turned out to be the first of a series of inguinal hernias that would plague my later life.

After finally getting down from the steep rock, I found Mary completely exhausted. By then it was early afternoon and we were hungry and tired, so we just rested since we had not thought to bring lunch. The trip back to our cabin proved more exciting than we had anticipated. We started to walk downhill and soon discovered that the terrain looked strange. We realized that we were lost. After some thinking, we decided to follow a small stream because it must lead down into the valley. That proved to be a wise move, but it led us to the main road several miles from where we had entered the woods. Footsore, exhausted, and hungry, we reached our cabin just as the sun was setting, plopped into bed, fell asleep immediately, and didn't wake up until late the following morning.

After a big breakfast, we entered Yellowstone Park, and spent the day driving from one feature to another. The park was quite crowded with tourists. At times this lent a carnival atmosphere to what was otherwise an extraordinary scenic wonder. We met brown bears on several roads. Motorists stopped their cars, and the bears went to the windows to beg for food. Although we enjoyed Yellowstone, we were anxious to get to the Tetons, which friends told us were more interesting and scenic.

The next day we traveled to Jackson Hole, just outside the park. We rented a small cabin and made plans to explore the wonders of the Tetons. Bill Dock had insisted that we take the hike to Lake Solitude. Early the next morning, we drove to Jenny Lake, a beautiful setting against the high mountains. It has been said—and I think truly—that the Tetons are the Swiss Alps of America. After parking the car, we proceeded to the resident ranger's office and got directions to the trail heading to Lake Solitude. The ranger warned us that it was nineteen miles one way and the trail was difficult at times. He recommended that we camp overnight and return the next day. Since we had no camping equipment, we decided to attempt the whole trip in one day. This time we brought lunch.

The start of the trail was quite pleasant and an easy walk for several miles. It was well marked and obviously well traveled, as it was a common path mostly circling Jenny Lake, but the trail to Lake Solitude split off and became obscure. The going got progressively more difficult. We crossed bogs, rock fields, and thick forests. The trail gradually became steeper, and the trees began to thin out. We were ready to turn back several times when we were stopped in our tracks by a final barrier—a deep ravine. I finally mustered enough courage to cross it by carefully walking on a log. Seeing how easy it was, Mary followed me. In another half mile we experienced one of the most wonderful sights either of us had ever seen—a clear, blue lake several miles wide and long, surrounded on all sides by snow covered mountains that reflected on the smooth surface of the water. The air was still with an aroma of pine trees in the quiet expanse of the wonderous scene.

We sat down at the edge of the lake and ate our lunch. Unfortunately it was already well into the afternoon, and we had to start back to get to the base before darkness set in. We were truly sorry that we had not arranged to stay overnight and experience sunset and sunrise in this extraordinary setting. We had counted on making the return trip faster than our ascent. But an immense porcupine delayed our return by insisting on sitting in a place in the trail that couldn't be bypassed. Eventually he ambled away with his barbs erect. We stumbled along as quickly as we dared and reached the ranger's cabin just as the sun was disappearing behind the mountains. Although we had many other adventures still to come, this was one that we have cherished our entire lives. The vision of Lake Solitude comes to my mind in serene moments, when reflecting on the wonders of our world.

We turned north next, crossed Idaho and into Montana. We were much impressed by both states. Their scenery was entirely different, but each had its inherent natural beauty. We followed the picturesque course of the Snake River. Its name was truly appropriate as it coursed a tortuous path through hill and dale. We eventually reached our destination, Glacier National Park. We found a cabin just outside the park and established a base of operations. The terrain was quite different and more foreboding than either the Tetons or Yellowstone. Craggy mountain peaks rose sharply on all sides. A good part of the park was above the tree line so there was less forest. Our first hike took us to the impressive Grenfeld Glacier. We had been warned about grizzly bears. Rumor had it that a tourist had been attacked and killed only a week before. We fortunately didn't see any bears but were delighted to watch a group of mountain goats frolic on the steep mountain slope. These animals are very shy and are seldom seen. Grenfeld Glacier was interesting, but we were anxious to get to our final western destination.

Before our trip I'd been in touch with my old friend Phil Kendall to tell him of our trip west and our intention to visit him and his family at Hanford in Washington State. After his residency and army duty, Phil became a full-time physician with the Atomic Energy Commission. By this time, everyone knew that Hanford was a large installation that produced plutonium for the atomic bomb. The government had built an entire town of 45,000 people—workers and their families, schools, entertainment facilities, hospitals, and ambulatory clinics. The community and plant were kept secret during the war. As we traveled toward Hanford, the terrain again became flat. Much of eastern Washington was really a desert. Irrigation from the Columbia River made some areas green. There were few towns, and the only city of any size was Walla Walla.

Hanford itself was in the middle of a desert, and its extraordinary size was an oddity. Phil and his wife greeted us enthusiastically. We spent the day and night at their home and spoke fondly of the "old times" at Kings County Hospital. We also compared each other's medical practice. Phil's was completely different from mine. The general population of Hanford was age 40 or younger. He saw little heart disease and stroke, but there were more gall bladders and acute appendicitis. Surgeons were kept busy. Phil seemed happy with his situation, but I soon decided that life in a place with little intellectual stimulation was not for me. The practice of medicine can become boring and routine unless there are new challenges. I felt that Phil, with his great diagnostic and perceptive skills, was being wasted in this isolated spot. I didn't express this to Phil, of course. This was my last contact with him unfortunately. He had a great influence on my medical training, and I was sad that distance and a change in professional outlook drew us apart.

If we were to reach Brooklyn by the end of July, it was now time to head east. The drive was much less interesting as we headed into less scenic areas. We took a more northern route to reach Niagara

Falls, the traditional honeymooner's hangout. It was worth seeing, although it was too commercialized compared to the national parks. As we traveled down the well-known W-9 route along the Hudson River, we soon encountered the sights and aura of New York.

Home meant an empty one-bedroom apartment in a cluster of new high-rise apartment buildings on Cropsy Avenue in Brooklyn. Coney Island could be seen in the distance. Our location near the water offered a better view and cleaner air than the interior of the city. We had no furniture so we borrowed the day bed from the office and spent our first night in our own apartment. It didn't take long before we acquired furniture and the inevitable phone line.

I was soon busy with my practice again and happy to see that my patients were glad I'd returned. It was still summer and my teaching duties were light so I had some time to help Mary fix up the apartment. Under her supervision, I put up wallpaper that brightened the living room. Mary took up her job with Jim Hamilton in the anatomy department and fully intended to continue working toward her degree.

Politics at the school were hot and heavy. Dock was having his usual troubles with the administration. Negotiations continued with the state to move the school's campus next to Kings County Hospital. Arrangements were made to buy the land. The group allied to the Long Island College Hospital was much opposed to the move. Alumni were unhappy because of the name change. Meanwhile, the place had to run. "Old Faithful" (me) kept his nose to the grindstone. It wasn't possible to do much serious research with my practice and teaching duties. Still, I had a research assistant, Tony Cacese, stationed at my peripheral vascular disease laboratory at Kings County Hospital. The intention was to develop new diagnostic and therapeutic approaches for this important clinical entity. The work languished, however, because I was unable to spend the necessary time and energy to get a research project off the ground. Tony also lacked the kind of innate drive and ingenuity essential to stick to a research project. I couldn't blame him. He was bright and willing enough but needed more direction and push than I could afford to give him. He spent his time pretty much as a substitute resident and probably learned a good deal of clinical medicine.

I drifted along, perhaps more occupied with my married life than intellectual pursuits. I organized a Friday night social club of Julie Stolfi, Bill Florio, Frank Guistra, a pediatrician, and Joe Cresci, an obstetrician-gynecologist. It was intended to be a kind of intellectual medical discussion group. We usually met once a month. In the beginning the discussions were lively and heated on subjects of medical politics and trends in therapy. Gradually, though, it turned into more of an eating society with the wives competed for the most sumptuous dinner. Mary won kudos for roast duck and lobster dinners. Florence Florio set forth a roast pig with an apple in its mouth. My best intentions to develop a group of high intellect succumbed to the lower merits of our culinary gut.

Television became available about this time. I visited electronics stores on Cortland Street in Manhattan until I was able to buy a TV chassis to be completed. It had a twelve-inch tube, which was considered enormous. I built a cabinet to hold what was then considered a "monster" TV. It worked quite well, and many hours were wasted watching the "Boob Tube." Before TV, we could read and think and listen to good music. Now, watching TV became a nightly habit that could be shared with your wife.

Adjustment to married life was difficult, especially for Mary. She resented being tied down to a routine of wifely duties and felt that her resolve to work toward a degree was fading. My occupation with professional duties left little time to relieve her of some of the domestic work. Mary became pregnant several times with subsequent spontaneous abortions that had a great depressing influence and brought resentment of the loss of her freedom. After two years of marriage, however, she bore us a beautiful baby girl. We named her Maria, but affectionately called her Bambi after the Italian "bambino" and the then popular Disney movie deer. The baby changed our lives, and we were now devoted to raising her with the best possible advantages. Mary gave up her desire to get a degree, decided to stay home, and take care of our baby. The instincts of motherhood are very great.

Our apartment, which had seemed spacious at first, now became crowded with all the things necessary for a baby. We began to look around for a house. This wasn't easy in Brooklyn where prices were high for anything desirable. Living out on the Island or in New Jersey was impossible because of my practice and the need to be available.

Meanwhile things were not going well in the Department of Medicine. In one of his numerous fights with the administration, Dock had written the dreaded letter of resignation. It was accepted, and we were faced with the prospect of a new chief. None of us was considered for the job because the administration felt strongly that outside talent was needed to ensure creativeness and prevent inbreeding. Since Dock was well liked by the faculty, this created an intense atmosphere of unhappiness.

About this time I received a letter from Hahnemann Medical School in Philadelphia inviting me to consider the position of Chairman of Pharmacology. I almost threw the letter away. I had never heard of Hahnemann. It certainly was not on the list of outstanding medical schools in the country. I found out that George Paff was responsible for this invitation. About a year earlier, Paff had resigned from the Long Island College of Medicine to take a professorship in anatomy at Hahnemann. He nearly doubled his salary and claimed that living conditions were much superior in Philadelphia. He called me soon after I got the letter to urge me to explore the position. After much hesitation, I finally succumbed and agreed to go to Philadelphia to explore this opportunity. It was not what I wanted, since it would mean giving up my practice that I'd worked so hard to build. I dreamed of a full-time teaching position, but one in internal medicine that would allow me to continue to see patients.

Mary and I finally made the trip to Philadelphia one Friday in the early fall. The school was located on 15th Street near Vine, not far from City Hall, Philadelphia's central landmark with a statue of William Penn towering above it. Aside from an impressive twenty-story hospital on the Broad Street side, the unimpressive campus was made up of some rather small red-brick buildings of Victorian vintage.

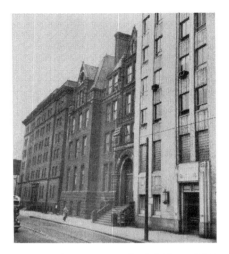

Figure 1. Hahnemann Medical College. This is what I saw on my first visit to Hahnemann in 1950. Location is the South East Corner of 15th Street at Vine Street. On the left is the old unoccupied nurses residence. In the center is the four story medical school building that actually was originally the Hahnemann Hospital. Note the Victorian architecture and the elegant brownstone stoop. Replacing a wing of the old building was the more recently built Khlar Building.

Charles Brown, the Dean, greeted me in his ancient office where a huge air conditioner was the most impressive feature. A rotund jovial man of about fifty, Dr. Brown had been a resident at Brigham at the same time as Bill Dock. They knew each other well. Brown had a reputation as a superb internist. He had been the chairman of the Department of Medicine at Temple University Medical School before coming to Hahnemann. He told me immediately that he had spoken to Dock about me and was very impressed with my qualifications. He wanted an M.D. rather than a Ph.D. to lead the Department of Pharmacology. He agreed that I could have hospital privileges, make rounds, and do as much clinical work as I wished, but I could not have a private practice. I liked the man. He inspired a considerable degree of confidence.

Brown called John Boyd, Chairman of Biochemistry and head of the search committee, to show me the school's facilities. Boyd was a short man with a boyish face and a stock of reddish hair. He came from the Medical School of the University of Cincinnati. An enthusiastic supporter of Hahnemann, he was gung-ho about the new young faculty, especially of the basic sciences, and believed that the school was "going places." Ray Truex, Chairman of

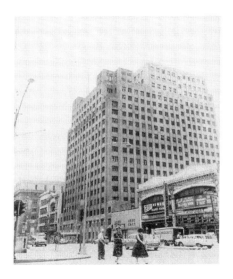

Figure 2. Hahnemann Medical College Hospital. On the Broad Street side there was the more impressive hospital building built in 1929. To the immediate left is the Gorson Chrysler-Plymyth Building that later became the Feinstein Clinic Building. On the right of the hospital was the Gorson's used car agency. This building was bought by the Cardiovascular Institute and remodeled into laboratories and lecture hall. Further on the right was Horn and Hardart Automat famous nickel slot restaurant much favored by students and faculty.

Anatomy, was outstanding. John Scott, Chairman of Physiology, was older and had been at Hahnemann for some dozen years. Boyd characterized him as "one of the senior physiologists" in the country. What Boyd didn't know was that I had worked in physiology myself and knew all the important physiologists. Scott was not one of them. Mede Bondi, the youngest of the Hahnemann chairmen and head of Microbiology, was very capable. The star of the basic science faculty was supposed to be John Gregory, Chairman of Pathology. Boyd explained how Dean Brown had obtained money from the state of Pennsylvania and had collected this brilliant faculty.

Besides being Dean, Brown also was the Chairman of Medicine and had revitalized the department by installing four young full-time internists. The other clinical departments were supposed to be stocked with equally qualified young men. Boyd didn't tell me that in 1944 the accrediting Liaison Committee of the American Medical Association and the Association of Medical Colleges had put the school on probation. Hahneman was one of the last surviving medical schools that taught homeopathy. It offered both a homeopathic and a medical diploma up to 1944. The Liaison Committee indicated that if Hahnemann wanted to continue to be accredited, it must give up homeopathy, reorganize and revitalize the faculty, change the administration, install a more responsible board of trustees, and in general enter into competition with the modern world of medical practice. There was no doubt that Hahnemann was a weak school, even though it had survived the famous Flexner Report that evaluated medical schools in 1910 and was financed by the Carnegie Foundation.

My experience at the Long Island College of Medicine had taught me that weak medical schools are hospital-medical school combinations, which are poorly endowed and operate marginally on tuition-generated income. Stronger medical schools are associated with a large university with adequate endowment. Less strong, but nonetheless stable, are schools supported by state finances. Philadelphia was unique in that it had three medical

schools—Hahnemann, Women's Medical College, and Jefferson—
that were hospital-medical school combinations. There was also
an osteopathic school that also derived its income from tuition.
These four schools competed with the powerful School of Medicine
of University of Pennsylvania and the Medical School of Temple
University, which was state supported. Thus, six medical schools
competed for the resources of a city of two million people. The
Long Island College of Medicine had a catchment area of Brooklyn,
a borough of three million people. The Philadelphia situation was
sure to lead to disaster for the weaker schools in time. I perceived
this and was not at all enthusiastic about the opportunity offered
at Hahnemann. In the ordinary course of events, it would have
been a case of "No Thanks."

One attraction of Philadelphia that is vastly superior to New
York City is its spacious, well maintained suburbs with excellent
schools and easy access from Center City. At George Paff's
suggestion, Mary and I took a ride around the city's suburbs and
were very impressed that we could afford a handsome house with
ample grounds. Despite this very tempting attraction, we returned
to New York convinced that we would remain in Brooklyn.

Back at home base, the situation was worse than ever. Dock
was sulking and did nothing but his main teaching duties after
resigning as chief of medicine. The Dean and he were simply not
talking. The administration of the Department of Medicine was
left in my hands but without the distinction of even being named
acting head. Everything was left in limbo. With the burden of a
private practice, I was having a difficult time without any help or
appreciation from the administration. I was simply the fall guy
who was there to fill in the gap until the situation could be resolved.
I knew that I did not have even a remote chance of getting a
chairmanship at the Long Island College of Medicine. While I was
admired, I was considered too young. And search committees always
think that selecting a local candidate is inbreeding. They are always
seeking the outstanding candidate with a national reputation who
is going to put the school "on the map." Our daughter was growing
meanwhile, and the apartment was becoming more congested. I

could do little research, and intellectually I felt a distinct decline. When another letter from the Hahnemann arrived a few weeks later and invited me for a second visit, I decided to accept the invitation. At the least it would tell the administration at Long Island that I was appreciated outside the institution.

This time I got the red carpet treatment at Hahnemann. Strong letters from Sam Reynolds and Gene Landis apparently made an impression. George Paff filled the ears of the committee with glowing accounts of my abilities, while the personal friendship between Dock and Dean Brown also must have helped. My impression was that they really wanted me and I could have the job if I chose. Ray Truex personally gave us a tour of the suburbs, which greatly impressed Mary. I had long talks with Boyd and Scott about the school's future that, they assured me, was bright because they now were receiving a subsidy from the state of Pennsylvania. I found that my main competition was a pharmacologist named Shideman. I looked him up, was very impressed by his qualifications, and was flattered that I was considered at least his equal.

The result of this visit was that I was more confused than ever. Although Mary tried to be neutral, I could see that she would be happier if I had a position where I could spend more time at home. As I expected, I received a letter a week later from Dean Brown stating that I was considered favorably for the position. There was merely the question of whether Hahnemann could meet my requirements for salary, departmental budget, and space. Now the decision was in my corner. I had to make up my mind one way or the other. I was torn between my allegiance to the institution that had given me my first breaks, my practice, and my close professional friends and the opportunity to chair my own department and be able to do decent research and teaching.

I consulted some of my older physician colleagues. They all warned against leaving the security of my own practice, but they agreed that with my talents, I would probably have a happier life as a full-time scientist. You'll enjoy your work more, they said, but you will make less income. As a result, you will have a smaller house, your wife will own a cloth coat instead of fur, and you will drive a less pretentious car, and probably have fewer children. I decided to consult Dean Curran who was friendly toward me. Perhaps he would make a counteroffer that would convince me to stay in Brooklyn. He was very sympathetic and certainly wished to retain me if at all possible. But he pointed out that because the school was getting a new Chairman of Medicine, he must wait for the new man before he could make major personnel changes in the department. He did offer, however, to raise my rank to associate professor with a modest increase in my part-time salary. This seemed reasonable enough to me at the time, but it did not convince me to stay put. Mary gave me the best advice. She suggested that I make demands of salary and departmental needs that were tops for what Hahnemann might be able to afford. If they turned these demands down, then I could remain in Brooklyn with dignity. If they accepted, then I had to make the move.

I wrote to Dean Brown requesting a salary of $12,000, a departmental budget for five full-time staff, 7,000 square feet of floor space, a research budget, and funds to remodel the assigned space into modern offices and research labs. I fully expected to be turned down cold. While today a salary of $12,000 sounds ridiculous, it was among the highest for chairmen of preclinical departments in 1950. I was sure it was considerably higher than any of the other preclinical department chairmen were earning at Hahnemann at that time. Yet if I stayed in Brooklyn, I would earn as much between my part-time academic job and my practice, so it was reasonable to me. The big difference lay in what that amount of money could buy in Philadelphia in the way of housing, schooling, food, and recreation, as compared to Brooklyn.

Several weeks went by. I had begun to forget about Hahnemann and Philadelphia. Events evolved as usual. The Department of Medicine situation was unresolved. On Dock's fiftieth birthday, the medical faculty and staff threw a big dinner for our favorite professor. The solidarity of support for our chief was gratifying to see, but it did not relieve Dock's problems with the administration. The search committee for a new chairman stalled as it awaited official word of a state takeover so it could attract a higher-profile candidate

I learned through the grapevine that George Paff was making a vigorous campaign for Hahnemann to hire me on my terms. I didn't put too much stock in this because I had figured I would stay in Brooklyn. To my genuine surprise, I received a letter from Dean Brown offering me the job on my terms. He asked when could I start—the sooner the better.

Now that I had a real chance to get out of Brooklyn and make a career in science and education, I was hesitant and undecided. A combination of Dock, Stolfi, and my wife convinced me to take this giant step. Dock said that Brown was a great person and would take care of me. He pointed out that in academics one should change institutions about every five years while young. Philadelphia was one of the great medical cities, and I was not going into obscurity. Stolfi, who'd become an intimate friend, knew me well and felt that I would be happier with a full-time academic position. Mary, who had been suffering the life of a wife of a practicing physician who made house calls, was enthusiastically supportive of the move.

My family, however, was quite negative. They would lose the weekly contact we'd maintained, as well as the medical attention my aging parents required. They could not appreciate why I would give up a private practice for a full-time teaching job. To them, it was a distinct step downward.

Only I could make the final decision in the end. I knew that opportunities for high academic positions were rarely offered to Italian-Americans. In the 1950s, American institutions of higher learning were practically all of church origin, particularly of the Protestant persuasion. All the staff, teachers, and directors were WASPs. It was extremely rare for outsiders, even if competent, to be offered such a position as a professorship or chairmanship.

Hahnemann had been established by emigrants of German origin. The Board of Directors was composed of local businessmen, bankers, insurance people, and a judge or two, all of whom were distinctly WASPish. Because of its recent difficulties, Hahnemann had become somewhat more democratic. Hahnemann had even made a few appointments of Catholics under Dr. Brown's administration. Compared to other medical schools, it admitted a relatively high proportion of Jews and religions other than Protestant. This cosmopolitan atmosphere was encouraging to me. I finally determined to make the move, which would be a decisive turning point in my life. Henceforth, my fortune would be locked in with Hahnemann's.

I immediately set about rearranging my affairs. I was fortunately able to turn over my practice and office to Monty Cohen who had finished his residency at Kings County Hospital. An ad in the local paper produced a tenant suitable to sublet our apartment for the remainder of the lease. Every weekend when I could get away, Mary and I traveled to Philadelphia to find a house. It was quite an exciting and hectic time, but somehow we got through it. The real estate market was somewhat depressed, but houses were rapidly rising in value. Mortgage rates were also increasing, but it was still possible to buy a very good house at a reasonable price in the Philadelphia suburbs.

We explored the whole region and decided on the Main Line just west of Philadelphia. We looked at every available house in our price range. After much debate, we settled on a fifteen-year-old house in Wynnewood, a beautifully built brick colonial on a 60-by-130 foot lot—enormous by New York City standards. The house had five bedrooms, four bathrooms, a two-car garage, and an enclosed porch. The garden was nicely landscaped. Its major disadvantage was that it was about 150 feet from Haverford Road, an alternate truck route that could be quite noisy. We paid $26,000 for the property, of which $16,000 dollars was a twenty-year mortgage at 4.5 percent. The $10,000 cash down payment was nearly my entire savings and was more than I'd wished to risk. But the forecast of steady employment encouraged the investment. Mary was pleased with the new house and busy with plans for furnishing it. We moved in shortly before Christmas.

On January 1, 1951, at the age of thirty-four, I started an entirely new life as professor and chairman of the Department of Pharmacology at Hahnemann Medical College in Philadelphia. It was a giant step that changed the rest of my life. I had the feeling that I'd abandoned my family and friends and betrayed the institution that had given me my education and academic opportunities. The new situation and challenges of a new environment, however, left little time to rue the past. I was determined to make a success of my position. Hahnemann was going to have one of the best departments of pharmacology in the country, with a national and international reputation. This was a grandiose ambition, considering the resources available and the competition of the other medical schools. Yet it was a time of post-war optimism and a general feeling of great oncoming medical advances with increasing government support. The question was, who could grab the most significant piece of the pie? I had no reason to believe that I—and Hahnemann—could not grab our fair share.

CHAPTER V

Academia

1951-60

"If development of your mind is your true desire, then be a teacher and a researcher."

Rupert Black, M.D.

The Pharmacology Department was on seventh floor of the newest Hahnemann building. Built in 1942, the Klahr Building was the gift of a patient of Harry Eberhart, a gastroenterologist who'd been a driving force on the Board of Trustees. The building had a nice façade, but little internal structure. The school had apparently run out of money before the building was finished. It was intended mainly to house the basic sciences. Each floor centered on a large student laboratory that could accommodate about 100 students.

Student enrollment was eighty five to ninety students so each laboratory exercise could be taught to all students at once. This was a vast improvement over the Long Island College of Medicine where laboratories could only accommodate half the class and required that each experiment be taught twice. When the students were not in session, these labs could be used as research areas. A centrally located service room housed the diener and the various pieces of equipment loaned to students for each experimental setup. At each end of the floor, two or three office-laboratory rooms were available for the faculty. There were staircases from floor to floor but no elevator.

To reach pharmacology on the seventh floor, we could take an old elevator that usually didn't work in an ancient adjacent red brick building, but it only went to the fourth floor. The rest of the hike involved an externally added stairwell up the remaining levels. The arrangement certainly could not pass a fire inspection, especially because all the staircases were wooden, but this was compensated by a steel fire escape along the exterior of the Khlar building. Reaching the pharmacology department was a feat of athletic prowess. Consequently, we didn't have many visitors. Brute strength was required to haul oxygen tanks up the stairs. Despite these disadvantages, the space was adequate and even airy just underneath the roof.

Laboratory benches for the students were new and excellently constructed of metal with synthetic stone tabletops. The laboratory equipment for instruction was antiquated and primitive, however. There was a paucity of research equipment, such as a research kymograph, respiratory pumps, and any contemporary electronic apparatus. Reinhard Beutner, the previous chairman, had been trained as a physical chemist and apparently had no taste for animal experimentation. He left behind a few ancient galvanometers and resistance boxes of little use in pharmacological research. A scattering of homeopathic and modern drugs had to be mostly discarded. Much work and good planning had to be done to bring the department up to date with its contemporaries.

Tom Barnes was the senior member of the department and held the title of associate professor. A tall, scholarly man, he was the son of a distinguished Canadian physics professor and the sole accomplished scientist in the department. His main specialty was electroencephalography. A special screened room was built in his laboratory for recording brain waves in animals and man. Barnes in fact did all the clinical electroencephalography (EEGs) for the hospital. He received no compensation for this, nor did the department, a future source of controversy between the administration and me. Beside his mainly clinical research, Barnes had some claim to fame as the originator of a theory of drug action based on phase boundary potentials. He and Beutner were able to show that neuroactive drugs like acetylcholine and epinephrine would alter the potential at the boundary of an oil water phase. This was supposed to explain the physiological activity of these potent neurohumors. While the theory was interesting, and perhaps even pertinent, it was an over simplification and non-specific. Barnes and Beutner attended various neurophysiology meetings and made pests of themselves promoting their theory. By some, they were almost considered quacks.

Ben Calesnick, a Hahnemann graduate six years out of school, had been a fellow in the department and gradually worked himself up to assistant professor. He had a private practice on the outside, but managed to spend his time in the department. His research program appeared sound and he seemed bright enough.

Jens Christensen was a refugee physician from Germany. A Swede, he had helped Jews escape the Nazis and finally had to flee himself. About fifty years old, Christensen had been unable to get a license to practice medicine and took a teaching job as a stopgap. He was a very cultured, intelligent person but was shy and unsure of himself. His title was that of instructor. Harry Pratt was supposedly a Ph.D., with the degree having been conferred by the Department of Pharmacology at Hahnemann. But because Hahnemann had no graduate school organization at that time, there was no way to determine the value of the degree. Pratt was only a part-time instructor who was also associated with an animal supply dealership, which was clearly a conflict of interest. Ray Siedel and Ed Messey were practicing homeopathic graduates of Hahnemann who lectured on prescription writing. Both showed up only when they had lectures and were on a volunteer basis.

In my discussions with Dean Brown, I had obtained the condition that I could remove any or all personnel of the department if I felt they were incompetent. I had the further option of filling two additional slots in the department at the associate or assistant professor level. Dean Brown assured me that there was no tenure at Hahnemann, only yearly appointments. Faculty served at the discretion of department head and Dean. It didn't take me long to determine that Pratt was incompetent and interested only in his animal business. He resigned quietly after I gave him a teaching assignment he knew he could not fulfill. After I sat in on lectures by Ray Siedel and Ed Messey, I simply cancelled their assignments. They were both fine gentlemen and took this graciously. I remained friendly with them, but the prescription instruction was completely changed to conform with modern approaches to therapeutics.

Despite what I thought were generous budgetary demands, I soon found that I would have to be resourceful in order to build a sound department. To be fair, my first order of business was to improve the salaries of the staff who would remain. Then I needed to add at least two additional members to create a diverse scientific expertise. Calesnick and I were primarily in cardiovascular and general pharmacology. Barnes might pass as a neuropharmacologist. Christensen really didn't have any specialty, although he had done some nice work on the toxicity of alcohol. My work on antiarrhythmic drugs had impressed upon me the importance of organic chemistry in the design of and comprehension of the actions of chemicals on living systems. Therefore the priority was to bring an organic chemist, especially expert in theory, into the department.

The second item on my wish list was to find a biochemist who might be interested in a pharmacological approach. Many new and exciting medical science discoveries were biochemical, and advances in the mechanism of drug action were based on biochemical interpretation. As far as teaching was concerned, I needed a biochemist to do conference-type instruction and staff an ambitious laboratory instructional program. I also wanted to attract graduate students to the department. This would require a diversity of instruction and an active research program.

Securing a jack-of-all-trades type of diener was as important as finding faculty. To run the ambitious laboratory program in both research and student laboratory instruction, I needed a man who was handy at constructing equipment, knew electronics, and could interact with professional staff and students. Such a person was hard to find, and the Hahnemann personnel office was not much help. It happened that I became friendly with a clerk in an electronics store across the street on Broad. I described my needs, and asked him if by chance he knew anyone who might fit the bill. Sure enough, he knew an electronics whiz who was house painter tired of his painting business.

John Dukirk proved to be exactly what I wanted. A bachelor, about fifty years old, an excellent painter, he also very handy with tools. He had studied electronics on the side and hoped to change careers. I easily convinced him to come on board at a reasonable salary. Dukirk developed into a first-rate diener who managed all the research apparatus of a pharmacology lab. Over the years he became of invaluable service by devising new solutions to research problems.

The curriculum of the pharmacology course was based on a minimum of lectures. Anesthetic agents introduced the course, followed by autonomic drugs, then central nervous system, cardiovascular, endocrine, and antibiotic and chemotherapeutic agents. This made a logical selection and correlated well with the laboratory exercises. The first laboratory exercise, for example, consisted of anesthetizing a dog with a volatile agent such as ether or chloroform. This type of general anesthesia was then current with human anesthesia and enabled the student to become familiar with the technology and the actual physical sign of the achievement of the unconscious state with loss of pain sensation that allowed operations to be performed. With cardiovascular drugs, students were able to simulate heart failure in the cat and treat it in a manner that simulated what was appropriate in humans. There were also laboratory sessions in which students worked on each other, involving sedative, analgesic, and mood changing drugs. Students thus had ample opportunity to observe first hand the effects of drugs on themselves and in animals. Each laboratory session ended with an analysis of the data collected and a discussion of what this data might mean.

Two hour conference sessions were held on Fridays. An agenda of topics and questions was prepared ahead of time so that each section of twelve students would have uniformity of subject matter. On occasion the session would start with a ten-minute written quiz. Between the laboratory exercises and the conferences, the faculty had maximum exposure to each student.

The lectures were divided equally among the professional staff, which came as a surprise to the faculty because the previous chairman had given practically all the lectures himself. I insisted that everyone attend the lectures. This was the only way the conference sessions could be of equal value, and it meant that every instructor had to know all subjects beyond his own field. To enrich the instruction, special weekly lectures by invited clinical faculty correlated with the current instruction.

An optional research program was available for extra credit and to obtain honors in the course. Two students were assigned to an instructor and allowed to select a research project, which usually required weeks of observation. Students performed the experiment during their spare time. Their work was written up as a paper and presented before their classmates on a special research day. About a third of the class volunteered for this special assignment.

Examinations consisted of a midterm and a final. Essay exams were not given. We used only objective National Board-type exams. These exams, plus performance in the laboratory and conferences, determined the final grade on a numerical basis with the passing level of 75 percent. Admittedly, it was not easy to pass the course because instruction and grading were set at a high level. Ordinarily about 10 percent of the students failed the course. Those who just barely flunked were allowed to take a makeup examination. Those who flunked by a wide margin had to repeat the course or take a make-up course during the summer at another medical school acceptable to the department. Under these stringent conditions, performance of the students on the National Boards and State Boards improved dramatically.

Hahnemann students on the whole were of a lesser academic level than what I'd been used to in Brooklyn and Boston. They came from smaller colleges and had not been subjected to the fierce academic competition of the large New York colleges. Because of the state subsidy it received, Hahnemann had to take a minimum of 70 percent of its students from a pool of Pennsylvania residents. The other seven Pennsylvania medical schools, drawing from the same pool, tried to skim off the most able students. Nevertheless,

Hahnemann was able to recruit a good proportion of very able students.

The other preclinical departments also had aggressive teaching and research programs. Each had a relatively young, energetic department chairman. Physiology was the exception. John Scott, an older man about fifty-five at the time, was more in line with the older school of medical scientists. He ran a very standard course with an extensive laboratory experience. Like the old timers, he gave practically all the lectures himself. His staff was unimpressive. I liked Scott nevertheless. He certainly was a dedicated and sincere individual. During Hahnemann's difficult time with the accrediting agencies, he was a stalwart and plausible defender. To his merit, he fit in well with the younger group of professors and got along exceedingly well with the clinicians.

John Boyd, Chairman of Biochemistry, also ran a standard course. It was much improved over the previous instructional program, which was run by the perennial dean of Hahnemann, William Pearson, Ph.D. Boyd was an enthusiastic researcher with an active staff of younger professors. Joseph Defrates, a superb educator, was one very popular teacher in his department. Boyd was very dedicated to graduate students and, without doubt, was the mainstay of the efforts of the faculty to put together a decent graduate program.

Ray Truex, who headed Anatomy, was an outstanding individual, excellent teacher, and even a better researcher. His specialty was neuroanatomy, a tough subject for most medical students, but he made it interesting and pertinent to clinical medicine. He had recruited George Paff, who in turn had interested me in Hahnemann. Paff was an excellent gross anatomy instructor whom students either loved or hated. An ingenious researcher, he devised many diverse experiments using embryological techniques. He was one of the first to describe the action of autonomic drugs on the embryo heart of the chicken. Oddly enough, Truex later became an expert on the anatomy of the whale heart. Thus, the largest heart and one of the smallest were studied in the same department.

Amedeo Bondi, only a few years older than I, had been the youngest of the fellow chairmen prior to my arrival. He headed microbiology and had collected a fine group of young investigators. Microbiology offices and research labs were in the basement, but the student labs were shared with pathology on the second floor. Bondi was a reasonable, sensible individual who had done very credible research. We became close friends over the years.

Pathology was considered a preclinical subject, although it related more to clinical matters. John Gregory, who headed the department, kept to himself and was not really an integral member of the preclinical chairmen. Dean Brown was said to have made a special effort to recruit him by giving him special concessions to secure his services. Perhaps this was a factor kept him apart from the other chairmen. It was still the age when pathology was considered the pivotal subject in medicine, and the pathologist had the final word on the diagnosis and criticism of the clinician. Good hospitals were supposed to have autopsy rates of at least 35 percent, which made it possible for the pathologist to determine if diagnosis and therapy were being done according to acceptable standards. The pathologist was a respected figure, although he may not have been liked personally.

The classical clinical departments of Medicine, Surgery, Obstetrics-Gynecology, Pediatrics, Radiology, and Preventative Medicine, together with the preclinical departments, totaled only twelve units. This was a happy situation compared to today when the average medical school has at least twenty-four departments competing for space and other scarce resources.

Dean Brown was also Chairman of Medicine. His reputation as one of the most able internists in Philadelphia allowed him to put together a very strong department. Before coming to Hahnemann, he held the chair of medicine at the Temple University School of Medicine where he was very highly regarded. He had established the full-time system there, which was the preferred organization of the country's most prestigious medical schools. Another major factor in his favor was the fact that he had some of the most important business and political people as patients. Most medical schools of that era operated their clinical departments by the use of volunteer physicians. Only the chairman, and perhaps one or two others, received nominal salaries on a part-time basis. The volunteer staff supported themselves by private practice. Their academic work of teaching and research was done purely on a volunteer basis. Full-time clinical faculties were not allowed to have private practices. The fees they earned seeing patients on the premises accrued to the institution and were used to pay salary and fringe benefits. Any surplus was used to finance other projects in the department. Full-time faculty did not make a comparable income to physicians in private practice, but supposedly had benefits of security and academic advantages that made up for this. A total departmental budget of $50,000 went a long way under these circumstances.

Brown recruited three outstanding board-certified internists to form the backbone of the full-time clinical faculty. The senior person was Al Lupton, who everyone agreed was an excellent clinician and a sound investigator of atherosclerosis. Bob Fitch was a snappy general internist in charge of the medical clinic. Ray Joyner was eccentric and kept to himself, but had no equal at bedside teaching. All three were young and energetic. Together with the older, very able volunteer physicians, Hahnemann attracted a high quality resident staff. There was no doubt that Brown's influence had a salutary effect on the reputation and functioning of the department of medicine. I was pleased to be part of this group and took my turn of service on the ward and in the medical clinic. In this manner, I maintained my clinical skills and was able to relate better to the clinical staff.

Bill Martin, a very capable, practical general surgeon who had spent time in the Navy and had a military bearing to show for it, headed surgery. He was a good administrator. He realized that he was no researcher and was wise enough to surround himself with young enthusiastic well-trained surgeons. The foremost was Paul Grotzinger who, besides being a good surgeon, knew a good deal of internal medicine and consequently could be involved in erudite discussions of disease. Other interesting surgical faculty were Frank Tropea and Al Pearce.

Ophthalmology, Otolaryngology, Orthopedics, and Thoracic Surgery were all divisions of Surgery but acted as separate departments in most ways. They were small units with usually no more than two or three people. Thoracic Surgery, the most interesting, was headed by Charles P. Bailey who had already achieved international fame as the originator of dramatic heart surgery. Early on, he had established a training program and was followed about by a retinue of admirers. There is little doubt that Bailey's daring and brilliant exploits put an obscure homeopathic medical school on the map. (I got to know him well and will describe in detail the man and his works as my career at Hahnemann progresses.)

Newland Paxson, a confirmed Quaker, chaired Obstetrics and Gynecology with skill and efficiency. He was an excellent, shrewd politician. He could not be called brilliant, but he was a valuable asset in any medical school. I liked him. In fact he delivered four of my five children. There were other capable physicians in the department but none who were research oriented. Carl Fisher, easily the most distinguished of the clinical professors, most ably chaired the Pediatrics Department. Soft spoken and sagacious, his presence in any conference insured that the discussion would be fair and to the point. With a wonderful command of the English language, he could stand up and expound on any subject with ease. The son of a physician, he was very loyal to his alma mater, Hahnemann. Fisher commanded respect in the national medical community as past president of the American Academy of Pediatrics. Horst Agerty, a volunteer in the department, was highly regarded as a teacher and physician.

In addition to the mainstay departments of the medical school, the subsidiary departments were important because a medical center could not function without them. Jay Stauffer-Lehman, a highly capable diagnostician who was very interested in cardiology, headed radiology. He and Bailey did some pioneer work in human cardiac catherization. Henry Ruth, the director of anesthesiology, had a national reputation for his work in the subject. He started the journal *Anesthesiology* and was responsible for anesthesiology becoming a boarded discipline. Mention must also be made of neurosurgery, directed by Alex Olsen, very capable surgeon known for seldom uttering a complete sentence. He answered most queries with a grunt or two.

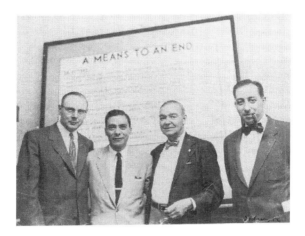

Figure 3. Cardiovascular Institute Founders. Some of the earliest members of the Cardiovascular Institute. Starting on the left is Charles P. Bailey followed by William Likoff, George Geckeler and Joseph R. DiPalma. There was no contest that Bailey and Likoff were the driving force in this enterprise.

For this period in American medicine, the faculty at Hahnemann compared most favorably with most medical schools. Considering that the school's annual budget was not much more than a quarter of a million dollars, Dean Brown had done an exceedingly brilliant job of collecting a young, energetic faculty who were congenial and loyally bound to the institution.

Dean Brown was also aided by the post-war aura of the nation's return to peace and industry. There was a general shortage of doctors at the time. Both federal and state legislators were liberally disposed to aid higher education. Spurred by technology developed as part of the war effort, an intense effort was applied to use this new information and expertise to develop science and industry. Television was an example of electronic technology that had many applications to science and education. Companies sprang up to supply advanced equipment that surpassed existing methodologies. Diagnostic radiology apparatus became much refined. The development, for example, of the image amplifier made possible catherization of the heart under direct view. Electrocardiograph equipment became direct writing and portable, replacing the bulky prewar photographic recorders. New technologies related to the development of physics' theoretical knowledge about the development of the atom bomb made possible the construction of such powerful therapeutic radiation devices as the linear accelerator and the cobalt bomb.

The National Institute of Health, started by President Roosevelt in the 1940s, now became the darling of Congress. Invitations to do research of a basic nature went out to investigators. Competition to get these grants was slight so most scientists were able to get generous support money.

As a matter of course, I applied for support to continue my work on cardiac antiarrhythmic drugs and cardiac electrophysiology. A movement was under way at Hahnemann, started mainly by Charles Bailey and his medical associate William Likoff, to form a cardiovascular institute. The goal was to establish a laboratory and research group of all workers in cardiovascular diseases so that cooperation could be engendered for the solution of major problems. Other members recruited into the group were John Scott, George Geckeler, head of medical cardiology, Stoufer-Lehman and Ray Truex. I enthusiastically joined the group myself.

The Institute was called the Mary Bailey Institute for Cardiovascular and Blood Vessel Research. Bailey and Likoff were adept at raising private money from a retinue of grateful patients, largely a Jewish group who were intensely loyal and supportive. They raised enough money to purchase a one-story used car showroom just north of the hospital on Broad Street. Enough additional private funds were raised to construct and equip laboratories in the rear half of the building, with the front end left vacant for future development. The group organized a large grant application for support and expansion of the institute, and application was made to the National Institute of Health (NIH). The major thrust was coronary artery disease and arteriosclerosis.

We were visited by an NIH-appointed site team of outside referees, a very distinguished group of eminent cardiovascular scientists headed by Irving S. Wright, known for developing oral anticoagulant therapy for the prevention of heart attacks. He lauded our efforts but could not be persuaded that a cooperative institute working on a single problem would be effective. He encouraged us instead to each apply for our own component of the project in separate grant applications. Reflecting retrospectively, I think he was right, although in later years NIH encouraged such institutes, notably in cancer. In any case, I applied for a separate grant and duly received it. I consequently had two NIH grants at the same time, which was more research support than I ever had before.

With this money in hand and assurance of continued support for three years, I began to put out feelers to bring on a very good technical assistant. I eventually settled on a young, black Bachelor of Science from Lincoln University. Bob McMichaels was actually a premed who had applied to local medical schools and had been turned down. This was no detriment because black students were rarely accepted then unless they were very exceptional. McMichaels turned out to be a great find. He was extremely good with his hands, intelligent, patient, loyal, and had a pleasing personality. Until I became Dean and even after, he has been my collaborator in practically all my research efforts.

We had sufficient research money to buy necessary equipment and support summer fellows and graduate students. In those happy days, NIH was very lenient about changes in budget categories. Institutions did not expect us to support our own salary from our research grants. Most importantly, we were allowed to budget money for travel to scientific meetings. To this may be attributed the great expansion of scientific meetings of all kinds—some of them in exotic places. It turned out to be a great boon for air travel and hotels. A great deal of the money was undoubtedly wasted, but on the whole the NIH granting program was extremely successful in stimulating fundamental medical research that has led to practical applications. It is not beyond the limits of reason to attribute the enormous growth of healthcare as a service and an industry to this substantial research support. While the United States has clearly been the leader in this, other countries such as England, France, Italy, Germany, Sweden, and recently Japan have also made important contributions.

My early years at Hahnemann were very productive because of research support and relatively few administrative duties. I was attuned to the science of the times and had the energy to pursue novel ideas. I didn't make any phenomenal discoveries, but my work was substantial, added to the general knowledge, and has stood the test of time. I gradually reduced the amount of my clinical work when departmental duties grew and my research program expanded. I nevertheless maintained an interest in application of basic knowledge to clinical problems and collaborated whenever I could with clinicians attempting to find solutions to disease situations. My background in practicing medicine allowed me to be equally facile with clinical as well as purely laboratory entities.

With five regular medical schools and an osteopathic school, Philadelphia had a fine scientific community. I soon became a member of the Philadelphia Physiological Society, one of the oldest in the country. Through its meetings at various medical schools, I got to know most of my confreres in pharmacology and physiology. The University of Pennsylvania School of Medicine had one of the best pharmacology departments in the country headed by Carl Schmidt, who had succeeded the very famous A. N. Richards. Schmidt was very kind to me and invited me to give a seminar at the University soon after I arrived in Philadelphia. Other members of the department were George Koelle of cholinesterase fame, and Domingo Aviado, a prolific researcher and writer. Later I got to know Christian Lambertsen, the foremost deep-sea diver physiologist in the world. Bob Forster was chairman of physiology at Penn. Since he had worked at Harvard with Gene Landis, we had a common bond. These scientists plus many others were very stimulating, and I enjoyed an intellectual atmosphere that I didn't have in Brooklyn.

My research and writings about cardiac antiarrhythmic drugs had given me some notoriety in this field. Sam Bellet an eminent cardiologist at Philadelphia General Hospital sought me out and we became quite friendly. When he held informal parties at his home in Center City, he invited his cardiac fellows and various cardiologists. He invited me to many of these meetings at which there were heated discussions on cardiological subjects. Through Bellet, I was invited to give talks before local and national cardiology meetings and came to know many of the foremost cardiologists in the country. Meanwhile my former colleagues, Chandler Brooks and Brian Hoffman, were doing pioneer work in cardiac electrophysiology. My former intern at Kings County, Jerry Stamler, who had gone to Chicago to work with L. N. Katz, was at Northwestern University Medical School and fast becoming a leader in atherosclerosis research and as an epidemiologist of coronary artery disease. I had some feeling that I was part of the national scene and was a component of a developing body of knowledge that would greatly advance diagnosis and therapy of cardiac disease.

My greatest satisfaction perhaps came from the long series of student fellows, graduate students, and research collaborating colleagues who were my pleasure to sponsor. In my first summer at Hahnemann, I was able to take on two second-year medical students as summer fellows. Both had the first name Frank: Burstein, a native Philadelphian, and Burno, a WASPish New Englander. I put them to work on assays of antifibrillatory compounds that I had left over from my work for Sterling Winthrop. We used cats to do the assay, and we soon ran into a shortage. Burno lived in a tenement house that he claimed had plenty of nightly howling cats. He volunteered to catch some for our experiments. The next night he was in the back yard, about to put one of the cats into a burlap bag, when his landlady stuck her head out of the window.

"Mr. Burno, if you don't desist immediately I shall call the cops and have you arrested," she yelled in a raucous voice. "These cats are all pets and are not to be harmed in anyway." Needless to say, Burno quit on the spot and never volunteered to catch a cat again. The work progressed despite this episode, and we did find some worthwhile results that were eventually published. Both students did exceedingly well. Burstein ended up with a fine family practice in Philadelphia and Burno in internal medicine in Vermont.

In the fall of 1951, I taught the first full-time course in Pharmacology to the class of 1953. It was a grand class of first-rate students. Strangely I recall more of those individuals than more recent students who came under my aegis. Like the first born, perhaps, they made a deeper impression. The experience gave me great confidence, and I was pleased to observe that this class performed better in pharmacology than any of the other basic sciences. Unofficial testing of student opinion was that I was a tough professor but fair and willing to work with the students. My own immodest opinion was that I had brought to Hahnemann a new, higher level of academic performance. To the credit of the institution and the other professors, they took this graciously. There was a great spirit of camaraderie and a sense of progress and achievement, which was never exceeded in subsequent years despite tremendous improvements in facilities and personnel. Part of this elan was universal throughout the country as the nation emerged from the Great Depression and the horrors of World War II. Many students were veterans who had gone back to college by taking advantage of veterans' benefits. They were older and more motivated than prewar classes.

To my surprise, the faculty governance at Hahnemann was more liberal and democratic than I was accustomed to in Brooklyn and Boston. While there was no tenure and no faculty senate, individual faculty members had more rights of appeal than if such supposed protection had been in place. The main academic governing body, the College Council, consisted of all Chairmen of Departments, the Dean as Chairman, the Associate Dean, and four faculty members-at-large, two from the basic sciences and two from the clinical sciences. The faculty members were elected at a yearly faculty meeting. Very well conceived faculty by-laws dealt with problems of rank, promotion, dismissal, grievances, and other items of interest to a faulty employee. John Scott, who had taken great pains to ensure maximum benefits for the faculty, had mostly constructed the by-laws that were jealously followed and served to keep Hahnemann on a straight and narrow path. Dean Brown reported directly to the Board of Trustees, as there was no president at this time in the long history of the institution.

The Board of Trustees, considered mediocre by any standards, was completely reconstructed since the probationary period. It now consisted primarily of Philadelphia WASPs from banking, insurance, business, and industry. The only difficulty was that they were mostly the lesser able of successful families. Frederic H. Strawbridge, Jr., for example, was considered by some to be a nice gentleman, certainly no blockbuster. Though the son of the famous Strawbridge family who, with the Clothiers, owned one of Philadelphia's largest department stores, he had never finished any decent education but was well-mannered and made a good appearance. His family used him to fulfill their community obligations.

The banking and insurance members of the board were there to protect the investments of their firms in the institution. The Hon. L. Stouffer Oliver, a very respected lawyer and judge, headed the board and made all-important decisions that the trustees rubber stamped. The Liaison Committee on Medical Education had insisted that there be two Alumni Members on the board, which was a good idea because there were few others to represent academic expertise. Very few board members had college degrees. The two alumni members of the board were retired from distinguished careers as members of the Hahnemann faculty and as professionals. Charles Hollis had been head of Otolaryngology and was a highly respected teacher and physician. Joseph Post was formerly head of Preventative Medicine and active in Philadelphia community health programs. Both were very capable speakers and served the faculty and the academic interests of Hahnemann well.

William Goldman was the most active and aggressive, and a rare Jewish member of the board. A patient and close friend of Dean Brown, he had given considerable money to Hahnemann so the board could not refuse him membership. Goldman owned a famous, extensive line of opulent movie theatres in Philadelphia. A powerful community figure who knew everyone in City Hall, he was an important addition to the board. Faculty and students loved him because he regularly provided free tickets to new movies. As part of the fanfare of a premier movie, he occasionally held luncheons with invited faculty and the visiting movie stars. I was lucky to have luncheon with Charles Laughten and Harry Bellefonte. Such touches made me feel that I had arrived and had some contact with the highest administrative level. In retrospect, such memorable interludes were of little consequence, and I'm sure that I made little impression on these famous performers.

Socially I gained more from interaction with the younger clinical faculty. I soon formed a small club that met at each other's homes once a month during the academic year. It was fashioned after the Friday Night Club that I'd organized in Brooklyn. I made sure that it didn't degenerate into an eating society by insisting on a scientific presentation at each meeting. The members included young internists from the department of medicine: Joe Gambesia, Danny Marino, Don Fitch, and Scotty Donaldson. From pediatrics, we had Dan Downing; from surgery there was Paul Grotzinger; and from pathology, Joseph Imbriglia. Because of its predominant Italian membership, the club was called the "Chircolo" an internal joke between us. We later added more members, but the original members bear some description, as they were all interesting characters.

Joe Gambesia, a short stocky man, was primarily interested in gastroenterology. He was a devout Catholic and distinguished himself by eventually having sixteen children! Tall blond Danny Marino was originally from Brooklyn so we had a common bond. Danny liked to bait people and lead them into embroiling arguments. Don Fitch, a dark haired Irishman, had a very sharp mind and could pepper any conversation with facts. Scotty Donaldson was born in Scotland. Tall and with a brogue, he was a natural comic who without doubt could have made his living on the stage. His claim to success was an ability to be liked by important people like Dean Parkinson at Temple University Medical School and later Dean Brown. Still, he had much native ability and was no slouch as a physician. Dan Downing came close to being an iconoclast and was one of the most astute in the group. His specialty was pediatric cardiology. He was one of the foremost experts in cardiac catherization in children. Paul Grotzinger, a skillful general surgeon, was unusually intellectual for one in a technical line. Paul was very well informed on any subject and could put most internists to shame. Don Fitch and he had many savory arguments on medical problems. Like many pathologists, Joe Imbriglia had a tendency to have a final, rigid opinion on any subject. The boys would plan to bait him into an argumentative field and get him hopelessly mired in impossible solutions to problems. After a few drinks with such a group, the conversation grew animated and many memorable debates occurred. At the end of the evening, good fellowship prevailed and everyone went home convinced that he had won all the arguments. I don't think that Hahnemann has ever had a finer group of young men on its faculty.

Meanwhile my home life was very satisfactory. My family was growing with the addition of two more daughters, Dorothea and Joan. The colonial house on Arbordale Road in Wynnewood proved to be most satisfactory. I made many improvements with the help of my wife who turned out to be quite an ingenious interior decorator. The cellar was spacious enough for me to build a woodworking and metal workshop as well as a recreation room. The land was adequate for a small vegetable garden and annual flowerbed. We yearned for more land area and made overtures to the owner of the lot next door, but he apparently had other plans.

As it became clear that we liked the area and that my position at Hahnemann looked rather permanent, we began to look around at other houses. Our search became a game, and we became experts in real estate values. Because we were in no hurry, it was possible to make some ridiculously low offers on some very attractive properties. In that time of post-Korean War depression, there were some realty bargains to be had. Among the many properties was the mansion of Alan Reed son of Jacob Reed owner of the fine men's clothing establishment on Chestnut Street in Philadelphia. The Price brothers designed the main brick and stone house, famous

Philadelphia architects. A Victorian Gothic in style, it had over five thousand square feet of living space. Built in 1898 on ten acres in Wayne, it also had a large carriage house that accommodated horses. Alan Reed died soon after the house was built, and one of his daughters took over the property. She married a Moulton who had claim to fame as an original member of the Lafayette Escadrille in World War I. The estate became known as the "Moulton House." Mrs. Moulton entertained and took an active interest in community activities. She in turn had four daughters who lived in the house until 1950 when Mr. Moulton died. The property proved to be too much for Mrs. Moulton, who was about to be married again, so the houses and land were sold to a developer named Fuchs. He divided the land into sixteen half-acre lots for new houses, a half-acre for the carriage house, and 2.3 acres for the main house. He put the later two up for sale hoping to get enough money to finance the building of the new houses, but they didn't sell. Meanwhile he had completed six new houses that were very sluggish in selling. By 1953, the main house had not sold. Vandals had invaded it and caused much destruction and deterioration. I boldly offered a bid of $35,000 but was insultingly turned down by an irate real estate agent. Mary and I pretty much forgot about the house and went about our other interests.

The next year was a busy one for us with three daughters and another one on the way. My work at Hahnemann was progressing satisfactorily and with no imminent calamities. By this time, my father and mother had both passed on within a year of each other. Parkinson's disease killed my father at age eighty-six, while multiple strokes and diabetes took away my mother. My two sisters and brother never married and were left together to carry on as a family in Queens. I received $3,000 from my mother, with the rest of the estate going to my sisters and brother. This was entirely fair as any money that had accrued to the estate was the result of the earnings of Mary, Kate, and Al. My other brother Frank who had left the family years before also received a negligible amount.

One day early in 1954, Mary noticed that the Moulton house was again up for sale. It was almost sold to someone who wanted to use the house as a dancing school. The deal fell through, however, when the township refused to allow this use. The house meanwhile had suffered further damage by vandals who, in addition to tearing all the electric fixtures from the walls, had turned on the fire hose on the top floor and flooded the whole house, causing extensive damage to all the plaster ceilings and walls. We found out from the new real estate agent that Mr. Fuchs was willing to consider any reasonable offer. Meanwhile we had found a very desirable English Tudor house on three acres in Devon that we could have for $35,000. But Mary still liked the Moulton house better so we made a ridiculous bid of $18,000. After some bickering, we agreed to $21,000, which was accepted. On one fine day in late April, 1954, we took possession of the grand mansion of Alan Reed, son of Jacob Reed the famous Philadelphia clothier. It was on 2.3 acres in south Wayne. We still had the house in Wynnewood that we had to sell. We were fortunately able to buy the Wayne house without a mortgage by borrowing $10,000 from the in-laws, so our financial burden of owning two houses was not so great. We did face extensive expenses to fix up the Wayne house and make it at least livable. It took us an entire year to make the necessary repairs and alterations before we could move in the following April. Ironically, a popular song had just come out titled, "This Old House Is A Needing Fixing," which seemed to play incessantly on the radio. The Wynnewood house meanwhile proved not too easy to sell, but we were eventually able to get rid of it at a very modest profit.

My full-time position allowed me time at home to make improvements and entertain the children. I felt somewhat guilty about this because years before I had been advised by C. J. Wiggers, the eminent physiologist, that to be a success in science one had to restrict family life to no more than two children and a small, easy-to-care-for house. Yet here I was with three offspring, a fourth on the way, and one of the biggest private homes on the Main Line. Down deep, this gave me twinges of conscience. I often had occasion to cogitate the question that, if I spent less time at home and more in the lab, would I accomplish more in science? Now only thirty-eight years old, I was supposedly at the peak of intellectual productivity. If I was to produce a substantial contribution, it had to be soon.

Every faculty member was required to serve on committees—another bothersome complication. As I became better known, I seemed to be more relied upon to serve on sensitive committees. The admissions committee was considered especially important. It consisted of five members headed by Nat Ludwig, the head of therapeutic radiology. Nat was an old time Hahnemannian and without doubt a very capable, shrewd operator. Like the other local schools, Hahnemann had to compete for a relatively small pool of Pennsylvania residents and tried very hard to convince attractive candidates to choose Hahnemann over Jefferson or Temple. I was recruited to serve a three-year term and soon learned all the tricks of the medical school admissions process. We had about 1,500 applicants for eighty-five places. Miss Britt, the Dean's secretary, also served as the secretary for the admissions committee. As the applications came in they were screened by Nat and the committee members and graded by a formula based on their grades at college, the score on the medical aptitude test, and the recommendation of the premed advisor. Those with the highest scores were selected for an interview. No applicant who wasn't recommended by his premed advisor was ever admitted. Close relatives of alumni were always interviewed, no matter how mediocre their grades. Veterans were given special considerations. There were few women and practically no minority applicants. I soon discovered that there was a "green" file," which meant that the applicant was Jewish. Nat was quite cagey about this, although we admitted Jews as about eleven percent of each class, which was consistent with the policy of other medical schools. Committee members conducted interviews, sometimes alone and sometimes jointly. Most of the time we knew which applicants were desirable so the purpose of the interview was a selling job to convince the applicant to choose Hahnemann over another school. Another important aspect of the interview was to determine that the applicant had the finances to attend medical school. Some applicants thought that they could work their way through medical school as they did through college.

Watching Nat work the admissions process was most educational. I don't believe he received any salary for his services, yet he devoted at least half his time to the job. This involved much paper work, many phone calls, and getting on a personal basis with premed advisors. He also made visits to feeder colleges with members of the committee, interviewed students on the spot, and practically admitted desirable candidates although they always had to be approved by the whole committee. He surely made deals with premed advisors along these lines: If you steer this desirable candidate to Hahnemann, we will consider taking one of your candidates who's having a hard time getting in. Dean Brown divorced himself from the committee and claimed that only the committee could admit students and that he did not have that power. There was no doubt, however, that he worked closely with Nat in regard to candidates who might influence financial or political considerations. Overall, the admissions were quite fair and above board. No member of the committee was in any way dishonest, played favorites, and certainly took no bribes. There really was no way to buy your way into medical school if you were not qualified. I didn't like the Jewish quota bit and was happy to see it abandoned in later years.

College Council met every month except August. The meetings were held in the library reading room on the first floor of the old college building. They started at 5 p.m. when the library was closed to the students. Dean Brown assisted by Associate Dean Harold Taggart ran the meeting. The proceedings usually dealt with mundane academic matters such as setting of schedules, promotions, appointments, retirements, and student and faculty affairs. Most meetings lasted until 7 p.m. when the group adjourned and went to supper at a local restaurant. This was a great opportunity to get to know our fellow department chairmen more intimately. Sometimes the meeting continued after supper if there was additional business to discuss. One such incident was the famous "Froio Affair" that led to much agitation in the institution.

Froio, an associate professor of pathology, did most of the surgical pathology. He was well liked by the surgeons who felt that he had sound judgment. The event in question was judgment on a breast biopsy for cancer diagnosis. John Gregory, the department chairman, was given the specimen to analyze first. He declared it to be free of cancer. The surgeon was suspicious of the diagnosis and passed the specimen to Froio for a second opinion. Froio's opinion was that it was definitely cancerous. In order to settle the matter more definitively, Froio sent the specimen to an eminent New York surgical pathologist without informing Gregory. The opinion came back that the lesion was definitely cancerous. When the whole clinical staff learned of this, it was very embarrassing to Gregory who was furious. He called Froio in and fired him on the spot for insubordination. Gregory claimed that Froio should have come back to him and Gregory instead of Froio should have sent out the specimen for a third opinion. Technically and ethically, Gregory was right, but whether this was cause for dismissal was the question before the council. Most members of the council liked Froio and didn't like Gregory, but they voted in support of Gregory because Brown wanted it that way. Froio found himself another job, but for Gregory this was an empty triumph that completely discredited him. All the clinicians avoided him, and he soon found it expedient to leave for another position. This imbroglio didn't do Brown any good both because his favorite chairman was discredited and the critics began to question his judgment.

Actually Dean Brown had done a magnificent job of earning Hahnemann a respectable place in the medical community. He had as much interest and respect for the porter as for the most distinguished faculty person. Perhaps, this was his undoing as his "friends" took advantage of him. Ray Truex, the anatomy chairman, for example, did not hesitate to make demands that were perhaps justified yet strained Hahnemann's limited budget. Charlie Brown earnestly tried to answer every demand. Hahnemann at the time had a financial officer, George Long, who was very accommodating. When Brown went to him, he seemed able to find money to finance extra budgetary demands. Long was honestly (really dishonestly) making the seemingly innocent mistake of spending money that the institution didn't have. In this case, it was money that needed to be set aside to pay the federal income tax money that had been withheld from employees' salaries for this purpose. The Feds descended on Hahnemann one day and wanted to know where the payments for 1952 to 1955 were—a total over $700,000. Not a very great amount by today's inflation, but a staggering blow at the time—enough to bankrupt the institution. The trustees, who were mostly of bankers and insurance people, were greatly alarmed and blamed Brown for this error because he was the CEO. They put Brown on ice and fired Long. Goldman, Brown's friend on the Board, tried to salvage the situation but to no avail. Brown became a lame duck Dean and a new hospital administrator was brought in to manage the corporation. As usual, the Board of Trustees cared little for the medical school and were primarily interested in the major income producer, the hospital. From a financial point of view, this was probably correct but was most demoralizing to the academic side of the corporation. This was only the first of many financial crises that Hahnemann was to weather in succeeding years.

Brown did what he could to control the crisis. His friend Goldman tried to get the board to refinance the corporation. The newly assigned chairman of the board, a banker named Barnes, was adamant that strict economy measures had to be installed and the debt had be paid to the government over a period of time. Brown was not even invited to the board meetings and thus was completely ineffective as a Dean. Faculty and staff had to go to Madison Brown, the newly appointed CEO, to get anything done. Morale deteriorated. Many faculty started to look around for other jobs. I had grown to like Hahnemann, and I had a big house and five children, so I decided to stick it out. Brown eventually got the job of establishing a new private medical school in Newark, New Jersey, sponsored by the Catholic Church, to be called Seton Hall after the university of that name. Brown offered to take me along in this new, exciting venture. In some ways, it was an attractive offer because I would be within commuting distance of New York

City where my relatives and friends were. This was to be the first medical school in New Jersey and was likely to receive state and federal support. I decided to stay in Philadelphia despite these attractions and never regretted my decision.

When Harold Taggart, the Associate Dean, became the acting Dean, things began to settle down somewhat. CEO Madison Brown ran a tight ship and faculty had little contact with the Board of Trustees. Mr. Goldman resigned from the board after Charles Brown left so we didn't get to see the latest movies anymore. A committee of three members of the Board of Trustees and two faculty members was named to search for a permanent dean. One of the faculty members was George Tedeschi, the newly appointed Chairman of Pathology. Tedeschi was entirely different from Gregory, his predecessor. Openly flamboyant and politically inclined, he soon became friendly with Madison Brown. They supported, a pediatrician at the University of Pittsburgh, as a candidate for the deanship. Burke's(not his real name) qualifications seemed satisfactory, at the least on paper.

Scotty Donaldson, acting Chairman of Medicine and the other faculty member of the search committee, were not too happy with the imminent appointment of a Pittsburgh pediatrician as Dean. Whether this was due to a genuine suspicion of some inadequacy in the candidate, or because he sensed that the candidate would not favor him for permanent chairman of medicine, is a moot question. Donaldson decided to investigate the candidate's past performance on his own. He found one Pittsburgh University executive who—on the phone but not in writing—gave Burke exceedingly bad marks and declared him to be incompetent. Armed with this information, Donaldson started a campaign among the faculty that led to the rumor that Madison Brown and Tedeschi wanted a weak dean so they could control the school. True or not, the rumor found attentive ears, particularly by Taggart and the clinical chairmen who were not especially fond of either Brown or Tedeschi. Taggart called an emergency meeting of College Council.

After much discussion, it was decided to inform the Administration that the faculty had no confidence in the prospective candidate's appointment as dean. This was most embarrassing to the Administration because the candidate had already been informed that he could have the appointment if he wished. The end result of this imbroglio was that the candidate didn't get the job, Tedeschi resigned from the search committee, and I was appointed in his place.

So began the Donaldson-DiPalma search for a suitable Dean. We never met with the board of trustee members of the committee, and indeed I didn't even know who they were. If Donaldson knew them, he never let on. I made a serious attempt to find a plausible candidate whom I could sell to the faculty and the board of trustees. Naturally I contacted all my friends at Harvard and Penn and soon found that very few capable teachers or scientists were interested in becoming a dean. The general feeling was that only someone who was a failure in medical practice, was an incompetent teacher, and could not do research was likely to want a dean's job. The marginal financial status of Hahnemann was also not an inducement. Some of the more attractive candidates suggested were Jewish or Irish or Italian Catholics who were out of the running in an era when WASPs dominated American educational institutions.

I told Taggart that Donaldson and I should attend the annual meeting of the Association of American Medical Colleges (AAMC) to sharpen the hunt. All the deans and personnel interested in medical education attended this meeting so it should be possible to find a likely candidate. That year's meeting was in Swamscott, Massachusetts, and a lovely resort spot with reasonable hotel rates in the off-season October. The first evening, a mixer affair gave us the opportunity to meet many attendees. Donaldson and I decided to work separately in order to cover as much ground as possible. I didn't make much headway and found that few people were interested in Hahnemann's problems. Donaldson, on the other hand, seemed to be getting along famously with one group of people in particular. Later that evening when we met in our room, Donaldson was highly agitated. He claimed he had received a fabulous job offer as chairman of medicine at a prominent southern school. He was very flattered and surmised that he could use this as a lever to force Hahnemann to give him the Chair of Medicine. He'd forgotten about the purpose of our visit, and all he could think about was his own career development. Our visit with the AAMC proved to be devoid of suitable candidates, although Donaldson made a great catch.

It turned out not to matter because, when we returned to Hahnemann, we were surprised to learn that the Board of Trustees had settled on a suitable candidate, Charles S. Cameron. A 1935 graduate of Hahnemann, Cameron was a trained and boarded surgeon who had become interested in cancer and had written a popular book entitled *The Truth about Cancer*. The book became a best seller, was translated into several languages, and secured great notoriety for Cameron as a cancer expert. The American Cancer Society, then starting its national campaign to raise money, made him director. Cameron was certainly a distinguished and accomplished person, but Donaldson and I could not perceive any qualifications that would give him experience in academic medicine. He had never held a position as a teacher or researcher in any medical school. This did not disqualify him, of course, but Donaldson and I wished to find out more about him because there were no letters of recommendation or even a formal *curriculum vita* available to us. I was selected to go to New York City and consult with Dusty Rhodes, one of the main movers of the American Cancer Society and a highly respected cancer researcher.

My interview with Rhodes was one of the most memorable of my career. As I was ushered into his cluttered office, he hastily pulled a screen in front of a blackboard behind his desk. I got enough of a glimpse to discern some chemical structures that were obviously variants of anti-cancer drugs. He was a tall, somber man who looked like he meant business. Motioning me to a chair and looking me straight in the eye he said, "So you're considering Cameron as Dean of your school. Don't take him. He will be a disappointment and a failure. He is no administrator and has certainly not been responsible for the successful money raising campaign of the cancer society.

"Besides, he hits the bottle, and you will have problems with his alcoholism," Rhodes continued. "Whenever a problem arises, he disappears and only returns when someone else resolves the situation. The only good thing I can say about him is that he makes wonderful speeches and charms the ladies. No one is equal to him in this respect. I cannot recommend him for this position."

Flabbergasted at this outburst, I could not think of any comment or any question to ask. Rhodes didn't offer to put his remarks on paper, and I did not expect him to do so. I thanked him and said that I would convey his feelings to the proper parties. When I returned to Philadelphia, I kept what I had learned to myself. Frankly I didn't know what to do with this most embarrassing information. I had never met Cameron and had no desire to do him an injustice. I did confide in my teammate Donaldson who was no help.

Even though it might be detrimental to my own career, I finally decided to inform the board of my information about Cameron. But rather than going to the committee that had never met, I arranged to meet with Watson (Pat) Malone III, the newly elected Chairman of the Board. Fortunately, Malone was a "regular guy" who was willing to listen to a young, inexperienced faculty person. He listened attentively to my story and smiled knowingly from time to time. When I was finished, he commented, "I appreciate your going to the trouble of furnishing me and the Board with this information. Rest assured that it will be taken into consideration when a final decision is made." I shook hands and parted, greatly relieved that I unburdened myself to capable hands. A few days later, Cameron's appointment as the new Dean was announced.

Some weeks later I learned through the grapevine how Cameron got the job. Jack Davies, a cardiologist at Hahnemann and a classmate of Cameron, was both friend and physician to Pat Malone and his family. Cameron's ability to imbibe enormous quantities of alcohol was well known even when he was a student. Notwithstanding, he was admired for his command of the English language and his intelligence. Davies talked Malone into accepting Cameron. I don't believe that Cameron ever knew that I had talked to Rhodes or Malone. As it turned out, Cameron was a pretty good dean and later an excellent president. Pat Malone, whom I became friendly with in later years, drew me aside from time to time and inquired, "What do you think of Cameron now?" After subsequently serving on many search committees, I realized that even the most astute and sagacious don't, on the average, do better than about 50 percent of really good selections. Even so, I have come to believe that in most cases one person, or at best two or three, can make a better selection than a large committee composed of different elements of the university, which has become the custom in recent years.

During these political engagements, I did not neglect the department. My own recruiting efforts for the department fortunately were quite successful on the whole, despite the lack of adequate funds. I scouted the local universities for an organic chemist who was ingenious and resourceful. From students who were Villanova graduates, I learned that Alex Gero, a Hungarian immigrant, was an excellent teacher of organic chemistry with a tendency towards research, which was unusual in a college instructor. I called him for an interview and found that he had worked in industry and knew a considerable amount about drug chemistry. He was receiving only a modest salary so it was not hard to convince him to join my department. He turned out to be a great find and developed into a leader in the field of theoretical pharmacology, which I don't think he or I anticipated. Gero was indeed one of the most cultured men I'd ever known. An accomplished cellist, he could have had an equally successful career in music as in chemistry. He was fluent in seven languages, which came in handy when we needed to translate foreign articles into English. When we later established a graduate program, Gero managed the foreign language requirements.

Meanwhile Ben Calesnick was called to do his two years of

army duty and had to take a leave of absence. This conveniently left a faculty vacancy that I could fill on a temporary basis and the opportunity to bring some biochemical talent into the department. When I put out feelers, I found that Morris Spirtes, a young biochemist who was actually an M.D., was unhappy working at the Fels Institute of Temple University Medical School. I called him for an interview and was impressed with his enthusiasm and energy. He did have a tendency to exaggerate and inflate his own work, and he had an almost pathological paranoia that the head of the Fels Institute, a Doctor Weinstock, was stealing his research findings. Because of his experience with recent biochemical research and with the Otto Warberg technology, the rage at the time, I overlooked his deficiencies. I offered him an assistant professorship on the basis of a two-year contract because when Calesnick came back, I would have to restore his position. To my surprise Spirtes was anxious to take the job on this basis.

Spirtes settled in fast and soon had a Warberg set up and running. To his credit, he secured an NIH grant and attracted a graduate student to work with him. He was a positive addition to the department and a good proponent of the emerging field of biochemical pharmacology. On the negative side, he soon made an enemy of Tom Barnes who had an adjacent laboratory, and the two never spoke to each other. Borrowing a scrub suit from the operating room, he walked around to the library and even the Dean's office in this pajama-like garb. This was against the rules of the operating room, and perhaps excusable behavior for surgical residents, but certainly not for faculty and especially preclinical faculty. Why he persisted in this irritating behavior was puzzling because otherwise he was friendly and even at times very considerate. Nevertheless, his uncouth behavior came to the attention of Dean Cameron, and I received many complaints from this and other sources. I was never able to correct this fault, and I suspect that the underlying reason was the resentment that although he was a physician and a veteran, he had a lowly position at a modest salary. There was no doubt that Spirtes was a capable and even talented researcher, a good teacher, and a stimulating individual, but he was also what can only be described in general terms as a trouble maker. When Calesnick eventually returned, I asked Spirtes to leave, as our contractual agreement provided. He pleaded to be kept on because he liked Hahnemann, had done good work, and did not have prospects of another job. Against my instincts I scrounged around for funds to him keep him on as well as restore Calesnick to his former position. Spirtes stayed but at no salary increase. I knew he was unhappy and looking for another job.

Chairmen don't like to fire faculty, I discovered then and became even more convinced later when I was Dean. The most unpleasant part of being a chairman is the responsibility for the welfare of everyone in the department. Even in a small department like pharmacology, this can become a burden. Between Spirtes' uncouth behavior and Barnes' alcoholic escapades, my time was occupied with matters that added nothing to intellect or grant-securing ability. I found myself spending much valuable time giving individual moral support to other department members. Despite my aversion to this role, I became a sort of father image to my faculty as well as secretaries and technicians. This was in addition to serving on more committees than I could reasonably manage. I soon decided it that being a department chairman was no fun.

I recall that Cameron called me aside one day to ask why so many basic scientists were rather queer individuals. Was he was referring to me or at the least to members of my department, I wondered. Recalling that he was a surgeon before becoming an administrator, I replied that many thoughtful persons felt that surgeons were oddballs in their own way. Scientists, I pointed out, are creative people. Like artists and poets, they often think and act in unconventional terms. Most are underpaid and need a kindly society that subsidizes their activities. But I don't think Cameron was satisfied with this explanation. He walked away shaking his head.

Despite a large house and garden to care for, and committee and research duties beyond the ordinary, I managed to find time to return to a former interest in art. The works of the surrealistic painter Salvador Dali fascinated me, although I realized their nonsensical nature. I imitated him and other surrealists in an oil painting that portrayed the ideal experimental animal for pharmacological research. The central figure was a humanoid with large buttocks—for intramuscular injections—and a rooster's head for vascular observations in the cockscomb. It was quite colorful and startling. After suitable framing, I hung it behind my desk in my Hahnemann office. The offices of preclinical department chairman were quite drab in those days. Mine had a plain concrete floor that I soon had my denier, John Dukirk, paint in colorful squares, each of which had an alchemists symbol inscribed in it. Imagine the surprise of the occasional visitor who had the sensations of standing on a weird floor and confronting a bizarre painting behind my desk. The effect was to put the visitor at some disadvantage. In the ensuing conversation about the floor and the painting, he often forgot what he was about to ask me. Some students informed me that a rumor was circulating that I marked exams by throwing the exam books on the floor. Their grades depended on which square the book fell upon. Not true, of course, but it did indicate that people noticed some eccentric nature in my character.

With five children at home, it was not easy to take a vacation, but this was convenient for my artistic tendency. Our home had a large cathedral hall with a grand staircase. An expansive blank wall provided a setting for either a large tapestry or a mural painting. Mary and I decided that a tapestry was too expensive, so we chose a mural, especially because I had the desire to paint one. As the house was castle-like in architecture, we chose a subject from the age of chivalry. What better portrayal than the Knights of the Round Table? Images came to mind from my childhood reading of Sir Lancelot, Lady Guinevere, and the dark knight, Mordred. The illustrations of N.C. Wyeth also sprung vividly to my mind. By combining three of his illustrations, I managed a dramatic battle scene complete with horses and armor with Lady Guinevere and a medieval castle in the background. The ten-by-thirteen-foot painting dominated the hall and made quite an impression on visitors.

The most difficult aspect of making this painting was that its large size required a multi-storied scaffold constructed to fit the staircase. There was no way for me to step back and view the work in progress and estimate color and perspective. Mary passed by frequently with the children and made remarks that, although irritating at the time, were very helpful in attaining the proper color tone and shadow-highlight intensity. For example, I had finished the whole sky background when Mary informed me that the blue I'd chosen was not sky-like. After much experimenting, I repainted the entire sky with a predominantly cerulean blue that merited Mary's approval. Of all the many varied projects I have successively completed in my lifetime, this painting has brought me the greatest satisfaction, although it is really only an enlargement and copy of the works of N.C. Wyeth, the famous illustrator.

Although, I never played a musical instrument, I was very fond of listening to classical music since childhood. Thank God for radio stations WQXR in New York City and WFLN in Philadelphia. These stations were always on when I was awake. All the great composers became my favorites, and I acquired some considerable knowledge and appreciation of music. Mary had done credible professional singing in her younger days and was interested in opera. Through her, I also acquired an interest in opera. She even gave me some singing instruction and thought I had a fine base voice. All this interest in music fed into my interest in electronics, and I invested in the best electronic receivers, amplifiers, and speakers that I could afford or build myself. Our interest in music had a profound effect on our children. All five of them play and enjoy a musical instrument. My oldest became a singer and the next one is a pianist. Yet I have never regretted that I did not play a musical instrument myself. There are only so many things one can do in one lifetime.

Our pharmacology department had a preponderance of relatively young people with growing families, and it was appropriate for some events to emphasize social intercourse. We had acquired graduate students and some technicians, and a yearly get-together event was in order. This initiated an annual picnic at my house in Wayne. The grounds were fortunately ample enough to allow soft baseball, badminton, and even an aboveground swimming pool. On the extensive porches, we had ping pong and other games, plus lounging space. From the outdoor barbecue, the aroma of steak and turkey added to the atmosphere of fun and good fellowship. Faculty members of other departments and administrative people were also invited with their wives and children. A gathering of nearly 100 people was not unusual. Over a span of fifteen years, these picnics did much to enhance the spirit of the department, our relationship to other departments, and the school as a whole, as it continued the friendly, optimistic atmosphere characteristic of a small school.

About this time Mary's father retired and needed a place to live because he had sold his home in the Bronx. He and Mary's mother first moved in with Mary's sister who had a small house in Great Neck, Long Island, N.Y. That arrangement did not work out. Our house in Wayne was large enough to allow a complete, separate apartment, so we invited Grandpa and Grandma to live with us—a very convenient arrangement as it allowed built-in baby sitters for our five children.

Grandpa was a very capable and resourceful handyman who loved to work on projects. He was of great help to me in maintaining such a large home and grounds. As my scientific activity increased, it became necessary to take trips to other cities and sometimes even abroad. With Granny and Grandpa at our home, it was possible for Mary to accompany me on most of these trips. These were really our vacations. We enjoyed Atlantic City, Boston, Chicago, San Francisco, New Orleans, and many other cities because the great expansion of air travel made possible such national and international intercourse. What a contrast to our immediate forebears who spent their entire lifetimes within a radius of a few miles!

After six years had passed since we moved to Philadelphia, I had occasion to reflect on my academic life. Never once did I regret my move from Brooklyn. I did miss my friends, particularly Julie Stolfi, Bill Florio, and Joe Cresci. I also felt the lack of intellectual stimulation that Bill Dock provided. Although I was a conscientious physician devoted to my patients, I confess that I did not really feel a vacuum in this regard. This surprised me because I always felt great satisfaction in human contact. Perhaps my contact with students, particularly graduate students, replaced the satisfaction I'd had from patients. I also kept up with developments in internal medicine, still made rounds, and took a turn at clinic duties.

My greatest concern now was my development as a scientist and a teacher. Although I was still doing frontline research, I had the feeling that I was falling behind and that obsolescence was setting in. What I clearly needed was a sabbatical and the stimulation that comes from contact with other minds. Bill Dock had advised me that in academics one should move every five years. But how could I manage it? A chairman cannot easily leave his responsibilities. On top of that, I'd acquired a large house and grounds, and my five young children could not be left to fare for themselves. So I delayed any drastic move from year to year. Besides, I was quite happy at Hahnemann and felt needed and fulfilled. It would have taken a very attractive offer to encourage me to move on to another medical center. Few cities could match Philadelphia for scientific, medical, and academic resources with its five medical schools, many outstanding nearby universities, the Franklin Institute, the Academy of Natural Sciences and the famous Philadelphia College of Physicians with its excellent medical library.

Having made a firm decision to stick it out at Hahnemann, I made haste to adjust myself to the personality and whims of Charles Cameron, the new dean. The former dean, Charles Brown, was a warm and very considerate person, and every department chairman felt a distinct personal attitude toward him. Cameron in contrast was a cold, fastidious individual with obvious traits of perfection in dress and behaviors. In the five years he was dean, he devoted himself mainly to hospital affairs. Harold Taggart, the associate dean, managed most of the work of the dean's office.

To Cameron's credit, he decided that the institution needed

superior people to head the two most important clinical departments, medicine and surgery. He went headhunting himself instead of relying on a search committee. For reasons only he himself knew, he chose Texas for his fieldwork. He took the aggressive step of going to Houston to personally invite John Moyer to become Chairman of Medicine and John Howard to assume the Chair of Surgery. Both men accepted the opportunity. Moyer became a very competent and constructive department head. While Howard never developed into a really good chairman, both men had a very large influence on Hahnemann's history.

Moyer was of Pennsylvania Dutch stock. His father had a farm in Lebanon where he grew up in the atmosphere of the thrifty, make-do country folk who populated that area near Hershey. He was used to hard work and the assumption of responsibility. His uncle, whom he greatly admired, was Carl Schmidt, Chairman of the Department of Pharmacology at the University of Pennsylvania. His uncle was his model and he aspired to emulate this famous scientist who discovered ephedrine, a very useful drug. From his earliest memories, he always wanted to be a physician and a scientist like his uncle. At Lebanon College, he studied hard to further his ambition. He was fulfilled to get into the University of Pennsylvania School of Medicine. Perhaps not a brilliant student, but certainly a satisfactory one, he completed his graduate training in internal medicine.

Eventually he landed at the Baylor School of Medicine where he held faculty positions in both medicine and pharmacology. Carol Handley, a very competent renal physiologist, was in the department of pharmacology at that time, and Moyer became friendly with him because they shared common research interests. Handley was working with a new group of oral diuretics related to carbonic dehydrogenase inhibitors that showed unusual promise. Moyer did some of the original clinical investigation with the new diuretics later called thiazides, which gave him a reputation as a great researcher. Moyer's ability to work hard and be persistent, along with his uncanny capacity for organizing clinical research and analyze data stood him in good stead. During a nine-year period, Moyer had his name on over 200 original research papers, a good many of them as senior author.

Donaldson was greatly disappointed that Moyer was made chairman because that left Donaldson in a subordinate position. Moyer, however, soon showed his mettle and set into place administrative functions that made the department more business-like. He brought on a financial manager and set up a practice plan that greatly expanded the department's financial base. He wasted no time recruiting capable young internists and required them to participate in a vigorous program of teaching, research, and practice. Among them were Lew Mills, a young internist from Baylor, and Morty Fuchs, a brilliant Hahnemann graduate. With these and other rising stars, Donaldson was side tracked. He soon decided that there was little future for him at Hahnemann and left for a better opportunity at Temple University School of Medicine.

John Howard was an entirely different type than Moyer. Tall, with a premature baldness, and white hair, he looked much older that he was. He had the charm of a Southerner and was a most attractive personality. As a surgeon, he was demon in the operating room where he antagonized nurses, residents, and colleagues. This was aggravated by an extremely slow, fastidious technique that psychologically seems always to cast an aura of incompetence on a surgeon. His major experience was in the army where he'd made a name for himself handling and researching traumatic shock and blood transfusion. In contrast to Moyer, he was a poor organizer and his staff had little respect for him. At that time thoracic surgery, headed by Charles Bailey, was only a division of the surgery department, which led to a turf question between the two men. Bailey, then a rising star with a national and international reputation, felt that he should have been made head of surgery and was openly critical of Howard. Cameron did his best to calm the troubled waters. Bailey was given his own department, but this didn't solve the problem because Bailey and Howard had to share the same surgical facilities in the hospital. Bailey eventually left to become Chairman of Surgery at the New York Flower Fifth

Avenue Hospital Medical School. This turned out to be a sad mistake both for Hahnemann and Bailey.

I got to know Bailey very well. He was about six-foot-two with an aggressive posture and step. His skull was round and somewhat cone shaped, which gave the impression that he must have a small brain. He was not an intellectual type, yet in a group he was able to dominate the conversation. Bailey's talent resided in a great drive and guts to explore where others feared to tread.

He came to me one day and said, "Joe, you know that Baine (not his real name) a cardiac surgeon from the South is starting to explore hypothermia as a means of performing extensive open heart surgery. I am going to beat him to the punch. Will you help me to get the basic animal work done and train some fellows in the required techniques so we can start to do some clinical cases? I need a lab and some senior person to collaborate with Brian Cookson, whom I have talked into assuming the role of investigator."

I was not too keen to take on this responsibility because I suspected that my standards for physiological research were far more rigorous than what Bailey expected for a hurry-up job to apply the knowledge in the surgical theater. I immediately questioned how the work was going to be financed. Bailey claimed that he had a grant, but I suspect that he financed the work out of the division's budget and what he could scrounge from grateful patients. I knew that his budget was strained at this time because he was also working to design an extra corporeal pump and oxygenator. Eventually John Gibbon, his competitor cardiac surgeon at Jefferson Medical College, designed a superior device that made open heart surgery practical. The hope at the time was that hypothermia would prove to be simpler and safer than the mechanical solution. Hence the urgency to develop new technology. As a pharmacologist, I was interested in the hypothermia approach. Smith Kline and French (SKF), a local pharmaceutical company, was also interested and had approached me (as I'm sure they did others) to explore the virtues of a new drug with unusual central nervous system depressant effects. The drug was thorazine that, among other actions, induced a hypothermic state in animals. Remarkably, thorazine failed for this use but became one of the first drugs to be effective in the therapy of schizophrenia. SKF made a fortune from it, but it was a washout for chemically induced hypothermia.

Despite all these misgivings and perambulations, I dropped some research I was doing and plunged into hypothermia research. I assigned a laboratory next to mine for the work. Brian Cookson turned out to be a fascinating character. He was short statured and rotund with a pink baby face and very black hair. His marked British accent gave away his origins. With my Brooklynese and his English, our conversation must have been most amusing to an observer. His father was a prominent pathologist at Edinburgh University in Scotland, and I had the impression that young Cookson was trying to outdo his dad. I soon grew fond of Cookson for he had a fine mind and a wonderful sense of humor. He was sloppy and untidy, however, and soon we had cockroaches all over the lab. Sometimes he left dead dogs in the lab over night, which created a dreadful odor by the next morning.

The work proceeded rapidly. We soon settled on a blanket that was perfused with ice water to cool the anesthetized dog. It took several hours to get down to a body temperature of twenty-four degrees centigrade. Observations were made of blood pressure, pulse, respiration, and electrocardiogram. When lower than twenty-four degrees, the heart was likely to go into arrest or more likely to fibrillate, a fatal arrhythmia. There was little doubt that the metabolism of all the body's organs was lowered to a minimal level. This was the gamble that, at this state of depression of life processes, it would be possible to operate on a nearly quiescent heart with the circulation arrested, and it would be able to recover without incurring appreciable ischemic damage to the brain and other vital organs. We soon learned that healthy dogs could be cooled to a temperature of twenty-four degrees, Centigrade, kept at that temperature for an hour, and then rewarmed as rapidly as possible and allowed to recover. Most animals seemed to withstand the hypothermic episode without apparent deficits. Some did not, depending on the state of health, age, and the complication of heart arrhythmias. This was without the insult of any operative procedure. When we added sham cardiac operations, the mortality was greater than expected. It was obvious to us that hypothermia was not going to be a panacea for the performance of open heart surgery. We struggled to find means of perfecting the technology. More rapid cooling? Lowering the body temperature to only thirty degrees and using some pump assistance? Using antiarrhythmic drugs to forestall ventricular fibrillation? As we became more skilled, our success rate improved, but there was still an unacceptable risk of failure.

Bailey visited the lab on occasion, but after about six months he seemed to have lost interest. Yet he came dashing in one day with the news that he'd learned through the grapevine that Baine was about to try an operation in a human using hypothermia. Bailey announced, "I'm going to beat Baine to the punch. I have a female patient who needs difficult heart repairs that can't be done with the available technology. Cookson, I want you to work with my fellows to prepare for the operation that is scheduled for early next week."

We immediately tried to dissuade Bailey from plunging into an area which was still highly experimental and which we felt we had so far failed to iron out all the bugs. Bailey, however, was insistent. Against his better judgment, Cookson went ahead to prepare for the operation. No mechanism such as informed consent existed at that time, much less a human research committee. Malpractice suits were rare and hardly ever settled in favor of the plaintiff. To make matters worse, Cookson and the surgical team decided that the cooling blanket method was too slow. They chose instead to first anesthetize the patient, then pack the body in ice. The problem was that there was no bathtub or receptacle in the operating room suite to carry this out. Not discouraged, they secured a small aluminum dinghy and used it as a kind of bathtub. It was quite messy but served the purpose.

Despite taking advantage of all the skills and information that had been obtained from the dog experiments, and despite Bailey's and his team's great surgical skill, nothing went really well. The patient never came out of the depressed hypothermic state despite adequate warming procedures. There was no doubt that the patient did not have long to live. The operation was a last chance, yet Cookson and the surgical team were profoundly depressed. Not so Bailey, who was soon planning another human venture into hypothermia.

Rapid progress was being made meanwhile with extra corporeal pumps and oxygenators. The experience of other hypothermia investigators was much the same as ours—namely that this technology was not the answer to facilitate open heart surgery. More surgeons turned to pump devices and hypothermia gradually faded out from the picture. That's not to say that we did not learn a great deal. We even had some brilliant successes. One young surgeon was able to transplant the heart and lungs from one dog to another, and the receiver dog survived for three days. This was a remarkable achievement at the time and preceded the same operation in a human by some twenty years.

At the end of that year, Cookson was completely discouraged with research and decided to go back to clinical endeavors. He returned to England and attempted to get specialty training. After some stormy times, he eventually ended up in Canada as a psychiatrist. Now married with offspring, he apparently lived happily ever after. I've lost track of him, but he stands in my mind as an example of the disenchantment that takes place all too often when young, enthusiastic researchers put all their eggs in one basket in an attempt to solve a major, challenging problem. Very few ever hit the jackpot. In contrast, his many failures never discouraged Bailey. He simply moved on to the next adventure.

The Board of Trustees in its wisdom decided that Cameron should step down as Dean and assume the Presidency of the institution. This was a fortuitous move because Cameron's talents lent themselves to public contact and money raising. Hahnemann's finances were skimpy and precarious. Now that their homeopathic supporters had died off, trustees were competing with four medical and one osteopathic school for financial support. Most of the money raised from the Philadelphia community came from clinical contacts of staff physicians and hospital admissions. The alumni gave only modest support since most of them moved to distant communities where they acquired new charitable obligations. Certainly Hahnemann did not enjoy an affluent and generous Board of Trustees as did Jefferson and the University of Pennsylvania. Women philanthropists were apt to have affiliation with Women's Medical College, thus effectively removing an important source of support. Temple University School of Medicine had more secure relations with the state government and was able to get state support denied to the other medical schools.

Hahnemann was frankly a tuition-run medical school without endowment and very little state support. Such schools with limited finances in the long run survive only as long as the environment is expanding. They must be careful not to acquire too many non-productive programs that end up being a financial burden to the rest of the institution. With this in mind, large universities were reluctant to accept government money because they knew from bitter experience that, when the politics changed, the money would stop and the new programs would have to be financed by the university. Nevertheless, practically no institution can withstand the invitation to expand with the temptation of government money.

In the 1960s the federal government decided that there was a shortage of physicians, particularly in rural areas. Money became available to expand enrollment in existing medical schools. The concept of capitation was introduced—a certain amount of money for each warm body enrolled as a medical student. State governments followed suit, including Pennsylvania. Naturally not a single school turned down this bonanza. Despite recommendations of the Association of American Medical Colleges (AAMC) that no new medical schools were needed and that the existing schools could efficiently handle the expanded enrollment, new medical training centers sprang up like a prairie fire. States with no—or few—medical schools suddenly discovered that they needed one or more. As a result, the number of entering places to study medicine increased from about eight to sixteen thousand in the span of a few years. In this frenzy to produce physicians, even foreign medical schools benefited, while some opportunists started flimsy medical schools in the Caribbean.

There was a parallel increase in specialty training so that a hospital with five hundred patient beds might have as many as three hundred residents and as many fellows as it could afford. Divisions of departments now demanded to have their own departmental status. The average medical school in 1950 got along quite handily with about a dozen departments. In the 1960s, no self-respecting school had less than twenty-four departments. This meant that the number of department heads and faculty, most of whom were on some kind of full time pay, and an increase in accommodations and fringe benefits were so markedly increased that it put a strain on the annual budget. Practically, the major increase was seen in a proliferation of clinical departments, while the basic science departments stayed at about the same number. Politically, this meant that clinical departments had more to say about policy and money distribution.

Deans and administrators frantically began to seek practical, ingenious solutions to the financial deficits created by this rapid expansion. The easiest, most expedient answer was to increase tuition. But this had limitations because it would favor wealthy applicants. The government was quite generous, however, in providing student loans. Still, this meant that the less financially able had to go into debt in order to acquire a professional education.

Another economy move was to try to streamline instruction. The animal rights movement had by the 1960s reached a politically important position. The legislation that antivivasectionists had been able to get passed in federal and state governments made housing and maintaining animal colonies extremely expensive. Pound dogs and cats could not be used. Experimental animals of all kinds became very expensive. Medical schools found it expedient to eliminate animal experimental instruction and get rid of or markedly reduce their animal colonies. This delighted some students but was actually detrimental to their education. Everything they previously learned in the laboratory about handling living tissues and the experimental approach to medicine now had to be learned in the clinic and the ward. It also contributed to less contact between instructor and student. The faculty also liked the abandonment of the laboratory instruction because it eliminated much labor. All they had to do now was give a few lectures. But they did not realize that administrators would now estimate that a course of basic science could be taught with a minimum of instructors and the budgets of pre-clinical departments could be reduced.

Soon the concept developed of medical centers in which the academic enterprise and the clinics and hospital became a combined nonprofit-profit exercise. In other words, income from healthcare delivery (through clinics and hospital) would be used to support the academic endeavor. The academic side, in turn, was to provide services such as clinical pathology, chemistry, and microbiology. Providing instruction to residents, fellows, nurses, and allied health personnel was another convenient cooperative area. This modis operendi made the academic medical center very powerful as compared to the non-academically connected private hospital or clinic. The academic center had the capacity for many residents and fellows, which made it possible to perform operations and technologies that were impossible to deliver without such manpower. There were also full-time clinicians who saw few patients and could thus devote themselves to the development of advanced medical and surgical services.

A tremendous expansion of specialties resulted. Internal medicine, itself a specialty, had over a dozen subspecialties such as hematology, rheumatology, endocrinology, cardiology, and respiratory diseases. Today there are easily over a hundred specialties and subspecialties, most with their own boards. In the beginning of the twentieth century over 90 percent of graduates practiced general medicine; today only about 10 percent are attracted to a generalist career.

Why was there this decline in interest in general medicine? The growth of knowledge and technology made feasible the division of medical expertise and practice in special fields such as cardiology, gastroenterology, rheumatology, endocrinology, and many others.

Organized boards developed that dictated special training and spheres of practice. Obviously it was more practical and lucrative to restrict one's practice to a specialized field rather than attempt to be inadequately trained or competent to handle situations in diverse areas. This had a chilling effect on the generalist who now became a sort of triage officer. Once he made a tentative diagnosis he was obliged to refer the patient to a specialist for treatment.

The generalists fought back against this trend and invented the specialty of Family Medicine, which enabled them to create training and boarded prestige in this field. Although Family Practice has made a considerable contribution, it still is a general field not very different from general practice and not many of its disciples do obstetrics, pediatrics, psychiatry, and certainly not surgery to any extent.

The growth of the specialties of medicine caused profound changes in the structure of medical school administration. The Hahnemann Board soon realized that the usual functions of the dean, which in many private medical schools involved running a practice plan for its clinical full-time faculty, would have to change. There was also the need for more serious integration of functions of the hospital and medical school. Deaning had grown so big and complex that it required a more complex organizational structure. The Board decided to move Cameron into the presidency of the corporation and restrict the dean to academic affairs. Other medical schools made similar moves. Although in those that had already had a president, the change was to create a new officer, usually called Vice President of Clinical Affairs. This was also to happen at Hahnemann at a later date. Unfortunately, the creation of a more complex organization, with new areas of influence and new executives, brought about increased competition that, in turn, created an atmosphere of politics and underhanded maneuvers.

These events were unsettling for me. As a pre-clinical department chairman, I foresaw that the formation of new clinical departments would mean a diminished space and budget allotments for the pre-clinical departments. The curriculum would also end to change in order to stress clinical training at the expense of the more abstract and theoretical pre-clinical training.

The new dean would have to be a person who was well trained with exceptional managerial abilities. Indeed, some medical schools favored physicians who had an MBA. Deaning became more of a business operation.

CHAPTER VI

More Academia

1961-1967

*"Despite the alleged moral and ethical purity of academic
institutions, they are just as contaminated with all the Biblical
sins of man as any other less noble human endeavors."*

Rupert Black, M.D.

A Dean's influence on a medical school—in either a positive or
negative way—can be tremendous even though, by the 1960s, his
power was diluted by the appointment of administrative officers
superior to him. With Cameron advanced to the President's
position, Hahnemann needed a Dean who could aid in the
ambitious attempt to elevate its stature. It was obvious that Taggart
had neither the experience nor the stature for the job. A blue ribbon
committee was appointed. With my recent memory of the previous
Dean's search effort, I was grateful not to be on it. My buddy
Mede Bondi was a member and proved to be the one who hit the
jackpot. He had heard of a likely candidate from a former faculty
member who had moved on to Seton Hall Medical School in New
Jersey. They had been looking for a Dean after Charles Brown
died. Among the final list was William Kellow who was not selected
but was rated very highly.

Kellow had graduated from Georgetown Medical School and
trained there in internal medicine and pulmonary diseases. He
then went to the University of Illinois School of Medicine in

Chicago as an assistant dean and assistant professor of medicine. There he became involved in an innovative program that was called Research in Medical Education, which later attracted national attention and was an important factor in developing medical education. His experience and training made Kellow an unusually qualified person for a deanship. As an Irish Catholic, he had a disadvantage since most educational institutions still favored Protestants. Yet he was a very determined man and made an impressive presence with his piercing dark eyes. Another arresting feature was a deformed spine, a hunchback, apparently from tuberculosis. It somehow projected the feeling that here was a man who'd overcome great difficulties and who was bound to be successful. Kellow was easily the best of the candidates. Although I had a feeling that Cameron did not really feel comfortable with him, Kellow was offered the job.

When Kellow became Dean of Hahnemann in July, 1962, it marked the beginning Hahnemann's rapid rise in academic stature and the acquisition of badly needed facilities. Kellow's genius for organization and efficient management soon became evident. As a first step, he moved out of the antiquated Dean's office in the old Victorian brick building. He very ingeniously constructed a suite of offices on the balcony of the auditorium of the Klahr building. This was difficult because the floor was sloped and curved. The arrangements were nevertheless quite convenient and even included a conference room.

When Harold Taggart retired, Kellow replaced him with Hugh Bennett who came from Baylor in Texas and was experienced in deaning functions. A tall, thin energetic man with bushy eyebrows and a crop of thick brown hair, he turned out to be a workhorse with an around-the-clock work attitude. He was trained as a gastroenterologist but was actually more of a generalist. Kellow put him in charge of student affairs and student health. The faculty soon grew to dislike Bennett because he always took the student's view of matters. Notwithstanding, for the first time Hahnemann began to have efficient student services mainly due to Bennett's efforts and Kellow's strong backing.

Credit should not be taken away from other administrators who greatly contributed to Hahnemann's successful growth. Charles Paxson replaced the unpopular Madison Brown as the hospital's CEO. A small, energetic man, Paxson seemed to be able to make things work with a minimum of staff. He had an uncanny ability to get along with physicians as well as other executives. He revitalized the nursing school, which was then under the management of the hospital. The first facility improvement was the construction of a dormitory and classroom building for nurses. Garage and conference areas were also added to the complex. The team of Cameron, Kellow, and Paxson proved to be a highly effective combination. For the first time, some effective planning was instituted to take advantage of the growing expansion of the health services and sciences.

Kellow greatly improved faculty governance and made the College Council an effective body. He was a shrewd recruiter and brought aboard a financial officer, Thomas Murray, for the medical school. This proved a very wise move because the hospital finance department in particular poorly handled the grant finances. Another meritorious acquisition was Joseph Gonnella as an Assistant Dean. A Harvard graduate, Gonnella had trained in Medical Education at Illinois, as had Kellow, and was conversant with the latest trends. Gonnella filled in the gaps in Bennett's efforts, although the two did not get along. Despite this inconsistency, the Dean's administrative team made dramatic improvements in the efficiency and academic quality of the institution.

From the beginning, I got along well with Kellow. He was five or six years younger than I but had married earlier and had five daughters matching my own record. His wife, a former nurse, had a rather domineering personality although she could be charming. She and my wife got along fairly well—undoubtedly stemming from the common problems of raising five daughters. I recall having the Kellow family to one of our annual summer picnics, which they seemed to greatly enjoy.

Kellow insisted that I attend the annual meetings of the Association of American Medical Colleges (AAMC) although, I confess, I had no real interest. Since he paid my way, however, and Washington was an interesting city to visit, I did not at all mind. I must concede that I did learn from this and by an unconscious analysis of Kellow's strategies and the methods of control by which he got things done. Kellow was a master at planning. Once a plan was made, he moved it into action by a series of steps. He planned the first serious retreat to orient the faculty to bring about a change in curriculum. It was an eye opener for most Hahnemann faculty who had been used to doing things in the good old way. He was helped, of course, by the fact that he had a quantity of younger faculty who were amenable to change.

Perhaps the main contribution of Kellow's tenure was the establishment of a practice plan for the full-time clinical faculty. Cameron was instrumental in securing the Board of Trustees' cooperation to purchase and remodel the Gorson Chrysler Automobile Showroom next door to Hahnemann Hospital on Broad Street. The building was completely renovated to provide practice facilities for the main clinical specialties, including radiology. Financing was partially accomplished by general fund raising but greatly helped by a generous grant by Meyer Feinstein, then a member of the Board. The building became known as The Feinstein Clinic and provided the basis of the practice plan. Although the Kellow Practice Plan was far from perfect, it was an important start. The main features were that full-time clinical faculty had part of their salary paid by the institution, depending upon their teaching duties. Money generated in practice made up the rest to the previously agreed total salary. If the individual made more than the set limit, then 50 percent of the overage reverted to the institution for a discretionary Dean's fund, 25 percent was assigned to the department concerned and the remaining 25 percent was a reward for the individual physician. If the individual did not make the assigned amount, then it was up to the department to decide if the difference could be made up.

As it turned out, very few faculty failed to make the allotted amount because recompense was based on billings and not on actual collections. Since the institution was responsible for making collections, it was easy for practitioners to bill generously to make up enough for their salaries. It took several years for the institution to correct this major fault, which caused the practice plan to lose money. Neither the Dean's discretionary fund nor the institution made any money from this plan, and it's difficult to understand why full-time clinical faculty were never satisfied with these arrangements. Later plans were far less advantageous with no provision for overhead and a straight salary situation. A fixed amount reverts to the institution based on collections, and the cost of facilities, equipment, and personnel are all costs that have to be earned by the physicians in the unit. It was true in the 1960s, and is still the case today, that a physician on average can make more income in private practice than in full-time academic clinical practice. The latter may please the ego, but it is a high price to pay for contact with students and the academic environment.

Kellow had a keen interest in community medicine, which used to be called preventative medicine. Hahnemann had no such department. Its weak efforts in this regard were satisfied by a volunteer visiting professor who was usually a member of the City Health Department. By taking advantage of a federal government program, Kellow established a Department of Community Medicine with Patrick Storey as its head. Storey was an Irishman with a very fair, red complexion, an ever present smile, and a wonderful sense of humor. He had a flair for general practice but had a superior intellect that led him to do things beyond the routine. For example, he traveled to Russia to study the characteristics of Russian physicians and their medical education system, which resulted in an erudite paper published in the *Journal of the American Medical Association*. This established him as an authority on this subject. The job at Hahnemann served another of Storey's ambitions, namely to establish a self-sufficient clinic, related to the needs of the people at all levels, in a very depressed neighborhood. Sure enough, he soon got a grant from a private foundation for this purpose. An old former mansion was bought on Green Street, one of the worse streets for crime and drug addiction in North Philadelphia. The building was quickly remodeled into physicians' offices and staffed with younger Hahnemann full-time faculty, including pediatricians, internists, and gynecologists-obstetricians.

Storey tried hard to create a community spirit and enthusiasm for his clinic. It turned out to be a very difficult task because the population was half black and half Hispanic who hated and were suspicious of each other. The blacks naturally felt that the clinic favored the Hispanics, while the Hispanics didn't like anything that was done for the blacks, even though it was a case of share and share alike. In addition, this north central Philadelphia community had a number of Medicaid racket clinics that definitely did not like the idea of an honest clinic educating the public about the value of good medical care. As recipient of the more serious cases from the clinic, Hahnemann Hospital was unhappy because of patients' indigent and Medicaid status. Despite these difficulties and numerous fires set by irate, disgruntled patients, the clinic flourished for a few years as a tribute to Storey's persistence, patience, and dedication.

The budding Department of Community Medicine was rounded out by the addition of Dean Roberts, a pediatrician who was also trained in public health. Roberts had a very sound analytic mind and provided a measure of stability to the department. He was an excellent committee organizer as I was to discover later. Another interesting member of the department was Melvin Benarde who was trained as a microbiologist but had drifted into environmental and epidemiological matters. He had written a book on this subject much less influential than *The Silent Spring* but which had made *The New York Times*' best seller list. William Weiss, a part-time member, was an internist with a primary interest in pulmonary medicine and well acquainted with public health affairs of the city. Jack Salmon, the youngest member, was a bright masters in public health. All in all, quite a credible department run on a shoestring.

It was a time of great expansion of medical services. Many existing hospitals and medical schools expanded and new ones opened. The federal government started Medicare, which funded medical care for the aged and opened up a vast reservoir of health services. Congress greatly increased the National Institutes of Health budget, which stimulated medical research so that many diseases previously considered untreatable were now possible to repair and in some cases even cure. Money became available from the federal and state governments to fund new buildings to house the expansion of medical and educational services.

With its antiquated buildings, Hahnemann was eager to join the bandwagon. Fortunately, in Cameron and Kellow, it had leaders who were aggressive and sagacious in putting the show on the road. Charlie Paxson, the hospital's CEO, had received funding to build a new combined nurses' dormitory and teaching building on the corner of 15th and Race Streets. Cameron initiated the 21 First Century fund that eventually raised some $6 million of private funds. He also planned an ambitious building project that expanded the campus to encompass the whole block bound by Broad, 15th, Vine, and Race Streets. This included a clinical science building, a new medical school building, and a new hospital. There was room left for an ambulatory services building.

Kellow got to work immediately on a medical school building. Architects were hired and plans soon drawn for a twenty-story building to be joined to the Klahr building. It would occupy the corner of Vine and 15th Street and would house the library, an auditorium accommodating 630 persons, offices and laboratories for twenty departments, multidiscipline laboratories, three lecture halls, and six conference rooms. The Dean's office and offices for the bursar and registrar were also included. Executive offices for the President and the Board Room were on the top floor. The basement held a video studio and other functional offices.

I got involved in a lot of the planning for this building. Although, I didn't agree with Kellow's formula for assigning floor space, I must admit that it was very functional and served the worthy purpose of scaling down the ambitious, grandiose proposals of department heads. For example, eighty square feet of floor space were assigned for a secretary. This meant that a small department (like pharmacology) would end up with a closet for the secretary that would not have space for filing cabinets and supplies, let alone Xerox machines and other furniture, like chairs and clothes trees for visitors. Similar paltry assignments of space were assigned to instructors, assistant professors, etc. This resulted in ingenious plans to bypass the stringent regulations to get more space. Most departments ended up with between five and twelve thousand square feet of space inclusive of offices and laboratories. Teaching space was confined to the first four floors serviced by escalators and designed to keep major traffic confined to the lower floors. The building turned out to be quite serviceable but, of course, did not compare to some magnificent edifices, especially those of state medical schools where money and space was not limited.

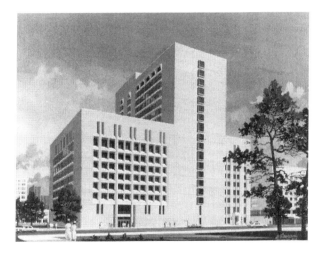

Figure 4. New Medical School Building. Architect's drawing of new medical school building on 15th Street replacing the old building and the nurse's dormitory. The Khlar building remains attached to the new building. In addition to a 630 seat auditorium the new nineteen story structure accommodates lecture halls, offices, laboratories and the Board Room of the medical center. There is access to both hospitals and the Feinstein Clinic on nearly every floor. It was completed and occupied in 1971.

Bids were let out and the building was projected to cost in the vicinity of $40 million dollars. Kellow worked on getting funding from the federal government by arguing that we could increase enrollment if we had modern facilities. Cameron himself applied to the state government by using a similar argument, adding that no new medical schools would be needed in the state and it would be cheaper and more efficient to enlarge the existing ones. The Feds soon made a site visit. As might be anticipated, they cut back the project by restricting the number of students to 135 in each entering class. Several floors that were to be added to the Klahr building were eliminated, and other trims were made. The leader of the group was John Deitrick, a well-trained internist and academician from Cornell University Medical School in New York City. He had spent some time as chairman of the Department of Medicine at Jefferson Medical College, so he had first hand knowledge of the Philadelphia medical scene.

As a New Yorker myself, I got along quite well with him. Although it's pure conjecture, this may have had a favorable influence. Luckily we were given an outright grant of some $18 million. By different tactics, Cameron got the state to grant us $12 million as a long-term loan that, with some private funds, made up the required $32 million that the architects and the contractor estimated would be the total cost of the project.

While all this was going on, I was not idle as a researcher and teacher. I was fortunate to be able to secure a training grant for graduate students in pharmacology from the National Institutes of Health. Among the students I was able to recruit were Paul Guth, Marvin Rosenthale, Morton Comer, G. John Digregorio, Frank Bove, and Vincent Zarro. There were others, but these stand out because they have had useful and brilliant careers, a source of great satisfaction to me. I shall have more to say about them as I touch upon various research projects going on in the department. There is little doubt that graduate students are stimulating to the research effort and also provide the manpower that's always a scarce commodity. A strong bond usually develops between the graduate student and his preceptor.

My friendship with John Howard, the chairman of surgery, gave me a lead to a Colonel Lindsey who was in charge of research activities for the Army. He encouraged me to seek out some opportunities for research with the Army Chemical Center in Edgewood, Maryland. This is how I came to know Van Sim, a civilian physician in charge of conducting clinical studies of antidotes to war gases. Volunteer soldiers were used who were exposed to small, safe doses of the milder types of war gases known as cholinesterase inhibitors. There was a minimum of symptoms but a measurable decline in blood cholinesterase activity levels. The antidote that had been developed by animal studies was an oxime known as 2-PAM Chloride. If this drug was given parenterally before exposure to the war gas, it prevented the decline in blood cholinesterase activity levels and hence symptoms of toxicity.

In the early 1960s, it was considered quite appropriate to use soldiers as volunteers for these experiments. I convinced Van Sim to let the Pharmacology Department at Hahnemann have an army contract to explore the feasibility of using 2-PAM Chloride orally. This involved giving the drug by mouth and doing studies of blood and urine levels, a technology now known as pharmacokinetics but then relatively new. It was highly secret work and classified, so everyone working on the project had to be investigated by the FBI, including all the officers of the corporation and even the members of the Board of Trustees. I put Ben Calesnick and Jens Christensen in charge of this project, and we all went through being fingerprinted and a thorough background check. We had to install a special filing cabinet in which all the data and correspondence was kept. Only Calesnick had the key to its lock. It was known that Russia had large stockpiles of war gases and was prepared to use them. If the United States could develop an effective antidote, it would be an important military advantage. I confess that I was less interested in this than in the pharmacology of the oximes and getting a contract that would allow the department to expand and do high level research.

The big problem was getting human volunteers to take the drug. It was a secret compound, so we could not reveal the identity of the chemical to the subjects. In addition it had no established clinical value. Nor could we appeal to the loyalty of the subjects because to do so would uncover the secret nature of the compound. For practical purposes, this prohibited the use of medical students or our faculty colleagues. Fortunately, 2-PAM Chloride had been given to humans before, and it had complete animal toxicity studies as required by the FDA. It was a relatively low toxicity chemical, but adverse effects on long-term administration to a large human population cannot be predicted for any drug. At the time, there were no standardized informed consent requirements or Human Research Review Boards as there are today. All reputable investigators, however, followed the procedures recommended by the Helsinki Commission. All volunteers were informed of the possible dangers of taking the drug, no excessive coercion or inducement was used, and withdrawal from the study was optional at any time.

Our first approach was to attempt to find men on skid row through interaction with several missions in the vicinity. We paid a small fee to the subjects and hoped that this would encourage them to volunteer. This proved unsatisfactory because many of the men were alcoholics, unreliable, and irresponsible. After much searching we chanced upon an Hispanic woman's club. These women proved most cooperative and reliable as subjects. Over the next year, accurate data was obtained that established 2 PAM Chloride as a safe chemical for oral administration and capable of achieving adequate blood levels by this route. Calesnick and Christensen did all the work on this project and deserve great credit for this effort under difficult circumstances. It remained for Sim's group at the Army Chemical Center to prove that oral 2-PAM Chloride was an effective oral prophylaxis for war gas poisoning. He did this using soldier volunteers.

My own contribution to this project was some animal work on the effects of 2-PAM Chloride on the circulation. This was followed by studying the effect of poisoning with the war gas Soman on the circulation to learn if the antidotal actions of 2-PAM Chloride might, in part, be circulatory rather than solely due to the restoration of cholinesterase. Vincent Zarro, a graduate student, and Robert McMichaels did most of this work. As a sidelight, both Zarro and McMichaels acquired mild poisoning from exposure to Soman that resulted in loss of visual accommodation for several weeks. The error they made was leaving a very dilute solution of Soman uncovered in a small beaker while they were doing the experiment. This illustrates the extreme potency of the war gases, and Soman is not the worst of these deadly agents.

Some years later 2-PAM Chloride was declassified and became available for marketing. Praloxime (its tradename) became a useful drug for the therapy of poisoning by insecticides such as malathion, parathion, and others widely used in agriculture and gardening. Undoubtedly it has been instrumental in lessening suffering and even saving lives. There is satisfaction in the thought that some of your research has had some practical outcome.

Graduate students need to be given interesting and challenging problems to work on, depending on their own inclinations and aspirations. They usually start out with an ambition to tackle a large comprehensive problem, such as the cure of cancer or heart disease. DiGregorio, one of the brightest and energetic graduate students, wanted a big problem to work on. I convinced him instead to work on a small but fundamental problem by promising him that its solution would lead to bigger things. The story of how I came to conceive this problem is of some interest.

I no longer recall the exact details of how or why Robert Mohl, a high school student, appeared in my laboratory some years earlier. Bill Likoff or Victor Satinsky likely referred him. Bob was interested in medicine as a career and wanted to volunteer to work during his summer vacation. Questioned about why he had such a research interest, he replied, "I grow goldfish, and I read that they have a small electrical potential that is located axially. That is, the head is positive with respect to the tail. It is generally believed that this potential helps the fish to orient itself with respect to the magnetic axis of the earth, although there is no substantial proof of this. When the fish dies, this electrical potential disappears. I should like to study this potential under various conditions to learn more about its origins and importance."

I was naturally quite impressed by this young lad's interest in a natural phenomenon. I explained to him that every living cell has a membrane potential the source of which is the difference in concentration of sodium, potassium, and chloride ions inside as compared to outside the cell. A sodium pump that requires energy to operate generates this differential in concentration. When the cell dies, the sodium pump ceases to function and the electrical potential disappears. This cellular potential is tiny, measurable in millevolts by very sensitive apparatus. The electrical potential of each of the billions of cells in the body can be hooked up to yield an overall body axial potential as he described in his goldfish.

Nature is much more resourceful than this, however, and uses the electric potential for many other purposes. A bizarre example is the electric eel. The electric potential of the muscle cells of its body is so arranged as to be able to discharge an electric shock of over 100 volts quite sufficient to stun prey or to repel predators. In cells that have an excitable function, such as nerve cells that conduct a signal, or muscle or heart cells that contract the stimulus causes the cell to depolarize. In other words, the positive outside potential temporarily disappears, which is characteristic of excitation of the cell. One of the most dramatic examples of this phenomenon is the electrocardiogram (EKG) that shows the characteristic depolarization of the heart with each contraction.

Bob seemed very interested and asked, "Can the EKG of a goldfish be recorded?"

"Yes it probably can," I replied, "but I have no immediate experience with this. Alternately, we can set you up to record the EKG of a frog." Over the next few days, recording the EKG of rana pipens, the common laboratory frog, fascinated Bob. He read all he could understand about the human EKG. He was so interested and helpful in our other work that I sought to find an interesting project that he could call his own.

Some time earlier, I had bought a venous fly trap (Dionea muscipula), a carnivorous plant that grows naturally only in North Carolina and is remarkable for the sensitive hair on its leaf surface which, when touched, causes the bivalve leaf structure to close and trap the unfortunate insect. I was less fascinated by the contraction of the leaf structure than by how the sensitive hair transmitted the signal to contract to the rest of the leaf. Was it purely electrical or was a neurohumor such as acetylcholine involved? The leaf has no structures analogous to nerves, but it does have a vascular system by which conduction might occur. I brought the plant to the laboratory and, sure enough, we were able to record the action potential of the leaf excitation and contraction. In amplitude and time sequence, it resembled the EKG. Bob was greatly excited by this and was convinced that we had made a significant discovery because a cursory search of the literature did not reveal any similar observation.

The famous Darwin had been much intrigued by the plant and had made important observations on the mode of contraction of the leaf. Lloyd's classical monograph on carnivorous plants made no mention of action potentials. I told Bob, however, that we must look further. Finally, in an old physiology textbook we found reference to a Burdon Sanderson, a British physiologist who had recorded the action potential of the Venus fly trap in 1890 by using a crude but adequately sensitive device known as the capillary electrometer. This was an amazing feat in view of the fact that devices to measure such small voltages were not invented until at least twenty years later and were certainly uncommon laboratory devices until the electronic age some sixty years later.

The summer period soon ended, and I urged Bob to attend the University of Pennsylvania instead of a less prestigious college as he'd intended. He did well in his undergraduate work and was later admitted to Hahnemann Medical School. He was an outstanding student, graduated with honors, and did his graduate work in internal medicine. Today he is a fine physician in practice in Ohio. I don't think that he has followed up on his research interest, finding that the practice of medicine satisfies completely his exploratory potential.

In retrospect, Bob did more for me than I did for him because this experience got me started on a long-term interest in plant physiology. I continued to explore the electrical activity of the

Venus fly trap and, although it was always a side line, in some ways it was among the most satisfying research that I engaged in. I was able to publish several papers in *Science* showing that hypertonic solutions of saline or of glucose would cause the leaf to close. Such solutions indeed caused a repetitive action potential that kept the leaf closed. I was also able to define a conditioned reflex of the leaf that is remarkable, considering that there is no nervous system. My failure to find any chemicals in the plant that might mimic neurotransmitter activity was a challenging question that kept on irritating me.

It dawned on me one day that the green leaf blade was actually red underneath the green chlorophyll. I looked up the subject of plant pigments and soon learned that the red pigment was an anthocyanin, a dye-like chemical with the ability to shift its resonance from one phase to another. The antocyanins give the colors of red, pink, blue, and purple to flowers, while flavones compounds with closely related chemical structures contribute yellow. Since only the contracting leaf blades of the dianea had the antocyanin and the flowers of the plant were white, I conjectured that it might be associated with movement. To further the concept, I needed to identify the exact anthocyanin and learn its exact chemical structure. In addition, enough anthocyanin must be acquired to test its activity in various appropriate biological systems.

This is where graduate student DiGregorio came in. I handed the whole problem to him. Fortunately he had majored in chemistry at Penn State and had some familiarity with analytic technology. Al Gero's knowledge of organic chemical synthesis also came in very handy. I advised DiGregorio that we must start with known facts. It was soon evident that a Professor Hargrove in England was the world's authority on anthocyanins. He was kind enough to send us samples of identified anthocyanins to compare with that obtained from the dianea. Using crude but adequate chromatographic methods, the dianea anthocyanin was characterized. It turned out to be not of unusual structure for an anthocyanin and probably was present in many other plants with red color but which had no extraordinary contractile properties.

This finding alone enabled DiGregorio to get a short paper in *Nature*.

With the suspect anthocyanin in hand, it was possible to make deductions about chemical structure and possible pharmacological activity. The seemingly unique feature was a ring structure that resembled quinoline, except that in place of the nitrogen, there was an oxonium atom. This suggested to us that the anthocyanin might have ganglionic or neuromuscular blocking activity. Tested in the appropriate systems, the dionea anthocyanin did have some activity but not enough to write home about. Unfortunately, little is known about the function of anthocyanins in plants apart from the rendition of color. Malvidin is an anthocyanin in grapes, and red wine has some antimicrobial activity. Not wishing to end up without reward, we decided to do a little chemical engineering ourselves. Substituting nitrogen for the oxonium oxygen gave us a 2-phenyl quinoline compound that proved to have both cholinometic and sympathomimetic activity. With the help of chemists at the Philadelphia College of Pharmacy, we were able to get synthesized some congeners that had reasonable activity. At this point, I tried to get some of the local pharmaceutical companies interested in these compounds without success. We published the work so it might be used and become part of the general fund of knowledge. DiGregorio, later a member of the faculty of the Department of Pharmacology, used the compounds as a project with another graduate student. Even my own daughter number three, Joan, did a summer project with the compounds as a premed student at Barnard College. Interest eventually dimmed in both the dianea and its anthocyanin derivatives. Such are the vicissitudes of the search for useful drugs. It's a case of "Many are called but few are chosen." I have kept the fascinating carnivorous plants in the back of my mind these many years, hoping someday to get back to them.

About this time I became involved in a big project that took up most of my spare time.

John DeCarville, a medical book editor for McGraw-Hill, called me one day to see whether I was interested in becoming editor of

Drill's textbook, *Pharmacology in Medicine.* Victor Drill, an outstanding pharmacologist, had started the book some years ago. It was quite successful and at the time in its second edition. I had written a chapter on antiarrhythmic drugs in both editions and so was well acquainted with the text. A third edition was due, but Drill had moved from an academic position at Northwestern University School of Medicine in Chicago to employment in industry at Searle, a large pharmaceutical company also in Chicago. He was no longer willing to spend the time and energy required to revise this major text. He wished, however, to maintain an interest in it. At Searle, Drill was in charge of developing oral contraceptives, and he wished to write the chapter on this subject.

I told DeCarville that I would have to think it over and would get back to him one way or another. To tell the truth, I really didn't want to get involved in a textbook. I had written chapters in several books including this one. I surmised that the meritorious quality of my chapter on antiarrhythmic drugs is what may have convinced DeCarville to ask me to take over the text. I wasn't foolish enough to believe that I was the first one asked. Publishers like to get authors from the top twenty schools in the country, and Hahnemann was certainly not one of them. He must have received a lot of turndowns before he settled on me. Nonetheless, writing one chapter is much different than the responsibility of organizing some forty chapters on different subjects and cajoling some forty authors to write a superior representation of their subject. There is no decent financial reward, and it usually does not benefit the individual in getting grants. The main detraction is that, once you become editor of a major textbook, you are married to it and revisions have to be done every five years and even more frequently. Since it usually takes two or three years to get a book of this size off the ground, you are pretty much occupied all the time with tedious details.

I talked it over with my colleagues, naturally. Al Gero was most encouraging and promised to write an original chapter on theoretical drug actions. Spirtes would do a chapter on drug metabolism, while Calesnick would handle toxicology. Friends in other institutions, meanwhile, seemed willing to lend their talents to the project. After a while, I grew accustomed to the idea of the feasibility of editing a massive text. Down deep I knew that it would have the effect of speeding up my demise from the cutting edge of science, although it undoubtedly would give me a broader knowledge of the subject and perhaps make me a better teacher. If at all successful, it might enhance my national and perhaps my international reputation.

So without fanfare early in 1963, at the age of forty-seven, I set to work on what was to be my Opus Magnus. On many occasions I rued my C grade in college English composition, my spelling inability, and my rusty syntax. Yet my experience with the many previous papers I wrote and many lectures and speeches came in handy. I soon found that the more I wrote and edited, the more skilled I became. Practice does make perfect! But no amount of practice can instill the poetic magic to words some gifted persons seem to have naturally.

At least a third of the previous authors of chapters retired, passed on, or just didn't want to continue as contributors, so I had to secure new authors. I wanted to get the best people in their respective field, of course. Not surprisingly, I found that most of the best were already committed to write for Louis Goodman and Alfred Gilman's text of pharmacology. Their text was the gold standard of pharmacology texts and had, up to this date, been written completely by the two original authors. With the rapid growth of knowledge, it became impossible for one or two people to write a whole comprehensive text. Victor Drill was on the right path when he chose the multi-authored route. So Goodman and Gilman had to convert to the individually authored chapters. Since they certainly commanded more authority and respect than I could manage, they were able to secure more experienced authors. I consequently had to use a good deal of ingenuity in finding and convincing talented people to write for my text.

Pharmacology as a discipline, it always seemed to me, had no structural theories of its own. Rather, it leaned heavily on disciplines such as chemistry and physiology. Texts of pharmacology prior to

1940 were largely descriptive and related more to materia medica or a pharmacopia than to a scientific rational. Goodman and Gilman revolutionized pharmacological thinking and teaching by using a physiological approach that drew heavily from the new discoveries in this field and newer mechanisms of disease. They called their text, *The Pharmacological Basis of Medical Practice*, borrowed no doubt from the well-known Best and Taylor physiology text, *The Physiological Basis of Medical Practice*. The important point is that an attempt was made to assign a mechanism of action to each drug and relate that mechanism to disease processes and further to indicate how the drug could favorably alter the disorder.

I determined to go one step further. In my reading I had come across the works of the Abbe Felice Fontana, 1750-1830. Mainly known as an anatomist in Florence, Italy, he also did many physiological experiments. In his study of snake poisons, he demonstrated that they were of two types; one type attacked the nervous system producing paralysis, while another affected the blood causing hemolysis. This led to his delineating the concept that poisons (and hence drugs) have a locus of action. Poisons or drugs seek out a particular site in the organism, and it is there that they exert their action. In turn, certain sites are attracting certain drugs. This was certainly one of the first attempts to unravel the mysteries of drug action. Later scientists further extended the locus of action concept notably Claude Bernard, Langley, and Clark. Paul Erhlich, of the magic bullet for syphilis fame, dramatized this theory by his lock and key concept, which explained that a drug must fit its locus of action, or receptor, as a key fits a lock.

In the early 1960s, no one knew what a receptor looked like. The drug-receptor interaction was purely theoretical, but all indications were that it followed the laws of enzyme chemistry— pretty much indicating that the receptor was a complex protein structure. The laws determining drug action could be worked out in a living system with a precision approaching that of a test tube chemical reaction. I determined to devote a whole first chapter to drug-receptor interaction in order to establish it as the core basis of the science of pharmacology. Fortunately, Gero was facile in chemistry and mathematics and well able to handle this task. A whole chapter was also devoted to the metabolism of drugs, a subject that was by now in an advanced state of development.

During the next two years, I spent most of my time cajoling authors to finish their assignments and send them in. I soon found that, if you give an author six months to write a chapter, he will take a year. If you give him a year, he'll take two years. How many times was I was told, "The manuscript is on my desk. It needs only a few final touches. You'll get it in the next week." Baloney! Months would pass, and I would not get anything. This would be unnerving because just one missing chapter would delay the publication of the whole book. To find another author always meant that I'd have to ask for a rush job and be satisfied with something usually short of what I expected. I then needed time to edit and revise most chapters to achieve some uniformity of style and content. I did most of the work in the evenings and weekends at home. My wife and family suffered, and I am indebted to them for allowing me this time without complaint. Luckily, most authors did a magnificent job on the whole. Victor Drill wrote his chapter on oral contraceptives, then a genuinely hot subject.

After correcting endless galleys, the third edition of *Pharmacology in Medicine* was published in August, 1965. I recall great elation and a feeling that this was the best thing I'd done. Looking back now after many years, I can modestly say that the book—while hardly a sensation—was well received. It was adopted as the major text in about twenty medical schools. Later translations into Italian and Spanish gave it an international flavor. It amused me to reflect that a school that only a few years earlier was homeopathic and considered marginal and backward, could produce a work that now was acceptable to more prestigious institutions. It certainly was good advertising for Hahnemann and for my department of pharmacology. At the national meetings, I began to be recognized and found it easier to recruit staff. Unfortunately, my research effort had suffered a price that one has to pay to produce a work of this size. I decided to concentrate on fundamental research in some new area in order to reestablish myself as an ingenious, resourceful scientist.

The technology of intracellular action potentials had been well established by this time, and we developed a capability in this area ourselves. It required drawing down in a small suitable flame a capillary tubing to a fine point in diameter of only one or two microns. This required great patience and skill. Soon laboratory equipment manufacturers came out with machines that did this automatically. Recording intracellular action potentials from the beating heart in the intact animal proved to be very difficult because the heart's motion would break the delicate tip. Most studies of the beating heart were therefore done on isolated heart preparations attached to a platform to minimize motion. Meanwhile, the electronic apparatus to record the minute potentials that had to be home built now became available commercially. As a result, most labs could now use the technology. Recording intracellular action potentials under all kinds of conditions became commonplace. Lenny Dreifus and Dr. Watanabe, a visiting Japanese physician, had a lab next to mine in the Cardiovascular Institute. They did yeoman work on conduction in the atrium and the atrioventricular node. This work was done on a rabbit heart in an isolated bath where movement could be controlled. Later the development of the intracellular pipette was most useful in transfer of genetic material from one cell to another. A most obvious application is the mechanical transfer of the sperm into the egg to make possible in vitro fertilization. Thus a technology that was invented mainly to study membrane electrical phenomenon eventually was an important factor in making some women fertile. The invention of one technology often opens up the development of even more ramifications. There are many examples of this in science.

Looking back now that many years have passed, I realize that I had a period of burnout about this time. Bored with cardiovascular physiology and membrane potentials, I longed to do some purely abstract research in a new field. Kellow was keeping me busy by putting me on many sensitive committees so I didn't have the leisure time to concentrate on the development of a new endeavor. I must also admit that middle age had set in, and I lacked the drive and enthusiasm of youth. All my daughters were now in their teens and required much attention. The large house and garden gave me much pleasure but also much work.

George Geckler called me one spring day and informed me that he had a dozen mature cymbidium plants that he was willing to give away to anyone who would care for them. I didn't even know what a cymbidium was, but I said I would think it over and consult my wife. After little scouting, I learned that Geckler had a patient who was a famous commercial orchid grower by the name of Fetzer. Through contact with him, Geckler had acquired an interest in growing orchids as a hobby and enjoyed getting discarded lines of orchid plants from Fetzer. Geckler had built a small greenhouse that soon overflowed. Hence his generosity. The hobby of growing orchids was not very common at that time because plants were expensive and relatively scarce. My wife was enthusiastic, and I succumbed to Geckler's offer. To my surprise, they were large plants in ten—to twelve-inch pots and barely fit in the back of my large station wagon. I had immediate misgivings. I had visions of trying to fit them in some sunny room indoors. Even in a large house, they would not fit anywhere. So I asked Geckler in some despair, "What do I do with these plants? Where can I put them? How do I care for them?"

Geckeler smiled a little slyly. "Don't worry. Just put them outside under an oak tree and fertilize them once a week with a very dilute fertilizer, such as the kind used for azaleas. Water them as much as you like. You can't kill a cymbidium by too much watering, which is what kills most other orchids."

Reassured, I did as told. Sure enough, the plants seemed to flourish. I meanwhile I bought some books on growing orchids and was amazed to find that there were some 30,000 species of orchids. Spring and summer sped by quickly. I began to worry that the orchid plants could not stand the winter freezes of our northern climate. Their original habitat was the Himalayan Mountains, and they did well outdoors in southern California.

"Would they survive temperatures down to zero?" I asked Geckeler.

"You need a greenhouse. Furthermore, be sure to keep the night temperature at fifty degrees Fahrenheit. Otherwise they won't bloom next spring."

There was little time before snow would fall, but I was undaunted and investigated the greenhouse situation. It would have been an unreasonable strain on the family budget to build an architecturally suitable structure to our mansion-like house. I decided on a modest nine-by-nineteen-foot aluminum and glass structure that I could buy in kit form and put up myself. It proved to be no easy task because I had to dig a foundation below the frost line, build forms, and mix and pour several cubic yards of concrete. My father-in-law and the kids helped some, but most of the tough work fell to me. I must admit it was fun because the foundation had to be made accurately and the bolts that held the house had to be located exactly in the concrete. Once the foundation was finished, the aluminum framework went up quickly. The glassing of the house was a delicate job, and I was glad that in my younger days I'd learned a little about handling glass. Next an externally vented gas heater was installed. Electricity and hot and cold running water was extended from the main house. As recommended, I also installed a fan ventilating system that worked automatically from a separate thermostat. Benches of redwood were finally installed, and I was ready to house my cymbidiums about the middle of November—fortunately before any damaging frost had occurred.

Now that I had a greenhouse, the bug of growing orchids became more of a passion. I soon acquired a small library of orchid and greenhouse books. The most fascinating challenge was to solve the mystery of what a plant needs in the environment in order to flourish. As I began to collect various species and hybrids of orchids with different requirements, I tried to form microclimes of temperature, light, and humidity that would suit each. I became a member of the Southeastern Pennsylvania Orchid Society, which was most stimulating because I met with experienced orchid growers who were most helpful with advice and tips. After a year or two, I became kind of an expert myself and was able to compete successfully at the monthly show table. My wife accompanied me to the monthly meetings, made many friends, and served her turn at providing refreshments. I found that orchid growers are nice, generally intelligent and interesting people. Many were physicians or teachers, while others were retired business people. A few were in professions that required travel or even residence in foreign lands, especially South America, where they had the opportunity to observe orchids in their native habitat.

The most outstanding character was Bill Wilson, a psychiatrist, who had easily the biggest greenhouse and the best orchid collection of anyone. A visit to his establishment allowed an orchid grower to view specimens of every available species and some known only to an ultra specialist. His first love was the paphiopedelums, which he collected and bred to produce new and superior hybrids. As a judge of the American Orchid Society and one of its officers, he enjoyed a national and international reputation. To have an orchid plant praised by Wilson was akin to winning the Nobel Prize because he knew the best specimens that existed and could compare it to your plant. Most orchid society members felt him to be abrasive because he always told it like it was and pulled no punches. As might be expected, there are many legendary orchid connoisseurs, but Wilson certainly heads the list.

For a period of some ten years, I had a most enjoyable time growing orchids. My collection grew; I built a second larger, more elegant greenhouse, entered my plants at flower shows, won numerous ribbons and medals, and even received an Award of Merit for an odontoglossum hybrid. My cymbidium crop was large enough to sell corsages on Easter and Mother's Day. My wife and daughters made the corsages, and I let them keep the income, which made everybody happy. Perhaps the most personally satisfying thing I did was to bring in plants to show in the Hahnemann medical library where many enjoyed my plants.

Now some thirty years later as I reflect on my past career, I recall a rather cynical remark an older scientist made on observing one of my orchid specimens, "Mediocre scientists sometimes make outstanding gardeners." While there may be some truth to what he said, I believe the reverse is true. Hobbies often give the scientist a body of knowledge or a way of thinking that contributes to their professional work. In my case, my childhood hobby of building and flying model airplanes gave me an early start in the application of the laws of physics and mathematics. Starting from seeds, it takes seven years for a cattlyea orchid to flower. If nothing else, one learns patience and skill in growing the plant to the mature reproductive stage. Darwin studied orchids in detail and made seminal observations about the complicated process of reproduction in cyanoches, a rare species of orchids. Yet the snide remark of my elderly colleague stuck in my mind, and there were occasions— such as, when a paper or a grant was turned down—when I wondered why I persisted in the research game. It would be easy to return to medical practice to make more income and at the same time gain satisfaction from my work. Physicians no longer made house calls, fees had been rising ahead of inflation, and work hours were shorter. I decided I was getting burned out and needed a vacation.

Providence came to my rescue. Out of the blue, Van Sim of the Army Chemical Center offered to send me on an extensive trip to Italy to visit all the University Pharmacology Departments and learn what I could about the work in progress in the chemical warfare field. All my expenses would be paid, but if I took my wife this would be on me. I naturally jumped at the chance and Mary was most enthusiastic. We had never been abroad and this was a wonderful opportunity. Aside from the expense of such a trip, we had always hesitated to leave the children to fend for themselves. Our live-in in-laws were willing to take care of the five girls, now aged five to ten—quite a handful even for experienced handlers.

Off we went to spend a few days at each of the universities in Naples, Rome, Padua, Bologna, and Milan. I had written ahead to each department head so that my visit was not unannounced. I soon discovered that departments in the Italian university organization are really separate institutes, often at a distance from the main campus. Some are located in villas or the equivalent of an

American mansion. Everyone was most gracious and hospitable. I spoke enough Italian to get along, and fortunately many of them spoke English. I also had occasion to speak to a few American medical students who were attending school in Italy because they had failed to gain admission in America.

From these sources, I gained a fair insight into the faculty and student life at Italian medical schools. Tuition is state-supported for Italian citizens. No one is denied admission, provided that they have had at least what would be the American equivalent of grammar school and junior high school. The medical curriculum is six years, or the equivalent of two years of college and four years of medical school. A student need not complete the course of study consecutively but can drop out and return when he feels able. Rarely does a student flunk out. If he fails a year, he can repeat as often as he wishes. Although the main lecture hall or amphitheatre may hold a maximum of three hundred, at least a thousand students are admitted each year. They only graduate about three hundred, however; the rest having gradually dropped out along the way. Even with this restricted output, there is an excess of physicians in Italy. Many end up in their father's business with their medical degrees wasted. The basic sciences are taught fairly well, but the clinical sciences are deficient. There is little if any bedside training, and rarely does a medical student actually get to see a patient because of the lack of any well-organized resident training system. Full-time physicians, who have little interest or motivation to teach medical students, staff the hospitals and clinics.

All the examinations are oral. This is in sharp contrast to the American system of objective, true-false type of exams where the student doesn't even have to know how to write to take the test. This system gave the American students great concern because they had to know the language in order to be able to perform. They also didn't know all the tricks of successfully passing oral examinations. They soon learned that they need to be fairly conversant with the questions the examiner is apt to ask. There is a veritable grapevine of informants who guarantee that they can give a student the right steer for a price. The most important person in this instance is the porter. As he shuffles about the room, presumably dusting during the course of an examination, he carefully memorizes key words. A sharp student can usually interpret at least what subjects were covered and fortify himself accordingly.

Contrary to the American dictate that all students must take the course exam at the same time, usually at the end of the semester, the custom in Italy is that the student takes the exam only when he thinks he is ready. While most students do take the exams at appropriate times, many students delay taking exams for months or years, thus extending the time spent attending medical school. They may repeat courses, hire a tutor, or even take the course elsewhere until they feel adequately prepared to face the examiner. The methods of grading are also strange, and record—keeping is the responsibility of the student. He carries a little book and, as he completes each required examination, the professor puts a grade in the book and signs it. When all the required courses have been accounted for in the little book, the student can present himself for graduation.

This system seems to work. Whether or not it relieves the pressure felt by most medical student is debatable. In American medical schools, students have insisted on a simple pass-fail system. Unfortunately this has degenerated into pass with honors, plain pass, and pass conditionally—so it might as well be the good old letter grades of A, B, and C. Combine a non-traumatic grading system with exams that don't require writing. Add adequate time to cram for exams, plus well-organized lecture notes, and no laboratory requirement. The natural result is that medical education becomes a lark. At least half the class attend no lectures and show up only for exams. With the introduction of minority programs, standards have been lowered for all. Rarely does a student flunk out of medical school. He or she may be forced to repeat a year or two but eventually they get their M.D. sheepskins.

To get back to our fabulous Italian adventure, we also found time to visit unforgettable Pompeii and, while in Naples, we made an excursion to the Isle of Capri. I couldn't help recalling Somerset Maugham's famous story of the man who visited Capri and decided to spend the rest of his life there instead of returning home to his job and family. He eventually outlived his savings and continued to live in this romantic isle even as a pauper and beggar. With its blue sky and azure sea, nearly always-perfect weather, and relaxed atmosphere, Capri does this to you. We all have the suppressed desire to escape from our humdrum lives and responsibilities and submerge into a primitive child-like state.

We gradually worked our way north and found that the people, language, and customs were markedly different from the south of Italy. Milan was as close to an American city as could be found in Europe. This was also true of the University where I met a chemist who was an expert in the chemical warfare of ants. He was a most interesting character and kind enough to invite us to his home for dinner. In his case at least, family and home life were not much different from that in America. In the Pharmacology Department of the University of Milan, I met an extraordinary character, Sylvio Garatino, who was known locally as "Il Cannone" or "Big Shot." A young man trained as a physician and pharmacologist, he had already made a name for himself as a researcher of great ingenuity and merit.

Charming and suave in appearance, dress, and demeanor, he gave more the impression of an actor than a professor and scientist. He and Poeletti, another pharmacologist, took my wife and me to dinner at a memorable restaurant in Milan. The dining tables were in the center of a large chamber, which was in effect the kitchen. Stations where cooks prepared various dishes simultaneously surrounding the dining area. When we sat down at a table, no menu was offered. Instead a waiter rushed to one of the cooking stations and immediately served a dish of whatever happened to be ready. As soon as we finished that dish, the waiter would rush to serve a newly prepared course. This went on as long as we sat at the table. The only way to stop the feasting was to get up and leave. Although Mary and I were astonished, we enjoyed the meal and all the good fun engendered by the unusual service. We also ate more gourmet dishes in one meal than we had before or since. Incidentally, the cannolis were superb.

As for Garatino, he was the full equivalent of any American physician-scientist and completely conversant with the cutting edge of pharmaceutical developments. He was scheduled to become director of the Mario Negri Institute, a multi-million dollar independent organization set up by the foremost drug manufacturers in Italy to foster the discovery and development of new chemical entities to cure and prevent disease. I have followed the course of the Institute over many years, and it has made significant and important progress.

Our first trip to Italy ended with a five-day sojourn to Bellargo, an isthmus in the center of Lake Como. It certainly is one of the choice vacation spots in the entire world. We enjoyed the wonderful climate that allows both tropical and alpine vegetation in the same vicinity. Returning to the States, I made a lengthy, detailed report to the Army Chemical Center about the state of and potential for research on chemical warfare in Italian universities. While I'm sure that the report yielded nothing of even minute significance, I'm equally suspicious that no one ever read it. Looking back now that many years have passed, the memory that most sticks in my mind is the pleasure of seeing my pharmacology textbook on the bookshelves of most university departments that I visited. That made me feel that I had achieved an international reputation. Such is the ego of man that there's no greater satisfaction than feeling appreciated for a good work by strangers, especially those in a foreign land, as well as your family and friends.

On our return to Philadelphia, Mary resumed her duties as a model mother. Our five young daughters appeared to have survived our absence quite well. Now the older ones were approaching their teen years and required more attention. The youngest, Mary-Jo, a lovely child, gave us the most worry because she was a slow learner and somewhat of a behavior problem. I resumed my habit of spending an hour or two each evening with each daughter individually in rotation. Together we worked on projects—some on handicraft, some more intellectual. As a scientist myself I naturally tried to stimulate their curiosity along lines of scientific inquiry. I made sure they actively participated in the science projects in school. Ironically, the result of this experiment was that none of them took any strong liking to science.

Mary had more influence. She insisted that all of them take music lessons, starting first with the piano. As a singer herself, she gave all of them singing lessons. This took hold. The oldest, Maria, became a singer. The next one, Dorothea, a pianist. The third daughter, Joan, entered medicine and eventually became a pediatrician, but the truth is that she would have been just as happy as a cellist. Number four, Yvonne, seemed at first to be taken with mathematics and physics but later dropped her physics major at Johns Hopkins to major in art. Eventually she became a sculptress. Mary-Jo loved jazz and ballet, but became a nurse's assistant. As many have observed before me, people end up being what they want to be no matter what forces are brought to bear to point them in different directions. Choosing a career primarily in science must be a rare quality because so few steer in that direction. They may indicate that they entered medicine or teaching because they loved science, but the reality is that they perceived that the possibility of making a living was better in these professions. Most scientists are considered to be eccentric and to be backward socially. It's a rare scientist who does not live a lonely life because of the dedication he must exert to be really good at his work.

Soon after our return from Europe, another event occurred that was to change the course of our lives. I remember the occasion vividly even after the passage of more than thirty years. I was giving a lecture on the life of the Abbe Felice Fontana before the History Section of the Philadelphia College of Physicians when I was handed a note to call the Hahnemann security officer as soon as possible. I naturally wondered what catastrophe could have happened in the laboratory or office. I didn't have the least inkling that someone in my family might be involved in an accident. I managed to finish the lecture and halfheartedly answer a few questions before rushing to the phone to contact the security officer. I could tell immediately from the tone of his voice and his hesitancy that something very grave had happened. Finally he blurted out, "Your wife is in Lankenau Hospital. She fell out of a moving train just as it was departing from the Overbrook Station. The doctor says she will recover. Call the neurosurgical resident at this number . . ."

Badly shaken I had visions of the track siding near the Overbrook Station. I pictured Mary falling headfirst on the sloping rough gravel surface. From the elevated platform, the distance to the ground must be at least eight to ten feet. I prayed that the train was not going very fast and that she missed hitting obstructions, such as switch boxes or support poles. Luckily, I had driven that day so I was able to reach Lankenau Hospital within fifteen minutes. Mary was lying on a stretcher with her eyes closed but I was relieved to see her breathing quite normally. The resident told me that she had come out of her coma and that I could rouse her. I took her left hand and said, "Mary, its Joe. Do you hear me?"

She opened her eyes slightly and whispered, "I don't remember anything, but they tell me I'm going to be all right." Then she went back to sleep. I learned from the resident that she had a fracture of the humerus of the right arm, which was set and explained the plaster cast. She arrived at the hospital in a comatose state, but her vital functions appeared normal. A head x-ray showed a depressed fracture of the skull with a spicule of bone impinging on the brain. Fortunately there was no sign of bleeding or a hematoma. She was scheduled to have a craniotomy in the morning to remove the bone spicule and help prevent the onset of seizures. I signed the necessary papers for this and thanked the resident for his good work.

I later found out the details of the accident. John Dempsher, M.D., was the hero of the episode. We knew him and his family because he lived in Wayne, and his children attended the Radnor schools with our children. At the time he was doing fulltime research at the Wistar Institute in neuroanatomy. He'd been sitting a few seats behind my wife and Mary-Jo on the train. Just as it started out from the Overbrook station, he saw Mary escort Mary-Jo to the entrance platform at the front of the train. The train lurched. Through the train window, he saw Mary fall out of the exit platform onto the siding. He immediately pulled the emergency rope to stop the train. Rushing out, he attended to Mary. An ambulance was called and he accompanied her to the hospital. He not only made certain that she was attended to, but also stayed by her side until it was clear that she was out of danger. This Good Samaritan act was exemplary and gave me esteem for Dempsher that I have for very few people. I have had occasion to wonder in later days if this experience had as much influence on his life and outlook as it did on mine. I imagine this because about a year later, as chairman of a search committee to find a new head of the anatomy department at Hahnemann, I tried to put his name on the list. He had excellent qualifications, and there was a good possibility of his getting the job if he wanted it. To my surprise and disappointment, he turned down the offer. He stated that he was quitting his scientific and research interests and going to take a residency in emergency medicine, then a growing specialty. He definitely felt that his future lay in the practice of medicine and not in academics.

Mary was home in a few days mainly because she could not stand the confinement of the hospital. This was a good sign, and fortunately she made a slow but satisfactory recovery. The only serious residual defect was a malfunctioning right hand that was the result of atrophy of the interosseus muscles that caused a weakness of the thumb. She also complained of the depression in her skull, but fortunately she did not have any seizures as might well have happened. We were so grateful that she managed to survive what could have been a fatal or very disabling accident that we did not actively pursue a reasonable settlement from the Pennsylvania Railroad that owned the ancient, rickety trains of the Paoli Local.

Other neighbors who happened to be on the train took Mary-Jo home. She was only five years old at the time, but I suspect that this episode had a profound psychological effect on her. She realized that her nausea caused her mother to take her to the exit platform in the first place. Later Mary recalled what actually happened: As the train lurched, she thought that Mary-Jo was about to fall so Mary instinctively pushed her back to safety. But in that act she lost her balance and fell out of the train herself. We never mentioned anything about the accident to Mary-Jo and tried as much as possible to downplay any role that she might have had in the accident. Even for a young child, it is still a heavy load of guilt to carry, imagined or otherwise. It happened that Mary-Jo developed a serious mental illness about two years later. Whether or not the accident was a factor will never be known.

The irony of the tragedy is that the Paoli Local kept on keeping the doors of its trains open between stations for many years after. Only when new cars replaced the decrepit World War I vintage cars were the doors kept shut between stations—undoubtedly only to preserve air conditioning, not for safety's sake. Any sensible person knows that if the doors of a moving train are left open sooner or later someone is going to fall out, and my wife proved the point.

Yet every unfortunate event has some favorable outcome. Mary didn't drive an automobile. I tried to teach her when we first got married, but I think she was intimidated and refused further instruction. After she recovered, I told her that she must learn because she'd be safer driving an automobile than riding the train. At the time we were the proud owners of a Buick Roadmaster, a good heavy car with automatic transmission. It was much easier to drive than the old gearshift Dodge that we owned when I first tried teaching her to drive. Sure enough, Mary took to driving like a duck to water and passed her licensing exam on the first try. It proved to be very convenient because now she could go shopping when she liked and didn't have to wait until I was free. How ingrained the automobile is in our daily lives and culture. Not to have wheels is to be imprisoned.

Mary's accident had a profound effect on my outlook about the present and the future. Now approaching the age of fifty, I had five children to raise and educate. Although my income was not bad, it was still difficult to set money aside for savings. Alfred Beck, my obstetrics professor at medical school, had given us the advice that if we could manage to save ten cents out of every dollar we earned, we would never want. Well, I had managed to do that, but old Beck had not calculated on Social Security tax, rising federal income tax, state tax, city wage tax, and sales tax. This and the beginnings of inflation made it virtually impossible to save much income.

As I look back from my present viewpoint, I perceive that any money we saved was due to our doing everything ourselves. We never hired a servant of any kind. Mary did all the housework in a very large house with five children. Her mother was some help, especially in baby sitting while Mary did the necessary shopping, cooking, and housework. I did all the gardening and repairs whether it was painting, plumbing, or carpentry. It wasn't long before I had a complete set of tools for every occasion. Mary's father was a tailor by profession, and he did most of the sewing and clothes alterations. He was also most handy with shoe repairs, and we rarely discarded any shoes. Actually we were only part of an era when "do it yourself" became popular. The increasing variety and utility of home appliances made it possible to accomplish tasks that previously required great tedious hand and back labor. I clearly remember buying my first power drill in 1951. It cost $21. I still have it and about a dozen others. Electric saws, routers, power lawnmowers, and every conceivable gadget soon followed. My greatest joy and pleasure was a power lathe for metal working with a twelve-inch swing and automatic feed and treading arrangements. With this equipment and later even a garden tractor, it was possible to handle practically any task.

In April 1967, Dean Kellow called me to his office to give me some surprising news. He announced that he was going to resign from Hahnemann so he could assume the Deanship at Jefferson Medical College on July first. I was taken aback, but I had the diplomacy to congratulate him on his good fortune. Although we Hahnemannians had great pride in our institution, down deep we had to admit that Jefferson was a richer, more distinguished a school. I knew that Kellow would be severely criticized for this lateral desertion to our closest competitor. Had he left to assume the deanship at Harvard or Yale or even Georgetown, everyone would have considered it a meritorious move. Will, I asked, "Why?"

He looked at me with dark penetrating eyes and replied with

a wry smile, "Joe, Jefferson is about ten years ahead of Hahnemann in planning, and I feel that I can achieve my true potential there. Hahnemann has a weak Board and its finances are precarious. Furthermore, I don't think they will ever improve. As you know, there are too many medical schools in Philadelphia."

I didn't want to agree with him, but there was no denying that what he said was true. I later found out the real story. Kellow and the President of Jefferson, Peter Herbert, rode into town on the train together every morning and became quite friendly. They were anatomically and personality-wise a symbiotic fit. Both were about the same size. Both had hunchbacks. When they were together, they resembled a pair of birds pecking at each other. Both were very ambitious and shrewd politically and knew how to get things done. When the Dean at Jefferson retired, Herbert invited Kellow to take the job.

Then came the real hooker. Kellow looked me in the eye and revealed the actual reason he wanted to talk to me.

"Joe, I would like you to take my place immediately as Acting Dean. As you know, I have started several large projects that are well underway, but I need to transfer a lot of important information to my successor if they are to materialize properly. Cameron and Paxson both agree that you're the proper individual to carry on temporarily. Of course, a committee will be formed to seek a permanent replacement but as you can surmise, this will take at least six months and more likely a year. You can be a candidate yourself if you wish."

I was frankly astonished at this offer, but it suddenly dawned on me that Kellow had been planning this move all along. Indeed he had been preparing me by invitations to attend the national meetings of the Association of American Medical Colleges (AAMC), which incidentally I found boring and infiltrated by a breed of professors who had mainly political ambitions. I made up my mind quickly and replied, "Will, I'll do it as a favor to you, but I've no interest in the Deaning business. I really should be taking a sabbatical to renew my research capabilities. Is there anything in it for me financially, and do I retain my Chair of Pharmacology?"

Kellow appeared to be relieved and smiled. "Yes," he replied. "There is provision for a substantial increase in your salary during the period of your tenure as Acting Dean. And you will be able to keep your Chair."

I hadn't expected much, but the substantial increase turned out to be a $2,000 increase in salary to do the work of both Chairman and Dean. I regretted making a hasty decision, but the tendency to refuse this unneeded burden of work and responsibility was counterbalanced by the realization that, if I didn't do it, one of my colleagues would. That person would gain the chance to make contacts and obtain leverage to do things for his department that I had passed by. This would not be so if the other person was someone in administration.

I asked Kellow why he didn't consider Joseph Gonnella or Hugh Bennett, both excellent associate deans, for the acting position. Kellow smiled and replied, "Gonnella is too young, and besides I expect to take him with me to Jefferson. I'll leave him with you long enough to get you started. Then I'll make him an offer he can't refuse. Incidentally, I'm also going to take the Dean's secretary with me. All's fair in love and war, you know. As for Bennett, I admit, he is a workhorse, but he's intensely hated by the faculty and the administration doesn't trust him." With this last statement, we shook hands and I was thus launched into an administrative career that I'd never had the least notion of achieving.

The next Monday I began attending the weekly meetings of the top executives: Cameron the President, Paxson the Director of the Hospital, and Kellow the Dean. Even though I had spent over thirty years of my life in medical institutions, I was surprised to discover that that I knew little or nothing about the fears and worries of the top executives. Even as a department head, I never had to confront the problems and daily pressures that CEOs had to deal with. It had never occurred to me that the situations that develop in a large institution are essentially never capable of complete and satisfactory solution. There is never enough money, the facilities are always inadequate, labor problems develop repeatedly, deadlines of financial obligations are ever present, competitors are always stealing your turf, banks are reluctant to lend more money, and insurance companies are raising rates. I learned businessmen's jargon: "cash flow . . . , bottom line . . . , point . . . man." But what struck me most impressively was the general paranoia of top executives. Anyone who might be in a position to criticize the President was scrutinized about what company he or she kept and what influence existed with members of the Board and the more affluent clinicians. The pettiness of high officials was indeed far greater than what was evident among the general faculty. The reasons for this paranoia became obvious to me as I began to get a feel for the function of the various officers.

The President relates to members of the Board of Trustees who depend on him to relieve them of their obligations. These consist mainly of raising money, whether by profitable operations, donations, or political subsidies from local, state, and federal governments. The institution must present a good front to the public and news media. Scandal is to be avoided at any price. If any unfavorable event occurs, even by the purest chance, it is always the President's fault. (He'd better have an assistant who can be conveniently blamed and severely disciplined—or better yet, fired.) To keep his position, the President must be careful to please those members of the Board who really count. This is usually the Chairman and one or two cohorts. The rest of the Board is usually ignored unless they are in a position to contribute substantially by way of finances or politically. In Cameron's case, it was soon evident that Chairman Pat Malone and Carl Vogel were the confidants and major supporters. I eventually got to know both of them quite well and shall have more to say about them.

Charlie Paxson, the Hospital director, related to the President but much more to the Board than the Dean because the Board inherently had little interest in academic matters. It was more intensely concerned with hospital finances. In the late 1960s, the medical school was a mere $3 to $4 million dollar operation compared to nearly $20 million for the hospital. The medical school, moreover, had a fixed budget that could be reliably predicted at the beginning of the fiscal year because it depended on tuition, the state subsidy and grants, and donations. On the other hand, the hospital had an unpredictable income that depended on what paying business it could attract that year. In addition, expenses could fluctuate widely because of the price of blood, insurance rates, and the amount of free care that had to be rendered. Nurses' pay and that of other help was always a problem because of strong union action. The Board's finance committee required monthly financial reports from Paxson that were carefully scrutinized. Because of the long delay in most hospital reimbursements, money had to be borrowed from banks in order to meet the payroll. This made the Board nervous because it knew well that millions of dollars could be easily lost, resulting in bankruptcy with default to the bank. Constant attention was paid to methods of insuring that cash flow would be adequate. Since the medical school and the hospital were one corporation with one Board, the finances were one, and all income went into one pot. The result was that, when the academic semester started and a big chunk of tuition money came in, it went to pay salaries, mortgage interest, and vendors' debts that were six or more months behind in payment. Thus in reality, the medical school did not have any control over its finances because the hospital ran the payroll and all other financial obligations.

It was always claimed that the hospital subsidized the medical school, but I could find little evidence of that. Kellow was the first Dean who managed to gain some control over academic finances. He did this by insisting that the medical school had to have a financial officer of its own. He appointed a knowledgeable, shrewd individual, Tom Murray, who attended all financial meetings and was at least able to have an accurate estimate of where the money was flowing. Paxson was honest, forthright, and conscientious. But in matters of finance, he naturally favored the hospital and, like all practical administrators, he wanted to treat the faculty as ordinary employees. He had been employed by the hospital before the Cameron era and had shown talent in running a tight, economical operation. Brought back as CEO, he had been charged with restoring fiscal responsibility and order to a chaotic operation. Cameron was no businessman and relied heavily on Paxson.

Kellow related very well to both the basic scientists and the clinicians on the faculty. In a strange way, they didn't actually like him but had enormous respect for his abilities. Unlike previous Deans, Kellow really knew the academic game and had experience in dealing with the American Medical Association (AMA) and the AAMC. He ran Academic Affairs Council, the highest academic decision making body, with great finesse. Among other projects, one of his major ambitions was to establish a practice plan for the clinical faculty that would generate income for the Dean's discretionary fund. He ran into some opposition in this area from Paxson who was more anxious to institute a plan with more juice for the hospital. Naturally, both Kellow and Paxson made efforts to make Cameron feel that all new plans and projects were Cameron's original ideas.

I soon learned that the President must always be made to look good. If anything meritorious eventuates, it is the President who must get all the credit and publicity. If a project fails or loses money, it is always someone else's fault. In no way is this meant to be derogatory of Cameron. He showed admirable insight on many occasions, and few people were as devoted to Hahnemann as he was. A man of great intelligence and sensitivity, he easily could have been an English professor. I always thought it strange that he chose medicine and especially surgery. I hardly considered him as a physician, in fact, for he never attended rounds or made any comments in a clinical sense. His greatest fault was a forgetfulness or abrupt change of attitude and mood. After much discussion and bargaining, for example, a final agreement would be reached on an important project and receive Cameron's full, enthusiastic approval. The next day he would call a sudden meeting, scowl, and call off the whole project as impractical and inconsistent with his thinking. There was a paranoid twinge that implied the CEO and Dean were conspiring to put the President in a bad light. Cameron was a bachelor who lived with his mother. She was a grand lady and an important stabilizing influence in his life. I never did find out if Cameron was a practicing homosexual and took the modern view that one's sexual inclinations had nothing to do with one's ability to perform in medicine or industry.

The indulgence in spirits was more serious and, although Cameron had the most remarkable ability to "hold his liquor," it may have impaired his overall performance. On the platform or in the presence of dignitaries, none equaled Cameron in ability to utter the "bon mot." His sense of timing was flawless and choice of language to suit the occasion superb. All the Hahnemann families were pleased with his representation of the institution, which suffered from an overcast of inferiority complex stemming from its homeopathic origins. One of his foremost masterpieces was a comparison of the careers of Samuel Hahnemann and his American contemporary, Benjamin Rush. Skillfully weaving parallels of the accomplishments of these two leaders working in the old and new worlds, Cameron convincingly demonstrated that Hahnemann was far superior in every way to the esteemed and honored Rush.

In two months with the executive group, I got to know the characters I had to deal with. I also became more familiar with the Dean's staff and other service people whom I would have to rely upon to get the daily business done. Ray Lear, a young man who was the Registrar and Bursar, covered perhaps the most important functions of the Dean's office, namely, officially enrolling students, knowing where they were, keeping their records, and making sure that tuition was collected. Faculty records also had to be kept as well as minutes of Academic Affairs Council and those of important standing committees, such as the promotions committee. Hugh Bennett handled the student health office and the admissions committee. The latter was perhaps the most sensitive spot in the schedule of duties of the Dean's office. More about this later. Unexpectedly, and to my surprise, the greatest daily burden of the Dean's office was answering the mail. A good secretary can separate the wheat from the chaff, but she cannot help with answering the volume of sensitive letters that require judgment and personal knowledge. Kellow soon unburdened himself of most of the mail by handing it off to me. He had a small recorder that he carried in his briefcase and dictated most of his mail at home for his secretary to transcribe the next day. I decided to follow this pattern, which ate up a couple of hours of my time each evening. Most of the mail that Deans receive is not worth answering, and I'm sure many end up discarding it. A good deal must be answered, however, such as requests for information from granting agencies, influential alumni, and local and federal governments.

As I became more indoctrinated in the Dean's routine duties and saw first hand the almost menial servitude of the office, I became firmly convinced that I didn't want this to become a permanent job. A Dean's search committee was soon formed with Carl Fisher as chairman. He was extraordinarily capable, and I was hopefully that the committee would soon find a replacement. Although invited to, I didn't put my name in the running. I made sure that I remained Chairman of Pharmacology to insure the temporary nature of my tenure as Acting Dean.

Inevitably July 1, 1967, rolled around and I was left holding the bag. The secretary, Jean MacArthur, a superb performer, soon joined Kellow at Jefferson, and I was in limbo to move even the most mundane matters along. It was evident that I must have an efficient secretary who could handle the irritating daily matters expeditiously and diplomatically. I implored the personnel department to find a suitable replacement. They sent me a good-looking redhead who was a fair typist but couldn't take dictation. She also lacked the maturity and backbone required to deal with irate customers. We staggered along for a couple of months before we mutually threw in the towel.

After trying a few others, I finally settled on a young lady of Italian extraction who fit the bill and worked out so well that she lasted for most of my Deaning career. Joanne Montecarlo was very presentable, perhaps a little on the sexy side, but with superb secretarial skills. She could take dictation as fast as I could deliver it, and her command of English was such that she could usually improve every letter or report. Joanne could get anyone I wanted on the phone despite all the subterfuges other secretaries used to protect their bosses. She maintained the dignity and authority of the Dean's office with uncanny finesse. Such ability costs a price and, as a consequence of her assumption of an authoritative position, she created antagonisms, jealousies, and even hatreds. It is evident that the success of many an executive depends on a capable secretary more often than is admitted.

If all I had to do was to be Dean, the job was not that difficult. But I had the pharmacology department to run. I appointed Warren Chernick as course director and acting chairman and skipped over Calesnick and Gero who were senior to him. The reasons were practical. Calesnick had a private practice and was only part-time. Gero, while very capable in his own field, did not have the depth in pharmacology that was required. My commitment to revise my pharmacology textbook was more troublesome. Three years were passing quickly since the last edition, and the schedule called for a new edition every five years. I had to get to work on it immediately if I was to make my deadline. From my past experience, I knew this would require at least three hours' work a day. This was not too difficult to fit in when I was a department chairman. A Dean's work schedule, however, requires his personal presence at more meetings than he can possibly attend. There are reports to make, faculty, students, alumni, and other administrators to interview, numerous lunches requiring speeches, and worst of all at least three dinners a week that kill evenings and often weekends. Without question, it's very difficult to keep up with intellectual pursuits while in an administrative position. This is undoubtedly one of the main reasons why most professors who become Deans don't last more than two or three years. There is little leisure time to think and reflect, as well as an emotional exhaustion from travails of the day that dull the mind and blunt creativeness. I nevertheless plunged bravely into the task of textbook revision, which proved to be even more formidable than I'd anticipated because of rapid advance of knowledge and the retirement and death of many of my chapter authors. Yet my textbook work was a release, in a way, from the pressures of the day. I think it helped to maintain some sanity from the vicissitudes that accrue for any Dean even if he is an angel.

The Dean's Search Committee began its work. Through the usual advertisements in the *Chronicle of Higher Education*, *Science*, and by word of mouth, candidates began to apply. The strangest people apparently imagined that they would make a very satisfactory Dean. A rear admiral thought that his successful Navy career entitled him to serious consideration. His only qualification was a medical degree. He had no experience in education or research, and his clinical training and performance were pedestrian. Some good applicants were associate deans in other institutions. For reasons not immediately obvious, associate deans seldom become deans. Hugh Bennett, for example, was highly qualified and certainly a very conscientious worker, but the faculty disliked him because he took the students' side in every dispute and the nature of his duties required him to tell the faculty to lay off on many occasions. He wisely didn't put his hat in the ring.

Few Hahnemann faculty applied, but one or two did ask my advice on the matter. One was a young internist who headed the Division of Rheumatology. Daniel McCarty was an excellent clinician with talent and performance in research. I had little doubt that he would have made an outstanding Dean, and I told him so. But also I informed him that becoming a Dean at his age, when he was just beginning to blossom, would deter his development and perhaps spoil his chances of ever becoming a department chairman. I illustrated the mundane and stultifying duties that I had to perform as Acting Dean. He listened carefully, but I had the feeling that he thought I was telling him this because I didn't want him as a competitor for the job. He didn't apply and left Hahnemann to become a Chairman of Medicine at another institution. He has had a brilliant career with significant scientific contributions.

A candidate was finally chosen who the committee thought was worthy of an interview. I no longer can recall his name, but he was from Chicago and had degrees in medicine and public health. Most of his experience was in the organization of programs designed to improve community health by education of the masses. Fortunately, he did not impress most faculty, and his name was put low on the list of candidates. The next candidate, Duncan Clark, was highly recommended by the AAMC. I knew him very well because he graduated a few years ahead of me from the Long Island College of Medicine. Like me, he had done his internal medicine residency at Kings County Hospital and had become a faculty member. His major interest was public health and community medicine. He became a protégé of Alonzo Curran who was then Dean. Curran appointed him Associate Dean, an office in which he served with some distinction while continuing his work in public health. When Curran eventually retired, Clark became Dean. His comparative youth and, perhaps naive behavior, earned him the nickname "Boy Dean." After serving in this capacity for only a couple of years, he retreated to a newly formed Department of Community Medicine. I admired Clark for his intellect and integrity, but I felt he lacked the kind of aggressive personality that Hahnemann required. His desire to undertake a Deanship in a poorly financed, struggling medical school when he was a chairman of a department in a well-financed, growing institution (Long Island College of Medicine was now part of the University of the State of New York) worried me. I saw myself in a similar position a few years hence.

I was by now fifty-one years old and my children were about to enter college. Although Mary and I had tried very hard to finance this, rising tuition and inflation had defeated our plans. Four of our children would be in college at the same time. I definitely needed to make more money, so I decided to look for a job in industry. I cast about and responded to an ad in *Science* for an executive position at a drug company. They responded to my curriculum vitae favorably and invited me for an interview. The company turned out to be Parke Davis, a respected, old company but by no means the largest. It was located in Ann Arbor, Michigan, a lovely university town. My visit was red carpet all the way. After interviews with all the senior scientists and learning what duties would be expected of me, I was offered a package deal with a handsome salary, generous fringe benefits, and stock options. I thanked them and said that I would let them know in about a week.

Mary said she would go along with the move if it made me happy, but I could perceive that she would be unhappy with the change. With the exception of summer, Ann Arbor possesses a cold, damp almost gloomy climate conducive to rheumatic diseases. The work itself was strictly a desk job, and Mary knew that my first loves were the laboratory and the clinic. Then there would be the problem of resettling five kids who had made bonds with friends and schools that could not be easily broken. We loved our house in Wayne and had our in-laws living with us who would also have difficulty resettling. I also had friends in industry who had the experience of early retirement at fifty-five, which was not far off for me. So after much soul searching, I turned the opportunity down. The situation might have been different if I could have found a similar opportunity in the Philadelphia area. Such was not to be the case.

Neither the committee nor the faculty liked Duncan Clark, although he was by far the most plausible candidate on the list. Mede Bondi and Carl Fisher encouraged me to put in my name as a candidate. Against my better judgment, I applied for the deanship and convinced myself that I could continue my teaching and research efforts and still do a credible deaning job. It would mean more income and solve my immediate financial problems. Inwardly I was hoping that I wouldn't get the job because I had pretty much figured out the ins and outs of the deaning business after nearly a year as Acting Dean.

Make no bones about it, deaning is a business. It has nothing to do with science and the humanities or research and higher intellectual endeavors. The power of the Dean lies directly in the control of the academic budget. Faculties support a Dean in relationship to his ability to increase their departmental budget or, better yet, their salaries and fringe benefits. They care little for a Dean's academic prowess or ethical distinctions. Kellow instinctively knew this. His increasing control over the academic budget through ingenious devices made him more effective and, as a result, more powerful. He also knew how to increase the institution's ability to get grants. But most of all, a Dean must know how to be comfortable relating to people. He must keep the President happy and impress the Board of Trustees with demonstrations of good management. On the other hand, the faculty and the students must be kept in optimistic good spirits. Not small tasks considering the diverse characters that infest the typical medical school. I learned these and other unsavory things as Acting Dean. Indeed, I longed to get back to the solitude of the laboratory. The distraction of working on the new edition of my pharmacology textbook kept me functioning, even though it was difficult being separated from my mentors in the department.

So the months passed as the search committee kept trying to find likely candidates. Hahnemann was not attractive either financially or academically and continued to suffer from the stigma of homeopathy even though it had been almost completely eliminated by this time. A very good candidate was identified and invited to visit Hahnemann. Robert Buchannan was a brilliant internist and Associate Dean at the prestigious Cornell Medical School in New York City. Every inch a WASP, he was tall, handsome, and already well established in national medical politics. At the time there were at least a dozen Dean vacancies, some in very attractive medical schools. I'm sure Buchannan was invited to consider every one of them. Why he even agreed to visit Hahnemann was a mystery. Great preparations were made to influence him to consider the position attractive. I was pleased that such a good candidate was at the least a possibility. In my interview with him, I did my best to present Hahnemann in the most favorable light. It was soon apparent that he was really not interested in Hahnemann or indeed in the other offers. He was holding out for the Deanship at Cornell, an institution where he had done most of his work and in a city that had been his home. His turndown of Hahnemann made the committee and administration realize that they were not going to attract a truly competent Dean from the outside unless the position was made handsomely attractive financially.

Meanwhile, some serious planning and operations had to be performed to get the new medical school building underway. From a practical point of view, my candidacy began to look more attractive to the committee. I knew the ropes by now, the faculty seemed able to tolerate me, and I was fairly popular with the students.

Under these circumstances, a committee and an administration often makes a stopgap appointment. A few days later, Cameron called me to his office and told me that the committee had submitted my name as a final choice. I don't recall his exact words, but I had the feeling that he might have wished that they'd been able to find a better choice. He went on to state that the school's finances were such that I could expect only the most modest increase in budget for the administration of the Dean's office. This was a way of telling me that I couldn't expect much increase in salary. I knew with considerable accuracy the salary income of most Deans in public as well as private medical schools. Mine was to be definitely in the lower level, averaging above the salary of a basic science chairman but definitely below that of the chairman of medicine and certainly that of surgery. The income that Parke Davis had offered me was much greater. Certainly with my training and experience, in full-time practice I could have expected to earn about double the Dean's salary. I told Cameron diplomatically that I was pleased and honored to be offered the opportunity, but I needed to think it over and especially to talk it over with my wife. Cameron said that he understood and would expect my reply soon. We parted with a handshake.

Mary was not opposed to my undertaking the Deanship, but I could perceive that she was not going to relish the additional social activities expected of a Dean's wife. The children were non-committal. I doubt they really thought that my assumption of this new position would materially change their lives. They enjoyed the large house and grounds and their local schools and friends and were relieved that no geographical change was about to occur. Mary's mother and father felt much like the children but were agreeable to any change that would benefit our family unit.

In the end, the Yogi Berra philosophy dominated my decision—"When you come to a fork in the road, take it." So it came to pass that I officially became Dean of Hahnemann as on July 1, 1968. There was little fanfare and some brief announcements in the local papers. My friends in academia congratulated me with reservations because they knew that most Dean's lives are short and unhappy. They pointed out that the average life of a Dean was only two and a half years. I had to give up the Chairmanship of Pharmacology, and I well knew that if I failed in the Deanship it would not be easy to slide back into a comfortable professorship. What Chairman wants an ex-Dean back in his department?

One aspect of the deal was personally amusing. The irony of the situation was evident. I was originally not interested in medicine and had a difficult time getting into medical school. My Italian origins and Brooklyn accent would ordinarily preclude my appointment in the Anglo-Saxon world of academia. Yet here I was, Dean of a medical school. Sure it wasn't Harvard or Hopkins, but Hahnemann was a respected medical school already 120-years-old and fully competitive in the esteemed atmosphere of Philadelphia medicine.

Now that the die was set, I decided to take stock of the situation and make definitive plans for the future. I naively gave myself five years to accomplish some lofty goals, after which I fully expected to step down from the deanship and retire to the laboratory. It didn't turn out that way, but nevertheless it was a practical way to plan. Finances dominated my everyday activities and determined what could and could not be done. Hahnemann was a tuition-financed school with little or no endowment and no substantial assets. Being part of a single corporation that was dominated by a large charity hospital also disadvantaged it. The Board of Trustees, more allied to healthcare problems and finances, had little sympathy for academic problems. Since the budget of the hospital was some ten times that of the medical school, the corporation could go under much more easily if the hospital and clinics ran at a loss. It was clear that the medical school could not be allowed to lose money. If any academic project was to be initiated, it could only be done if the finances were first obtained.

The hospital, in contrast, often ran into periods of financial deficit when indigent patients flooded the wards or when many patients failed to pay their bills. Money had to be borrowed from the banks to tide the corporation over these periods. To minimize borrowing with its costly interest, the moneys of the medical school that came in convenient blocks, such as tuition and the state subsidy, were used to pay salaries of technicians and nurses. In between such influxes of cash, it was a precarious struggle to meet the salary payroll every two weeks. Money owed to the hospital was always paid late, and many times proved to be uncollectable. Vendors' debts meanwhile mounted beyond the limited ninety days to six months and even a year. This was most exacerbating to researchers who had money in their grants and couldn't get supplies and equipment because the suppliers wouldn't deliver to an institution that had not paid previous bill for many months. Indeed when I first arrived at Hahnemann, I soon discovered that only one chemical company would accept orders. Others would only sell on a cash and carry basis. This cash flow problem improved from time to time but the institution usually seemed on the verge of bankruptcy. Undaunted, I plunged boldly into this tangle of financial inequities and a faculty with an insatiable hunger for more manna from above.

CHAPTER VII

The Deaning Business

1968-1972

*"Given that a medical school dean should have high ideals
and perfect integrity, what he really needs is a cast iron stomach
and a carbon fiber spine."*

Rupert Black, M.D.

As I began my term as Dean, Harvard Medical School announced in a money raising effort that it spent approximately $35,000 per year per medical student to provide each with a first class education. With about 130 students in each of the four class years, a simple calculation indicated that the yearly medical school budget must have been over $18 million a year. Tuition was about $2,000 a year, so only about a $1 million was contributed from this source. The other $17 million presumably had to come from endowment, government support, grants, and gifts. There are many fudge factors in such calculations, of course. How much was contributed by the expense of the gymnasium, the cost of the football field, and the university president's residence? More important in a medical school is, how much of the budget comes from the healthcare dollar? Nevertheless, simple comparisons like this are useful in a gross sense.

When I compared Hahnemann's yearly budget in the same manner, I soon found that it was approximately $3.5 million. Since we had only four hundred students, this meant that it cost nearly

$9,000 annually to educate a medical student—a figure only a fourth that of Harvard's. Hahnemann's tuition was the same as Harvard's, so only $800,000 was contributed from this source. Yet this amount contributed roughly one-fourth of the total budget. Compare this to the tuition component at Harvard, which was only an eighteenth of the total budget. This comparison is meant to indicate that Hahnemann was a tuition-driven medical school with tuition a major component of its annual budget.

Hahnemann survived, as did the other medical schools in Pennsylvania, because of a state subsidy that was voted on and allotted on an annual basis. Temple and Pittsburgh were state-related and received a bigger share. At Hahnemann, the state subsidy was $1.2 million, or about one-third the annual budget. The rest had to be squeezed out of grants, gifts, and where possible the healthcare dollar. Only the University of Pennsylvania School of Medicine had sufficient endowment and grant funds to make tuition a minor part of its annual budget. Yet even this prestigious school felt the necessity of the state subsidy. Good academic instruction can never be a self-supporting enterprise, much less a profit-making business.

Like any industry or business, the biggest budget item was salaries. Next in order were operation of the facility, heat, lights, repairs and maintenance, interest payment on mortgage insurance, and lawyer's fees. As the medical school was one corporation with the hospital, the expenses of the latter items were shared on an allotment basis, as were the president's salary and his office cost, the development department, and any commemorative function. Since the hospital was by far the bigger operation and the trustees were oriented towards the hospital, the allotments seemed to me to be distinctly favorable to the healthcare side. I could not understand, for example, why the medical school paid 40 percent of the president's salary when the operating budget of the medical school was less than a tenth that of the hospital. As for the development department, which the medical school had to support heavily, its activities concerned mainly creating publicity and raising money for the hospital. On the other side of the coin, the medical school maintained the medical library that was used by nurses, residents, and hospital staff without any financial support from the healthcare component. The dean of the medical school performed many services for the hospital and clinics yet received no recompense from this area. The combination of hospital and medical school is unhappy and cumbersome. Both are, or at least were, considered non-profit organizations and both are directed towards the improvement of healthcare. They can and do share many common facilities, and both the basic science and clinical faculty can operate in healthcare delivery areas in teaching and research. But combine two businesses that are genuinely non-profit, and you must expect financial disaster to be an ever-present danger. Both school and hospital are bottomless pits. How much free first-class healthcare and excellent education can you give away by soaking those who can pay? It can work on a small scale. As technology improves, however, it becomes more expensive to deliver services because much more can be done and expectations rise. The wonderful invention of the Xerox machine increased the consumption of paper not by ten or even 100-fold but by thousands. The imaging technology of ultrasonics, magnetic resonance (MRI), and x-ray computerized devices makes diagnosis exquisitely accurate but also prohibitively expensive.

With these simplistic concepts in mind, I boldly set about to solve them. My knowledge of accounting was mediocre at best, but I set about to replace Tom Murray, who as predicted was called to Jefferson by Kellow, with the best talent I could attract and afford. I asked around and found that the University of Pennsylvania's Department of Biology had a large program of research and education with a talented staff of technical support. One of the laboratory managers was anxious to make a move. I called and asked him to come for an interview. I surmised his rather tricky and ingenious ways during the interview. I hired him on the spot and was not disappointed.

John Deufel proved to be just what I needed to reorganize and reconstitute the finances of the academic side of the house. The first order of business was to manage properly the $1 million or so of federal grants so that income to the operations of the plant could be maximized. Until that time, the individual research investigators never knew the balance of money in their accounts. As a consequence, they often bought more supplies and equipment than their grant allowed. Extremely sloppy bookkeeping supplied from time to time by hospital personnel led to money being lost on every grant, sometimes in huge amounts. One aggressive investigator managed to overspend his grants by $200,000 year after year. Deufel said the answer to this problem was to establish a commitments section. This meant establishing an accurate budget for each grant with respect to salaries, equipment, expendable supplies, travel, and other miscellaneous costs and committing money to each category before it was expended. Each commitment was then followed on an annual basis, and the investigator was warned when there were under—and over-expenditures. The great advantage of this system was that both the institution and the investigator knew at any moment exactly where they stood financially with each grant. This was impossible to accomplish easily with a mechanical system of bookkeeping, of course, so Deufel soon informed me that I needed a computer and help to run it. Before he left, Kellow had fortunately established a computer division with money from a federal grant. He had recruited and appointed Perry Scheinok, a talented mathematician who was versatile at computers, to run the operation. Perry was a good resource person and very helpful in getting our operation under way. I told Deufel to find himself an assistant, who turned out to be Bob Walker; a former buddy of his at Penn. Walker was a great find. He considered himself to be a systems man, and this was no exaggeration. Walker was tall and thin with abundant gray-white hair, a mustache, and beard that made him look distinguished. When strangers saw us together, they thought that he was the Dean and I no more than an assistant.

In a period of some six months, this unlikely team turned out what was the first commitments section for grant finances of any medical school. It turned out to be a superb managing tool. For the first time, the Dean was in a position to know where the money was and what it was doing. It allowed the academic side to deal on an equal basis with the hospital's financial executives. It was such a good plan that it was soon adopted by many sister institutions. The financial personnel of the AAMC made a special visit to Hahnemann to examine its structure.

My attention next turned to the admissions procedures. From serving on the admissions committee for over five years myself, I was well acquainted with the process, its strengths, and faults. Many of the most distinguished Hahnemann faculty had served on the committee, an indication of the importance of attracting the best applicants to Hahnemann. I asked John Scott, who was retiring as Chairman of Physiology, to take on the committee. He certainly was experienced and about as sincere and upright an individual as one could find. I realized, however, that in order to compete successfully with other institutions, we needed to have a very efficient admissions process. We had over two thousand applicants for the hundred-odd places so speedy handling of data and rapid resolution of individual cases was essential. We needed a full-time person in the dean's office who was young and had some experience in the best methods of college admissions. After a thorough search, my staff located Gerald R. Hejduk who turned out to be just what we had wished for. Working with Walker and Deufel, he soon had the admission process computerized so we had the capacity to select the applicants with the best cognitive criteria. We were, in fact, one of the first medical schools to have a computerized plan for the admissions process. The AAMC, which later computerized its admission application procedures, studied our plan and learned from it, I'm sure.

Now the important question was, what was the role of the Dean in the admission process? I asked alumni what prior deans had done. I was told that Dean Pearson (1921-1942) interviewed and admitted applicants personally; there was no admissions committee. Dean Brown (1947-1956) established an admissions committee under Nat Ludwig. He divorced himself from the admission process externally, but I'm sure he worked with Nat on delicate admissions problems. Dean Kellow (1961-1967) played a strictly professional game and steered clear of the admission decisions. He agreed that President Cameron should have two or three candidates whom the committee should bend a little in favoring admission. I do not know whether he himself tried to use influence to favor certain applicants. Knowing Kellow's almost fastidious character, I doubt that he abused any privileges. At Temple University School of Medicine, Dean Parkinson personally admitted every applicant until the late 1950s. No wonder that most applicants and their families believe that the Dean or the President of an institution could get anyone into medical school if they wanted to. I firmly believe that the Dean's role is purely supervisory. He must certify and insist that applicants are admitted purely on their qualifications regardless of race, color, religion, or finances. The admissions process is a faculty matter, and the faculty must set the criteria for admission in a democratic fashion. Admissions committee members are to be elected for a term and the committee and its chairman are answerable to the highest academic body. The Dean is merely an executive who oversees the process and makes certain that no applicant falls through the cracks. Like any member of the faculty, he can communicate a recommendation to the committee about any applicant. The weight his recommendation carries should depend entirely on the judgement of the committee.

Despite all the rules and precautions, presidents, members of the Board, alumni, faculty, friends of the institution, and politicians all firmly believe that the Dean can get anyone into medical school. In my case, I was hounded almost daily from the beginning by people who claimed to be my friends and who just happened to have a candidate who was wonderful and guaranteed to become an outstanding physician. My standard answer was, "Send me a copy of his application, and I'll give you an estimate of his chances." Usually it was some poor soul who had applied to every medical school in the country and had been turned down by all. If the application was pending at Hahnemann, I would volunteer to look it up and give my estimate of the chance of being admitted. The applicant usually had a poor record and was not scheduled for an interview. The next question was always, "Could I get the applicant an interview?" No amount of explanation would appease the caller's conviction that the applicant would charm the committee in the interview so much that it would assure admission. Under pressure I would request the committee to give the interview, but I don't remember a single case where it did any good. Alumni, close relatives, and veterans were interviewed as a matter of courtesy, and I suspect that in a few cases the interview did improve the candidate's chances.

For applicants with excellent records from good universities, the interview can do more harm than good. The candidate might show great immaturity, a complete lack of interest in medicine, or be a bookworm with no capacity to relate to people. These cases give the Dean the most trouble. An irate parent calls and yells, "What's wrong with your medical school? My son has a straight-A record from Princeton (actually B- or C+) and you turned him down!" What sensible answer do you give this parent? I have never found out. The fact that it was a faculty committee decision never convinces a parent that it wasn't the result of racism or discrimination of some type. The scenario gets much more worse if the applicant happens to be accepted by another medical school. There's no explanation for that, and I have a strong suspicion that some deans got themselves fired under such circumstances. I could spend much time on the admissions happenings, but I will leave the more spicy stories to their time and place. As we shall see, a great deal depends on who the President or Provost happens to be and the attitudes of the Board.

Early in my career as Dean, I concentrated my attention on the problem of faculty governance. Hahnemann had no faculty senate and no tenure policy. For a Dean to function effectively, he must have the fidelity and support of his faculty. Smaller institutions are distinctly autocratic in governance matters, and even large universities pay only noblesse oblige to the democratic process. John Scott had put together a rather good set of faculty by-laws. They allowed for two faculty meetings a year that theoretically allowed individual faculty members to bring up matters of injustice or grievance. Nothing ever actually happened at these meetings,

and it was difficult even to get a quorum necessary for elections
and voting. The President and hospital administrator usually made
a report that was sullenly received. Emergency meetings of the
faculty could be called. (As we shall see, they were effective in
bringing about an important change at a later date.) The College
Council was the academic body with considerable clout. Composed
of all Department Heads and four elected faculty, it met monthly
to adjudicate all academic matters. This concerned the formation
of departments and divisions of departments, faculty appointments,
and all matters concerning curriculum, student affairs, promotions,
resignations, and dismissals. The Dean chaired the meeting and
was a voting member only when there was a tie vote. The President
was ex-officio. Cameron faithfully attended the meetings, but later
Presidents attended only when requested.

Since the Council was composed mainly of department
chairmen, it was aptly called the Chairmen's Club by junior faculty.
This was a significant concept because when there were only twelve
departments (six basic science and six clinical science), the Council
was an efficient, effective body. Later when the number of
departments increased to twenty three (seventeen clinical and only
six basic science), the balance of power reverted to the clinical
chairmen. This had a deteriorating effect on matters of academic
decision. The College Council reported to the Academic Affairs
Committee of the Board. This was a rather perfunctory exercise
performed by the Dean. Members of the Board assigned to this
body were generally the weaker ones except for the rare occasions
when the Board had a qualified person to assign to this task. With
a preponderance of clinical chairmen, there was a tendency to
discuss clinical accomplishments in lieu of academic ones.

In spite of these shortcomings, the College Council was the
base upon which the Dean could either stand or fall. In the ultimate
analysis, the Dean must be able to keep the chairmen happy and
satisfied in order to keep their confidence and support. The only
way to do this was to increase their annual budgets, their space
and facilities, their salary and health benefits, and other favors
such as free tuition for their children. I became convinced that any

longevity I had as a Dean simply resulted from the fact that during most of my tenure, the academic budget increased each year due to federal and state support, increases in the number of students, tuition increases, and the receipt of more federal grants. It was a period when medicine and healthcare greatly expanded and the need for more doctors and medical scientists was a priority item.

It was certainly a time when the federal government greatly increased its support of educational institutions so places like Hahnemann, that had little ability to raise private funds, could expand their sights. The AAMC wisely moved to Washington, D.C. to become a more effective lobbying organization. It was very helpful in convincing key members of Congress to support academic medical institutions. Deans began to plan expansion of their educational programs. The most obvious one (for which money was easy to acquire) was to start a College of Allied Health Professions. About this time it became apparent that delivery of healthcare involved many more personnel than the traditional doctor and nurse. Respiratory therapists, physical therapists, radiology technicians, medical laboratory technicians, physicians assistants, and many other forms of therapy and diagnosis specialists served very important roles besides sparing the physician's time.

Hahnemann already had a school of nursing with a three-year diploma program run by the hospital. It had little integration with the medical school. It was frankly an antiquated program designed to get some slave-labor advantages from nursing students. For the times, it was an expedient, effective method to educate and produce nurses. Many very excellent nurses were graduates of such programs, but they did not fit or satisfy more modern educational standards. It proved to be quite difficult to get the nurses to agree to become integrated into a college program. Nor did the hospital authorities want to give up what they considered their territory. The State Board of Nurse Examiners and the National League of Nurses were also a challenging hurdle. Nurses, I believe rightly so, have a strong sense of professionalism and feel that their delivery of healthcare is unique and quite distinct from that of physicians. With the help of some more favorably inclined nursing leaders like

Mary Schlosser, a two-year associate degree program was designed that finally gained approval. A very well educated and experienced person as Associate Dean of the College, Mary Schlosser managed to make the nursing programs successful, and they became an important sustaining factor.

To get the College of Allied Health Professions project off the ground, we needed a capable, resourceful dean. After some serious searching we were fortunate to secure the services of John Martin, a cheerful, enthusiastic man with political savvy and excellent qualifications in education. He was a driving force in securing a much-needed substantial grant from the Feds to get the college started.

Perhaps the most significant program in the college came a little later. The physician's assistant program was the brainchild of Wilbur Oaks, a Hahnemann graduate who also took his graduate training in internal medicine at his alma mater. Oaks was thin, boyish looking and with his horn rimmed glasses, appeared to be a scholar. He was actually a human dynamo who took care of an enormous patient load as well fully participating in teaching. Not a researcher, he had a dedication to healthcare delivery that was extraordinary. Concentrating on general internal medicine, he developed a concept of office practice that was consonant with the times. The first physician's assistant program started at Duke University School of Medicine. It was a considerable success and the federal government supported the introduction of similar programs. Oaks studied the Duke plan and decided to duplicate it while introducing some concepts of his own. I gave Oaks and his colleagues what support I could to get the program started. As might be expected, there was much opposition to a program that had a potential of infesting the medical profession with "second-rate doctors." There was also the question of state licensure. Would the State Board of Medical Examiners oppose the program? Nurses were naturally antagonistic because they felt they were being demoted in stature. In other states, nurse practitioner programs had actually been instituted that were similar in purpose and intent. All these obstacles were finally overcome and with the help of an

NIH grant, the physicians assistant program started. It was a success from the beginning and continues to this day to grow in size and quality. In fact it is the program that brings in the most tuition income.

That is not to say that the college didn't have growing pains. Dean Martin moved on to become Dean of a similar school at the rapidly growing New Jersey College of Medicine This left a serious void, and it proved difficult to attract a person of Martin's caliber. We decided that we would operate with a managing director until a suitable replacement could be found. This turned out to be Leonard P. Krivy who proved to be quite efficient in day-to-day operations. Professors in the medical school had little respect for Krivy's academic accomplishments. Aside from this difficulty, Krivy had a radio program that served very conveniently to recruit applicants to the various courses of the college. As a result of these activities, Krivy became a recognized expert in educational opportunities in the health professions. But Krivy's private practice, in which for a respectable fee he gave advice and instruction on how to get into medical school, became a source of embarrassment for the institution. I'm sure that there was nothing illegal about Krivy's practice, and he had no connection with the Hahnemann Medical School's Admissions Committee. Nevertheless, Krivy's practice gave the embarrassing appearance that there was a backdoor entrance into the medical school. The AAMC probably had complaints because they made discreet inquiries about Krivy's modus operandi. Eventually we came to a parting of the ways, which was unfortunate because Krivy was a good manager and a fine recruiter.

I twisted Tom Devlin's arm to take on as Acting Dean. Devlin had no intentions of becoming permanent dean because this could destroy a fine biochemical career. Devlin had a keen interest in education at all levels and contributed substantially to the development of the college. More about the college later but let it be admitted that the desire to have the medical school support an undergraduate program was part of an overall strategy to attain university status for Hahnemann.

After discussion with faculty leaders early in 1968, I appointed an Ad Hoc Committee on University Status with Mede Bondi as Chairman, and Tom Devlin and Dean Roberts as members. The committee's charge was to investigate the feasibility and desirability of Hahnemann Medical School and Hospital's becoming a university of the medical sciences. The fact that our sister institution, Jefferson Medical School, had moved in this direction was undoubtedly part of the motivation. More importantly, there was an ingrained desire to be part of a university instead of a medical school-hospital combination. Past rumors were probably plausible that Hahnemann made overtures to prominent universities to be taken over by them. To be realistic, however, I can't imagine any sensible university taking over the burden of a medical school and hospital. Cameron was not very keen on the idea that Hahnemann could achieve university status, but he went along with the concept as long as it did not dilute the operation of the medical school and hospital. I doubt that the Board even knew that such an undertaking was being planned.

At a special joint meeting of the Board of Trustees and the Faculty, the Ad Hoc Committee on University Status presented its findings in the form of an oral dissertation with arguments for and against presented by myself, Bondi, and others. There was considerable discussion, but I perceived little real enthusiasm. Most felt that it was too ambitious an undertaking without a promise of substantial financing. It would be better, most said, to be taken over by a large, affluent university than to attempt to attain such status ourselves. The matter was left in limbo. As usual it was decided that "If you can get sufficient faculty support and raise the money to do it, then go ahead. If you can't, then forget it." Members of the committee and I were not discouraged and proceeded to present the full, detailed report to College Council at its May 1968 meeting. Truthfully, it took energetic lobbying to get it passed by a reluctant faculty who saw no personal advantage to themselves in this venture.

As I scan its yellowed pages and faded print some thirty years later, I find myself forming a ironic smile. How naive we were. Little did we realize what time and effort would be required. Most of all, we little anticipated the ultimate effect it would have on the institution. The web of fate is indeed strange. What did the document say? It said we have made a thorough study of the situation, and we have come to the following conclusions and recommendations. I quote them directly from the document rather than summarize them:

Conclusions

On the basis of its study and the long and serious deliberations reflected in the preceding report, the Ad Hoc Committee on University Status for Hahnemann Medical College and Hospital respectfully presents the following conclusions:

1.   *That the emerging health needs of the nation today urgently require the teaching institutions of the country to gird themselves for an all out effort to find ways to meet them more effectively;*
2.   *That among the most critical needs is that for increased health manpower, trained in such numbers and of such types as to make it possible to meet changing health needs;*
3.   *That training of physicians and other professional personnel must go hand in hand with research and community service;*
4.   *That Hahnemann has a rich tradition and great resources of professional skills to bring to the solution of these problems; that its goals in teaching, research, and community service are inevitably related to the national task; and indeed that success in reaching those goals lies in identification with that task and initiating relevant plans for future growth and development.*

Recommendations

Therefore the following recommendations are made in the committee's belief that their implementation will enable Hahnemann to fulfill both its responsibility and the highest potential of its contribution:

1.   *That Hahnemann proceed promptly to develop and adopt specific*

academic goals in appropriate health science areas; that these goals include as a minimum:

A.   *A baccalaureate program*
B.   *Programs in selected allied health professions*
C.   *An expanded undergraduate medical program*
D.   *An expanded graduate program in the basic sciences*
E.   *An expanded graduate program and postgraduate program in clinical areas.*

2.   *That steps be taken to achieve university status, as essential to Hahnemann's future development and academic growth.*
3.   *That the evolution be toward a broadly based health sciences institution whose primary educational function would be the production of health manpower, associated with academic and research functions and appropriate service elements.*
4.   *That the two following approaches be considered as routes to the development of such a health sciences institution:*

A.   *Merger with an existing college or university under an arrangement whereby Hahnemann would become a Health Science Division of a University;*
B.   *Development of Hahnemann through growth from within into an independent Health Sciences University.*

5.   *That in addition, further study be given to the desirability of affiliation with the State Commonwealth System of Higher Education, if it develops that such affiliation is essential to the achievement of the objectives.*
6.   *That a joint Faculty-Trustee Committee be created without delay to pursue the most effective means for achieving the goal of a health science institution with university status.*

Respectfully submitted,
Amedeo Bondi, Ph.D., Chairman
Thomas M. Devlin, Ph.D.
Dean W. Roberts, M.D.

Quite an ambitious document, but obviously the committee clung to the premise that the shortcut might be merger with a strong existing institution. Such did not prove to be feasible. A true state university system does not exist in Pennsylvania as it does in New York State, which salvaged a score of medical schools including my alma mater, the Long Island College of Medicine. Pennsylvania does give affiliated support to three medical schools, one in Philadelphia (Temple). State legislators continually try to get rid of this obligation, and it would be extremely unlikely that they would support another medical school, especially one located in Philadelphia. So only growth and development from within, unfortunately, was the only possible avenue for Hahnemann.

Like many a meritorious document, the University Status Report was soon forgotten. Only the persistence of myself and committee members who would not give up brought this project to a successful conclusion—but only after many years and travails with four Presidents. Cameron should have picked up the challenge but let it die on the vine. The requested Faculty-Trustee Committee was never appointed. I do not blame Cameron for this. He had enough troubles on his hands just keeping Hahnemann above water without getting involved in what, by any measure, was a frivolous dream given Hahnemann's precarious finances.

My confreres and I realized that there must be a strong graduate program to become a university. In the early 1950s when I first came to Hahnemann, I recall frequent meetings of the basic science chairmen to discuss graduate education. The most enthusiastic member was John Boyd, Chairman of Biochemistry. Ray Truex, the anatomist, was much less keen but went along. Mede Bondi was a firm supporter. John Scott, the senior member, gave approval. I had never been involved in graduate education except medical school and residency, which are quite different, but I was willing to experiment. We discovered fortunately that Hahnemann had a charter from the state that was all-inclusive and allowed it to grant higher degrees, such as the Master and Doctor of Philosophy. This right had been wisely exercised only rarely in the past. What other educational body would recognize a Ph.D. in homeopathy?

We decided to design rigorous doctorate and masters programs in the basic sciences that, because of their excellence, would gain the approval of accrediting bodies and other universities. There was no financing for this, of course, but a sympathetic Dean Brown allowed us $30,000 a year, which we used as stipends of $1,000 or $2,000 to attract Ph.D. students to Hahnemann. While this amount was not much, the addition of the free tuition made it palatable. Paper work and records were kept in biochemistry where Dr. Boyd's secretary took on the burden of doing the necessary work. In view of this, we elected Dr. Boyd director of the program, a position that he greatly enjoyed and maintained until he retired. Strangely, the first few batches of Ph.D. candidates were the best we ever recruited. At least, it seemed that way to me. I was able later to obtain a training grant in pharmacology from NIH, and this enabled the department to attract some outstanding candidates. I never bothered with masters candidates but did award this degree to candidates whom the department felt did not measure up to the requirements of the Ph.D. degree. When the NIH money dried up, it became difficult to find good candidates. Minor league schools like ours attracted East Indians and Orientals who were trying to get U.S. citizenship or gain entrance into medical school. Nearly all medical schools were soon training graduate students, and the competition to get high quality candidates grew intense. Stipends were increased and opportunities for research made more attractive. Only well endowed universities with big research budgets got the first line applicants.

Hahnemann's graduate program would have died had it not been for the large, academically oriented department of psychiatry headed by Van Buren O. Hammett. In the style of the day, it was renamed Mental Health Sciences and dealt with a variety of psychological subjects as well as hard core psychiatry. Hammett himself was of the psychoanalytic school, having been trained before the discovery of potent drugs that were effective in the most severe mental diseases. Other prominent members of the department were Paul J. Fink, M.D., Director of Education and Training, and Clifford J. Bodarky, Ed.D., Executive Director of the department. Jules C. Abrams, Ph.D., a psychologist, was a most important member of the team because he designed a superior course of study that led to the Ph.D. in psychology. This course was very popular because it emphasized the practice of psychology rather than a research approach favored by other institutions. In contrast to the science degrees, this was one for which students paid tuition and thus was self-supporting. Other programs of the mental health sciences, such as music and art therapy, also were income producing. Although looked down upon by the hard-core scientists, the programs enabled the graduate school to survive and grow despite the competition of more endowed institutions.

When plans for the new medical school building were completed, it became necessary to evacuate the buildings that were to be replaced or restructured. We would lose all the basic science teaching laboratories and the lecture halls in the Khlar Building. The old building used as an animal holding facility would be demolished along with the old quaint Victorian medical school building. An ancient nurses' residence on the corner of 15th and Vine, unoccupied for years, was also to be razed. Much doubling up of offices and research labs was accomplished, but substitutes for the teaching labs and lectures halls had to be found. Fortunately, before the astute Kellow left, he made arrangements to buy the Eccles School of Mortuary Science conveniently located on 16th Street. It was acquired just in time to move in the student laboratories and the bookstore. Anatomy laboratories with their complement of cadavers fit in perfectly with some accommodations left behind by the morticians. One was an external pulley arrangement to lift cadavers up to the second floor since the building had no elevator. Pharmacology and Physiology shared a small floor that proved to be quite adequate. Lecture halls were rented in the Shriner's Building on the corner of Race and Broad Streets. The Shriner's Building auditorium had excellent acoustics, and we were proud to share it with the Philadelphia Orchestra that used it to make recordings. Bob Walker arranged many of these moves and was of inestimable help. As expected, there was much kidding about the medical school being located in a morticians' establishment. But it was a great investment. A few years later, when 16th Street was widened to accommodate traffic to the Schuylkill expressway, the old by-then unused building was sold to the state for a generous profit.

During these years of intense professional work, the support of my family was most important to me. Our five girls were growing and developing rapidly. They now were approaching the period of selection of a professional career.None of them showed the faintest interest. I helped them with science projects and they won prizes, but none of them showed any signs of mental stimulation by science. When they were old enough, I had them spend time in my laboratory and participate in the ongoing research. Despite these not too subtle intellectual stimuli, none of them demonstrated any leanings towards a scientific career.

When number three daughter, Joan, later became a physician, my influence played no role. She confided to me that her interest in medicine arose as a young child when she received routine examinations and vaccines from the pediatrician, Carl Fisher. He was a wonderful person who had a great manner with children, but it seems not plausible that a career choice is made on the basis of a few childhood contacts with a physician. Yet applicants in interviews for medical school do not infrequently mention this scenario. Maria, the oldest, had a very good brain and picked up new techniques quickly. I had her do a summer project on the Venus flytrap that involved making detailed measurements every day. The data turned out to be quite good and we were able to publish a paper in *Science*. I thought that this would be a great thrill for her, but it turned to be less than a small goosebump.

Mary had much more influence on the children than I did. She was herself quite a good singer having performed on the radio and other professional engagements. She insisted that all the children have piano lessons. She coached each of them in singing, but only Maria took to this. In fact she became a professional singer and teacher of vocal arts. Dorothea, or Dori, the next in line, hated piano lessons and gave them up only to beg to restore them later. She fell in love with the violin later, and eventually she became a pianist. Joan picked the cello as a second instrument and she derived great enjoyment from it although she chose medicine as a career. Yvonne had considerable talent at the piano but chose physics as a major at college. All along she had a natural talent for drawing, and midway in her college years she changed her major to art. She eventually became a sculptress. The youngest Mary-Jo didn't take to the piano but she developed an interest in ballet.

All of the above proves the old saying, "You can lead a horse to water but you can't make him drink." Since there is no practical way to predict what will interest a child, exposure to a variety of experiences is required. There is also the beneficial possibility that exposure to a subject might create a strong dislike for the modality. As a consequence of my childhood exposure to the grocery business, I decided that I didn't ever want to be a grocer. However, I did learn about hard work, profit and loss, marketing, and interpersonal relationships. My attempt to expose my children to science perhaps did the same thing for them. They probably realized the disadvantages of a scientific career much more clearly than those who drift into it only to find out that they are failures. Instinctively, an individual senses that mental and physical assets are not sufficient to assure competitive ability in a particular field.

I had a great interest in the outdoors and the beauty of nature. To impart this to the children, I planned a series of camping trips during summer vacations, which would be at least several weeks long to enable us to visit all the national parks of the U.S. and Canada. Scouting about, I found that the International Harvester Company made a large, sturdy station wagon, which could accommodate all seven of us as well as camping equipment. Our first trip was to Vermont and New Hampshire to visit the White Mountains and some of my old camp counselor's stamping grounds. The kids learned how to set up a tent, make a fire for cooking, and other skills for living outdoors. It was soon evident that the primitive toilet facilities were the least appreciated item. Daily hikes and bathing and swimming in cool lakes and streams were most popular. This first experimental trip was rated a success, so we planned to cross the country the next summer. On this and successive trips we were able to visit all the natural wonders, such as the Badlands of South Dakota, Yellowstone, and the incomparable Tetons. When we reached the West Coast, the children got the trill of dipping their feet in the Pacific Ocean. Then there were the Grand Canyon, the majestic redwood forests of California, Mesa Verde, Crater Lake, and the incomparable Mount Rainier—all these we saw and more, and wondered at their silent, stately beauty. Of all the places we visited I liked Glacier National Park the most, although I'm sure the children would not agree. To me it's a less developed tourist atmosphere. The presence of the glacier, grizzly bears, and mountain goats represented a more primitive, natural aura of how it must have been over thousands of years. Banff in Canada, which we visited later, was more picturesque, of course, and Lake Louise was as pretty a sight as any in the Swiss Alps.

After supper in the open air, we played games or just watched the setting sun. Nights in the mountains with the clear air made watching the stars tremendously inspiring, and the children were impressed with the vastness and mystery of the universe. Bedtime meant that we gathered in the tent and assembled in a circle. We told stories, recounted the day's experiences, and studied maps anticipating the next day's adventures. We often played bridge, keeping scores and cumulative averages for each team. I had the greater experience and usually won, which made the children try all the harder to excel.

These camping trips continued over a period of seven or eight years until it proved impossible to get everyone together, and as the children got older they developed their own interests. Once they finished high school, they began to scatter in various directions to prepare for college and polish their skills for their chosen careers. Dori, for example was keen on a musical professional future and obtained a counselor's job at a girls' summer camp teaching the guitar. Others took summer courses. We did take one final trip when I combined a family camping trip with the fall meeting of the Pharmacology Society. We had the opportunity to be housed in dormitories of Stanford University in Palo Alto, California. The children enjoyed this because they could imagine life away from home in a college dormitory.

I have wondered in later years what influence these camping trips had on the children. Some seemed to have derived great benefit, while others were just bored by the monotony of the long drives and not even appreciating the scenery. Maria gained the most. She became expert in reading maps, planning a trail hike, putting up and tearing down a tent, cooking on the open fire, and all the other skills common to camping and surviving the rigors of a primitive existence. The others could take it or leave it, and I observed that in later life they never attempted to duplicate the experience themselves. Of course, camping today has lost much of its charm because of the vast increase in tourists with their convenient recreational vehicles. Yet I sometimes notice traces of the camping years in all of them, faint as they may be. Dori likes to eat out in the open whenever she can and is a fiend for fresh air. Joan likes trees and has an appreciation for photographing scenery. Yvonne has bought a piece of land far from the city to expose her children to the wonders of nature. Maria is still an expert map reader and trip planner. She has taken a bicycle tour of French castles. So maybe it was all worthwhile, but I surely derived the most enjoyment.

As I reflect on my family life during the early Deanship years, I must admit that despite the intensity of my duties, I managed to have as much contact with my children as I would have if I'd stuck to private practice or a rigid schedule of scientific inquiry. Nor did I neglect repairs and upkeep on the big house. My father-in-law made rounds every day and greeted me in the evenings with news of urgent repair jobs to be done on the plumbing, the roof, and the masonry. We rebuilt a crumbling brick wall surrounding a porch one summer. Throughout the backbreaking labor, the only thought that sustained me was the story that Churchill had laid a brick wall at one time. If that magnificent statesman and intellectual could do it, then I could, too.

Physical labor relieves the tensions of the mind and spirit, and solid visible achievements reinforce the ego. Many of my friends and colleagues played golf, which probably served the same purpose for them. I enjoyed the few times I played the game, but I never felt that it was worth spending the time required to participate practically. A round of golf would take the better part of a whole day every week, an expenditure of valuable time that I could not afford to lose. I preferred playing croquet with my children. Our large lawn made it possible to enjoy croquet at home. The girls became quite skillful at this game. We were able to form teams and have some exciting matches. While golf is more challenging physically and certainly more glamorous, croquet requires just as much finesse and dedication to achieve perfection.

I relate these domestic experiences to illustrate that a Dean's life can be quite normal under the right circumstances. Looking back, the first three or four years in the deaning business were not too bad compared to subsequent years. Yet any Dean can only be as successful as the resources he commands. Hahnemann's facilities were quite modest, but there was a $50 million expansion program of which the $32 million medical school building was the main component. Hahnemann Hospital was over thirty years old and showed signs of obsolescence. Clinicians had a great desire for a new, modern hospital. Under pressure, the Board responded in a characteristic fashion. With Cameron nearing retiring age, the Board's pervasive thinking was, "Let's push him upstairs and get us a younger, vigorous president who'll stir up the institution and raise more money." Cameron was naturally not too happy about this but was assured that he would be made a paid Chairman of the Board with full control over the incoming president who would have to answer to Cameron. A search committee was formed, composed mainly of Board members. I was not on it, but my buddy Mede Bondi was so I was kept informed. I no longer recall the other members, but two who were board members, alumnus Charles Hollis and businessman Morton Jenks, were to play a crucial role in the selection. Little did I realize at the time that this committee would select a president who would change the whole course of Hahnemann and make my life miserable.

Times were changing, and the delivery of healthcare was becoming more commercial so the search committee looked for someone with business savvy. Perhaps a physician who also had an MBA might be Mister Right. It was a given that whoever was chosen must have contacts with wealthy people. By some such miraculous discovery, Hahnemann was going to get endowment it never enjoyed before. Never mind that Jefferson, The University of Pennsylvania, and other schools and hospitals had already tapped all available and likely sources in the community. When Morton Jenks suggested that he might be able to convince a very successful business candidate to consider Hahnemann, the committee listened.

Morton Jenks resembled a twin of Ichabod Crane. Tall, very thin, with a slight stoop, gaunt face, and long sharp nose, he was a member of a quite a respectable Philadelphia investment firm. It was rumored that his main involvement was seeking out wealthy old women and convincing them that his firm could make money for them by wise investments. It so happened that Jenks was also the Board member responsible for managing the relatively small Hahnemann investment account. In all the years he handled it, no money was earned; in fact, there was a considerable loss. His skinflint activities were legend. One example: He would buy the x-ray equipment of a retiring physician for a pittance then donate it to some hospital and claim a huge charitable deduction on his income tax. He would get the hospital administrator to write him a letter certifying the contribution, of course, so he satisfied his charitable obligation and made money on the deal at the same time.

The candidate whom Jenks recommended in glowing terms was Wharton Shober. Jenks claimed that Shober (His friends called him Wharty) was a financial genius who had made a fortune for himself. Now independently wealthy, he was considering devoting the rest of his life to philanthropic endeavors. Yes, he was interested in considering Hahnemann and indeed would work without salary for a year or two to straighten out Hahnemann's financial difficulties. Although the committee had some knowledge of Jenks and was naturally cautious, it agreed to consider Shober because, if it could be worked out, this might be the bonanza that Hahnemann was waiting for. There was a rumor that Shober was distantly related to Jenks, but that probably would not have prevented them for exploring the matter in more depth.

Who was Wharton Shober? A scion of a family that, while not exactly noble, at least was well settled in America as important immigrants dating well before the Revolutionary War. The original Shober forebearer was given a land grant that included most of the Pineys (or Pine Barrens) in New Jersey and its valuable water supply. Indeed, there was a plan to pipe the water to Philadelphia—at a price, of course. This never came to pass, but the descendants did well in various businesses. Wharty's family settled in Philadelphia and lived on the Main Line like other successful business people. Not extraordinarily wealthy, the family was very comfortable and easily fit into the well-to-do class of the glorious post-World War I 1920s. The young Wharty was a spirited maverick who liked to play jokes and indulge in exciting, daring activities. He became an excellent horseman and steeplechase rider, one of the champions of the Radnor Hunt Club. At the best prep schools, he was not an outstanding student but apparently did well enough to get into Princeton, his father's alma mater. He soon got into a fraternity of spirited lads who had the common aim of having as entertaining a time as possible. They were not interested in education in the least because all knew their future was assured, having come from affluent families. Most were endowed with enough native intelligence to skin by the minimum requirements for graduation. Not Wharty. It seems reasonable to assume that he flunked out for academic failure. He never admitted this but attributed his dismissal to playing practical jokes with his fraternity brothers. For whatever reasons, Wharty never did receive a college degree.

Young Wharty now cast about trying to find himself. He learned to fly an airplane and apparently had some jobs that involved salesmanship. He traveled to Central America, mainly Nicaragua, where he became acquainted with the notorious President Somoza. Wharty characterized this as his diplomatic service. During this period, he managed to become acquainted with a few Congressional leaders whom he glibly mentioned from time to time as if they were his intimate friends. He succeeded in a search for a wealthy, well situated Main Line debutante, and this was one source of his affluence. As long as he remained a respectable husband, he need not worry about his financial future. He eventually landed an impressive partnership with a reputable New York business investment firm where he would acquire contracts and manage important business deals.

My first contact with Shober was at a luncheon in his honor to make his acquaintance with the senior faculty and administrative officers. Tall, slender, with a fair complexion and light hair, he gave me the impression of an Aryan. Thinning hair made his brow high, but it did not make his facial expression intelligent as it does for some people. His bright blue eyes were neither piercing nor kind; his somewhat aquiline nose did not seem to fit his face. His mouth and chin were unpleasantly weak. From a distance, he fit the image of a German cavalry or airforce officer. Up close he lacked the charm and good grace of a cultured individual.

By chance Shober sat next to me at the head table. We made light conversation.

"How long have you been at Hahnemann."

"Twenty years."

"Where do you live?"

I explained that I lived in Wayne on the Main Line in a fine old mansion known as the Moulton House, formerly the estate of Alan Reed son of Jacob Reed owner of the famous Philadelphia men's clothing establishment. This seemed to strike a vibrant cord.

"I knew the Moulton girls and visited them frequently. In fact, my dog died in the basement of that house." I wondered briefly if the dog's ghost was still around. His next question astounded me.

"Do you ride to the hounds?" he beamed. Apparently he associated me with the Reed estate in its original state with its stable of fine horses.

"Look Wharty," I replied, "I'm a kid from the streets of New York City. The only horse I knew was Fritz who pulled my father's grocery truck. I used to feed him cabbage leaves and apples."

Shober turned his back to me. I don't think we spoke to each other again for several months. Much was to transpire, however, in those months that would change the course of Hahnemann and my role as Dean.

To understand Shober's impact as Hahnemann's new President and chief executive officer, it is appropriate to describe the administration as it existed just prior to his taking office. Robert Holmes, a new major player who was personally selected by Carl Fisher, was on the scene. On his retirement as Chairman of Pediatrics, Fisher had been appointed Medical Director of the hospital. Now retiring again, he wished to leave his alma mater with an outstanding, capable personality to step into his shoes. After a thorough search, Fisher was confident that he'd made a brilliant find in Holmes. On paper he did indeed have a commendable record that certainly qualified him as a competent candidate. Holmes was an M.D. who had graduated from the Tulane School of Medicine and subsequently trained as a pathologist. He entered the military and rapidly rose in rank. After the end of World War II, he was assigned to Japan to survey the effects of the atomic bomb at Hiroshima. His work was highly regarded by the military and was appropriately commended. On his retirement from the military, he became the medical director of the Miles Laboratories, an up and coming drug firm.

Holmes was short and stocky with a firm step and a dominant personality. Like most pathologists, he liked to have the final word on every subject. Despite his erudite quotations from Shakespeare and other sources, most did not consider him to be academic, perhaps because he put a military twist on everything. For example, when Shober became president, Holmes immediately offered his resignation because this was the custom in the Army. On assumption of his office as hospital director, he soon took command

and put everything "in order." Paxson, who really ran the hospital and had done a splendid job of economic recovery, was put on the back burner. Holmes' maneuvering must have impressed the Board because it elevated him to a Vice Presidency, which had the effect of elevating the hospital director to a higher position than the Dean. My friends on the Board fortunately insisted that the Dean be also made a Vice President, thus giving me at least equal rank to Holmes. This did not prevent the martinet from telling me on frequent occasions how to run the medical school.

Cameron didn't know quite what to do with Holmes because, I believe, he did not quite trust him. He had also become accustomed to working with Paxson in whom he'd developed great confidence. He nevertheless had Holmes join our executive group, so the four of us were the chief executive officers making the major decisions. This was to change drastically when Shober took office.

I discovered many months later what Machiavellian machinations Shober undertook long before he was installed as President. In the spring of 1971 when he ascertained from his internal source, Mort Jenks, that he was definitely going to be appointed, Shober immediately began a campaign of ingratiating himself with every Board member. He was ready with a plan of favors for each individual. For one, Shober knew a Senator who might be able to help with a legislative matter. For another, he had some trade maneuver that might help. Another had a favorite relative who was having trouble getting into medical school. Shober would try to get him in. Oh, yes, Shober didn't even have a bachelor's degree, but he was a master in manipulation. He knew that control of a corporation depends on being able to manage the Board. Once he was in power, he would get rid of any member who opposed him and would pad the Board with his own cronies. Shober knew that Cameron would be a mortal enemy, and he needed to defuse him and eventually get rid of him by forcing retirement. Cameron had the support of Board Chairman Pat Malone and Vice Chairman Carl Vogel, and their allegiance could not be directly assailed. Fortunately for Shober, both were going to retire in a year. All Shober had to do was wait and insure that the next Chairman would be his man. He was shrewd enough, however, to realize that in the beginning at least, he must give the appearance of working closely with Cameron.

Cameron had what he imagined was a winning agenda. Sure, he would play along with Shober and let him think that he was running the institution while Cameron would really pull the strings. After all, Shober knew nothing about a school of medicine and certainly had no skills to run the hospital, so he would have to rely on Cameron to tell him what to do. Cameron meanwhile would use Shober's superior contacts with wealthy people to bring in money. As paid Chairman of the Board, Cameron felt that he could get rid of Shober anytime should he prove to be unmanageable.

To insure his plan of action, Cameron needed strong allies on the faculty and staff. Charlie Paxson's allegiance to Cameron was unquestioned so he could be relied on to run the healthcare side. Cameron felt that I was a pretty good Dean and had done a credible job so far. Down deep, though, he had misgivings about my ambition for university status for Hahnemann, and he doubted that I had the aggressiveness and administrative ability to move the institution forward in a mainly clinical direction. His handpicked protégé, John Moyer, had more than proven himself in the past ten years as Chairman of Medicine. Not only had he managed to expand the department greatly, but by establishing a program of Continuing Education he also had put Hahnemann on the national map. Cameron was certain that Moyer was more than a match for Shober and could soon wrap him around his little finger. He slyly took Shober into his confidence and pointed out how he could greatly strengthen the institution by an internal restructuring of the executive table of organization. Moyer was to be made Executive Vice President for Academic Affairs, a position second in command only to the President. Thus as paid Chairman of the Board, Cameron could carry on his own master plan because he could control Shober through Moyer. The Dean would have to answer to Moyer and thus would be lowered to a minor echelon of executive power.

The stratagem should have worked under ordinary circumstances, but unfortunately for Cameron it was his undoing. He had overlooked Holmes who was Vice President for Health Affairs. Holmes hated Moyer and was not about to see him have any influence over Shober. Holmes was no fool. He realized that Shober was the means by which he could gain more support for the hospital side of the corporation. Using all the ingratiating tricks he had learned in the Army, he soon had Shober's complete confidence. It was also true that Shober was not going to have any reliance on Moyer, someone Cameron had recommended. Shober indeed had his own agenda for eliminating Cameron in a few months after his installation. He already had convinced a majority of the Board that Malone and Vogel must be retired as active members. This would undercut any remaining support Cameron could expect from the Board. Indeed, Shober had already picked the new Board Chairman—a surprising choice, Isadore Krekstein, a pillar of Philadelphia's Jewish community.

Krekstein was a CPA and founding member of the accounting firm of Laverthol, Krekstein, Horwath and Horwath, which served most of the large businesses of Philadelphia. He was a small man with a trim look. If you didn't know him, you might imagine him to be a haberdasher. I liked Krekstein because he was honest and had ideals of humble origins. As head of the Board's finance committee, he without doubt saved Hahnemann from financial disaster on many an occasion. Why did the Board go along with Shober's choice? Or did it in a moment of sanity want to neutralize Shober's suspicious business background. Whatever the reason, Krekstein made a fairly decent chairman but one who was unable to control Shober. Becoming chairman of a WASPish Board honored Krekstein himself, and Shober made certain to flatter his ego by allowing him to officiate at social and official functions.

Cameron was easily disposed of and made Provost, a meaningless position at that time. He was given a small office in a back room of the library without even a secretary. He soon found himself another job as a Director of the Papiniculau Cancer Institute in Florida.

A believer in instant starts, it didn't take long for Shober to take over. At a specially arranged faculty meeting, he allowed Cameron to officiate and introduce him. Cameron made his usual well-prepared, flawless address. There was little applause, however, as the faculty already had doubts about the capabilities of the new President. Shober's brief speech of appreciation revealed that he was a mediocre public speaker. He worked much better behind the scenes when he could consult others more knowledgeable than himself. Cameron announced organizational changes and introduced John Moyer as Executive Vice President for Academic Affairs. This went over like the proverbial lead balloon—stunned silence and no applause. I could see that Cameron was surprised. He hadn't anticipated that the faculty's intense dislike for Moyer.

Seeking to rescue the situation, he next asked me to say a few words because he knew that I had a degree of popularity with the faculty. Surprised and unprepared, I said the first thing that came to my mind. I began by praising Cameron for his admirable comments on this great occasion but added that perhaps he might have better spent his time tending to more mundane business. This obviously implied that Cameron, who'd been all powerful, was a dammed fool for allowing a man like Shober to become President. I could sense that Cameron was infuriated at my statements, which were certainly unwise and lacking in diplomacy. It was not until many years later that I found out that Cameron knew all about Shober and was caught in a no-win situation. He had actually gone to New York, interviewed Shober's business partners, and was told that Shober had been fired because he was a failure in every business venture he undertook. Cameron came back and informed the Board of his findings, but like my own experience when I returned with my information about Cameron, the next thing he knew, Shober had been selected as President. Such is the irony of fate that amuses herself by allowing a coincidence to seem like poetic justice.

Seeking to rescue the situation, I went on to try to make Shober look better than he was. I said that the greatness of an academic institution's president resides more in his ability to raise money than his academic and research prowess. This approach also did not ride well, and I hurriedly sat down wishing I could evaporate without leaving a residue.

It didn't take long for Shober to settle in. As soon as he took over Cameron's office, he hired new secretaries and several publicity agents whose sole purpose was apparently to build up his image and enhance his money raising capacity. Cameron moved down the hall to an unkempt storage room. He was able to keep a secretary, but she was at a distance because she didn't fit in the restricted space. Shober thus began the expedient process of eliminating his predecessor as his first step in a broader plan. For all practical purposes, Cameron no longer existed.

Whatever Shober's deficiencies, the ability to run an office was not one of them. He soon had secretaries humming, coming in early, and working into the evenings. He held daily meetings of the staff that included mainly Paxson, Holmes, Moyer, and MacArthur, the contemporary financial officer. Paxson soon became the butt of everything that went wrong—abetted by Holmes who had a grandiose solution for every problem. Moyer usually had a dissenting opinion to Holmes' views, and there was a continual crossing of swords. MacArthur (whose first name was Douglas; no relation to the famous general) was a patient and resourceful soul. He did his best to contain Shober's spendthrift ways. I'm sure he would have been fired had he not had Krekstein's complete confidence.

No one could claim that Shober was not completely dedicated and motivated in his work. Having failed in so many other endeavors, he was determined to succeed in this one. The trouble was that he lacked the experience and the sagacity that are acquired only by patient, prolonged study. In essence, Shober was a gambler. He plunged into major decisions with the reckless ardor of a steeplechase rider. Without doubt the most exuberant and ridiculous of his many misadventures was the carbon dioxide therapy (CDT) of opiate addiction. None of the many stories he told about how he became interested in opiate addiction seem plausible. He somehow came under the influence of a Dr. Albert A. LaVerne, a New York psychiatrist whose oddball therapy for treating alcohol and opiate addiction involved inhalation of 30 percent carbon dioxide administered by facemask until the subject became unconscious. While the subject had vivid dreams and entered a semiconscious state, the therapist gave a suggestive talk intended to reinforce the subject's conviction to cure his addiction. The claim for this therapy was that it enabled an addict to stop taking his drug cold turkey—without going through the debilitating, painful symptoms of withdrawal.

CDT was actually introduced in the early 1950s by a reputable clinical investigator, J. T. Meduna, who had to admit after careful study that it was ineffective. Other clinicians who tried the CDT therapy also confirmed its lack of therapeutic value and pointed out its potential toxic effects and disadvantages. The scientific basis for the therapy was obscure, and most qualified investigators considered CDT akin to quackery. This did not prevent offbeat physicians, however, from exploiting CDT for every ailment of the nervous system.

Without any visible experience, without any qualifying degree or training, Shober set himself up as a principle investigator of a CDT project to cure opiate addiction in humans—to the horrified dread of faculty and staff of a reputable medical school and fully accredited, nearly 125-year-old hospital. The project could not have been more wrong from a scientific, social, and ethical point of view. Why was it allowed to happen? Shober was smart enough, and on consultation with his personal lawyer, to set up a medical supervisory group. He first consulted VanBuren O. Hammett, the distinguished Chairman of the Psychiatry Department, who told Shober in no uncertain terms that CDT was unproven, unsafe, and certain to lead to disaster for Hahnemann. Not in the least dismayed, Shober turned to Holmes for support, which he got in spades. Holmes gave his unqualified blessing to the project and promised a whole hospital ward for this purpose, much to Paxson's dismay because the project was unfunded and most addicts were penniless.

Moyer was consulted next, but he was cagier. He offered to do some investigation before he would give an opinion. He sent his protege, Lewis Mills, to New York to view LaVerne's therapy first hand. Mills was a young, competent physician and investigator whom Moyer had brought to Philadelphia from Texas as his right hand man in the Department of Medicine. Mills was therefore subservient to Moyer and lacked the backbone to make a decision that should have been obvious. He came back from New York, reported that he was impressed, and said there was promise in the further investigation of CDT. That's all Moyer needed to override the faculty's negative opinion. But he shrewdly avoided direct responsibility for the medical and scientific aspects of the project by putting Mills in direct charge. Mills had no genuine interest in this haphazard research and was certainly no match for the domineering Vice President Holmes, much less the reckless President Shober. Besides being the poor fall guy, Mills had lost any respect the faculty and staff might have had for him. Most were after his scalp.

Shober now ran amok. Convinced that he had a sure winner and jubilant that he'd foiled an entire medical school faculty, he plunged ahead—without any funding—into what was a very expensive research project. Thirty hospital beds were occupied for weeks by non-paying patients who received expensive medical attention free of charge. The recruited addicts were most cooperative. They had never had such good food and lodging. They were getting their drugs smuggled in by their buddies. Shober made rounds every day and was extremely impressed with the favorable response. Nearly all the subjects claimed that their craving for drugs was disappearing and they weren't suffering withdrawal symptoms.

Not satisfied with the usual grant application to the National Institutes of Health (NIH), Shober started a publicity and lobbying campaign. Articles in the local Philadelphia papers were not completely laudatory but did attract attention. Weekly lunches were held in the Board Room, and prominent city officials and other dignitaries were invited to a three ring circus show with Shober as the ringmaster and selected addicts as the dancing bears. Trips were made to Washington to influence legislators to favor the grant application for a large-scale study. Shober persisted despite the universal protest of faculty, alumni, and friendly supporters.

To everyone's dismay, a site visit team from NIH was favorably impressed, probably under political pressure and the rumor was that the CDT project was about to be funded to the tune of over $1million over a three-year period.

Shober didn't bother with me during this initial period. Apparently he considered the Dean an academic nobody, little more than a gopher. But he was intensely interested in the medical school admissions process. He called me to his office one day to explain to me his plans for solving Hahnemann's financial problems.

"Joe," he began without the flicker of an eyelid, "I understand that we have six thousand applicants for the 150 students we take in each year. With such a pool, it should be possible to charge at least $100,000 for each candidate for admission, which would generate at least $10 million in new money annually."

I was astounded at the naiveté and lack of ethics of his statement. I imagined that he must be joking, but I hastily replied, "Wharty, you're not the first to think of this nifty idea. In Japan, I understand that some smaller private medical schools do charge $40,000 for admission. However, in this country it's considered unethical. We would lose our accreditation and might even be put in jail."

I went on to explain how the AAMC-AMA Liason Committee and the State Board of Education scrutinized the admissions process. To insure our absolute credibility, I had streamlined the admissions process and computerized it so that every applicant would have an equal chance. Furthermore, I had hired the best talent to manage admissions. Robert J. Boerner, Assistant Dean for Admissions, was nationally recognized for his work in this field. William C. Kashatus, the faculty Chairman of the duly appointed Admissions Committee, was a distinguished pathologist, a member of our faculty, and an alumnus. There were no selected lists, no discrimination as to race or sex. Applicants were admitted purely on their academic records in college, their scores on the Medical Aptitude test, recommendations, and the interview. Historically, Hahnemann in the early 1940s had nearly lost its accreditation because of dubious admissions practices. In the recent past, a prominent state senator had held up our state appropriation because we refused to admit a candidate he had recommended. Our above-board admissions procedures fortunately saved the day, and the irate senator had to recant.

Shober listened with a strained expression to my explanations. It was obvious that he considered me an obstructionist who had to be bypassed. Consequently, I didn't go on to tell him that, in fact, our admissions process, like all medical schools, was under inspection by the federal government and the Pennsylvania State Relations Committee. In 1968-69, student riots and confrontations in most colleges resulted in the formation of the Students for a Democratic Society (SDS). Many faculty were sympathetic with the movement to make educational opportunities more democratic. I was subjected to a confrontation of pigtailed, sandal-wearing, uncouth medical students who sat in my office with definite demands. The most prominent request was that the medical school admit African Americans as 30 percent of the class. No amount of explanation would appease them. They only left my office on my solemn promise that I would do my best to expedite their request. I learned later that the other medical school deans had been similarly confronted. Subsequently, deans of all the medical schools in Pennsylvania met frequently on this problem and eventually each school developed its own special program. Hahnemann did eventually develop an effective program that greatly enhanced the admission of minority students.

Shober finally cut me short by saying, "Despite your objections, I must have a political list and will deal directly with Boerner and Kashatus (Chairman of the Admissions Committee). I will send you memos about my actions, and you will deal with them accordingly."

The conversation was over. As I left his office, I knew that my days at Hahnemann were numbered. I felt a disturbing pain in the pit of my stomach and rushed to my office to find some antacid tablets. I immediately called in Boerner and Kashatus who fortunately understood the dilemma and promised to launder any selective lists and maintain the integrity of the admissions process.

Shober went right ahead with his political contacts and practically promised a place in the entering class for any applicant they might recommend. He wrote memos to Boerner and me, mentioning candidates and political figures by name. These indiscreet memos were carried open-faced in the elevators so that anyone could read them. This really created an extremely antagonistic atmosphere against Shober by faculty, staff, and students. Hallway and backroom conferences soon formed with the common focus that this arrogant, uncouth president must be eliminated.

As predicted, the CDT program got completely out of control. There was no adequate medical and scientific supervision. Patient addicts came and went as they pleased. It appeared that no one cared about the project except Shober who seemed pleased by its superficial success. To everyone's surprise and dismay, a rumor circulated that the project was apparently going to be funded by NIH to the tune of more than a $1 million for a three-year period. This alarmed me because anyone who had any experience with the treatment of narcotic addicts knew that the CDT project, as planned to be carried out at Hahnemann, was already a disaster waiting to become a catastrophe. It might well close the institution.

Without telling anyone, I decided to do what I could to bring an end to the project. It was already a serious financial drain. If outside funding were not available, it would have to be terminated. I knew William R. Martin, M.D., the Chief of the Addiction Research Center at the National Institute of Mental Health in Washington. He was author of the chapter on drug addiction in the pharmacology textbook that I'd edited. A distinguished clinician and scientist, Martin was recognized as an expert in drug addiction problems. I called him up and pleaded with him not to fund the project. I made the argument that it was so poorly managed and the scientific basis so tenuous that it was certain to end up as an embarrassment to the government and to Hahnemann. He seemed to agree with me, but I surmised that he must have had strong political pressure to fund the project. Shober had done his work well. I could only wish that he would exert the same energy to support other, more worthy projects. Events that shortly followed my phone call actually sealed the doom of the CDT project.

Ronald Brown, a young black patient who had a severe opiate addiction, was being aggressively treated by the CDT method. Resting quietly in bed at 6 a.m. with normal vital signs, he was found dead at 7:10 a.m. An attending physician, probably a resident, was called. He signed Brown out as, "Cause of death due to head injury with narcotic withdrawal symptoms as a contributing factor." This might be a reasonable diagnosis—except that there were no clinical signs of head injury and no observations of withdrawal symptoms, such as trashing about that could have caused a head injury. An autopsy performed by the chief medical examiner, Marvin E. Aronson, M.D., found no evidence of head injury. Brown had received several CDT treatments just prior to his death, but the details are obscure. Did he die as a result of this treatment? Several years prior to the Brown episode, two women in Maryland had died under similar circumstances, and the physician in charge was indicted by a Grand Jury. Although the involved physician was later declared innocent, these deaths were one of the important reasons why CDT was considered dangerous as well as ineffective.

My own conjecture about the Brown case is that he was having severe withdrawal symptoms, the CDT treatments were not giving any relief, and he somehow was able to secure some heroin and accidentally gave himself an overdose. Certainly this is one of the frequent causes of death in severe addictions. The nursing and medical attendance in the narcotics ward were sloppy, and this was also the opinion of the Pennsylvania Medical Society which investigated the Brown case.

This unsavory episode would probably have gotten little attention in the press if Brown had not already attained media notoriety. In a previous opiate binge about a year before his death, he'd been sent for rehabilitation to Gaudenzia House in West Chester where he met another patient, Fawn Pitcairn, heiress to the Bryn Athyn Pitcairns. The two fell in love in an atmosphere characterized as definitely Romeo and Juliet by the resourceful media. Both families were violently opposed to the marriage, which took place notwithstanding. Aside from this romanticized angle, the marriage of a black man to a wealthy white socialite created at the time a mighty stir of emotions fanned by the media. Apparently cured of their addiction, the couple moved to a modest apartment in Northeast Philadelphia where they made a modest living as animal groomers. They didn't live happily ever after, for Brown again became addicted and made the fatal mistake of entering Shober's CDT program. He ended up very dead, signed out as a, "therapeutic misadventure."

Shober shrugged off the bad publicity and boldly continued on as if nothing had happened. He simply hired more agents to brighten and sweeten his name. Another fatality finally put a quietus to the CDT project. Morris N. Kallen Jr., another opiate addict was receiving CDT treatments at Hahnemann on an ambulatory basis. He had a room at the nearby Philadelphia Hotel where, without medical supervision, he was apparently getting more and more addicted despite the CDT treatments. One night after receiving a shot of methadone (a synthetic opiate), he died suddenly. This second death attracted another flood of unfavorable media attention that lead to an investigation by First Assistant District Attorney Richard Sprague who charged Hahnemann with, "medical huckstering." The matter was smoothed over by the powerful law firm of Obermeyer, Maxwell and Hippel. Soon after Hahnemann quietly announced that the CDT program was terminated by a lack of funds.

I managed to stay clear of the whole CDT incident. As far as my knowledge goes, no one suspected that I may have had a hand in preventing federal money from flowing to Hahnemann. Nevertheless, all the good work I had done as Dean in the previous four years was being destroyed by Shober and the reorganization that had he forced. John Moyer, now in charge of all academic activities, made Wilbur Oaks the acting head of the Department of Medicine, while he moved his office next to mine and took over the sorely needed conference room. I welcomed Moyer and promised cooperation, but inwardly I knew that our relationship could never work for me or indeed for Moyer. Psychologically Moyer was in a no-win position because he was forced to be loyal to Shober, while he had his own agenda to take over the governance of the institution. He had to have a substantial base of support to achieve his goal. This could be the faculty and staff, but they hated and mistrusted him. Meanwhile, his previously loyal, large powerful department of medicine was glad to escape his yoke once he moved out of direct control. His Board support could only flow through Cameron, but Shober soon rendered this worthy supporter inoperative. With a very competent secretary and a new recruit, Earnest Kuhinka, Ph.D., Moyer began to set up a paper empire of grandiose programs and objectives that had no real prospect of realization. Every department had to submit an organizational chart with projections of their objectives. Moyer personally revised and modified these charts. He set up numerous committees outside those established by the bylaws and completely ignored College Council. Perhaps his biggest hope was to organize a School of Continuing Education, which would put Hahnemann on the map.

Moyer considerably eroded the position of Dean. If the situation continued, the Dean would be nothing more than a lackey to the Vice President for Academic affairs, which is probably what Cameron had anticipated when he made the organizational recommendation to Shober. As it happened, I retained considerable power politically because the faculty remained faithful to me in this time of crisis and looked to me to lead them in the effort to get rid of both Shober and Moyer. This was obviously an untenable position for me, and it had serious emotional conflicts that resulted in anxiety, nervousness, depression, insomnia, and even compulsive behavior.

By prodigious effort, I'd managed to get the medical school accredited for a seven-year period (the maximum) by the Liaison Committee of the AMA and the AAMC. Then only two years later, the faculty contacted the Liaison Committee to visit Hahnemann again in the anticipation that this would discredit Shober and hopefully force his resignation. This alone would cause deep, acute depression to a conscientious Dean. My commitment to the worthy faculty I'd recruited was even more serious. Two of the most important were Evangelos T. Angelakos, Chairman of Physiology, and Thomas M. Devlin, Chairman of Biochemistry. The loss of control of the budget and finances of the medical school would mean that I could not fulfill my promises to them and to others whose departments I'd anticipated needed help and development.

To make matters worse, Moyer made overtures to Deufel, my financial officer. Claiming that he did not want to work for Moyer, he boldly told me that he was going to desert the Dean's Office and work for Shober. He claimed that he could help the school more by being at the source of decision making. It didn't turn out that way. Shober was having trouble with his marriage and had hot pants for Deufel's secretary, a beautiful, shapely redhead. The poor girl had ulcerative colitis, and Shober's attention so disturbed her that she had to have a colostomy. Deufel did not fare any better. Shober got rid of him in a few months. My only consolation was that Bob Walker remained faithful to the school and me. With his help, I was able to recruit Frank J. Bachich who eventfully made a superb financial officer. I turned to my family for solace and their understanding and devotion kept me in a reasonable degree of sanity.

I decided to put the Deaning business out of my mind at least during those hours that were my own. This was Charlie Paxson's advice, and he had equal and even greater problems than I had. "When you leave the office at the end of the day, put all your problems aside and just concentrate on your own interests," he'd said. This was excellent advice but not easy to follow, especially when Moyer would call in the evening and engage in a lengthy, emotional conversation about a problem that had no realistic solution. I tried nevertheless to engage in absorbing, intricate pursuits so that my body and brain could use up all the adrenaline that I'd built up during the day. One particularly helpful avenue was the building of an authentic scale model of "The Bounty," the ship of the famous mutiny. The intricacies of the rigging and other minute details involved many hours of patient work. These were capable of solutions that seemed to ease the pain of my professional problems, which could not be solved satisfactorily.

I had little doubt that sooner or later Shober was going to fire me. I sensed that he felt that I was collaborating with those on the faculty who were running a campaign to oust him. Moyer was also unhappy with me because he couldn't seem to gain the confidence of the faculty, and he imagined that I was partly to blame. When a new management team takes over, it appears that they're suspicious of remaining administrators who had a modicum of success in the past. They feel that they are being compared to past accomplishments and customs, and their instinct is to eliminate the obstructing person and make a completely fresh start with their own ideas and fancies.

This air of suspicion and mistrust was augmented by the bizarre, mysterious appearance of poison pen letters that were very ingeniously written and extremely critical of Shober, Holmes, and to a minor extent Moyer. I was not mentioned in any of the early letters, and this cast some suspicion on me as a likely contributor. To make matters worse, the letters were printed and the envelopes addressed by a type and form that was familiar to the institution. Everyone was therefore convinced that a member of the faculty or administration was supplying the author of the scandalous missiles with pertinent juicy information from the institution's inner sanctum. The letters were signed, "The Hahnemann Faculty Committee of Nine."

Despite much amateur and professional detective work, the individuals' identity was never discovered. The style and characteristics of the writing changed with time, so it was assumed that different individuals did the actual writing and editing. The letters were extremely damaging to Hahnemann's morale, self-esteem, and especially to its reputation in the academic and medical world. They were mailed to every possible interested party, including faculty, students, and administration of Hahnemann, the AAMC, the AMA, other medical schools, affiliated hospitals, state and federal officials, and naturally all possible news media.

Indeed hardly a day passed without some lurid story appearing in the Philadelphia newspapers, *The Bulletin* and *The Inquirer*. Shober became a notorious character, hounded by reporters who sensed a story in his every move. Strangely, Shober seemed to enjoy the publicity. Some people suspected that he had even planted the poison pen letters himself. Notwithstanding all this unfavorable activity, which must have deteriorated Hahnemann's already shaky position with the banks, the Board of Trustees stood steadfastly behind Shober. He continued in his usual fashion to conceive and initiate new ventures almost every day.

It was obvious to me that I was in a no-win situation. Life as a Dean at Hahnemann had become unbearable. The faculty called for frequent meetings at which I could give no reasonable explanation for what was going on in the administration. Moyer was of no help because he was not trusted. All I could do was follow the bylaws religiously and allow each individual to air his thoughts and complaints in a reasonable manner. To insure compliance, I appointed Charles A. Snipes, an Associate Professor of Physiology, as parliamentarian. For unknown reasons, he had an extraordinary knowledge of parliamentary procedures and wasn't afraid to use it. He saved the day for me on many an occasion when unruly faculty members wanted to push through some resolution that was impractical and out-of-order. These meetings were so tension-filled and so consuming of time and energy that they not only gave me ulcers, but also prevented me from pursuing what little research and teaching I had been able to accomplish in addition to my deaning duties.

I felt trapped. My age was now fifty-six, which my experience on search committees indicated was too old to be attractive to prospective employers. In spite of this all too evident disadvantage, and certain that I would be fired soon, I determined to make an earnest effort to secure a full-time job in another institution. I'd retained my medical license and membership in the Philadelphia County Medical Society and the AMA. The most practical, feasible escape from Hahnemann would be to return to the practice of medicine where I could make a decent living and have much calmer living conditions. Since I retained my professorship, I probably would be allowed to return to the pharmacology department but at a much-reduced salary. An ex-Dean is rarely welcome in his former department, particularly when he was originally the former chairman. In weighing these considerations, I chose first to try to gain a high administrative position and keep the return to medical practice as a retreat position.

In retrospect, my experiences in seeking a high level administrative position were revealing and instructive, but at the time they were most depressing to my ego. I naturally contacted all my friends and related my difficulties. They were most sympathetic and solicitous. Very few had any decent opportunities to offer me, although I knew that some did have influence on search committees for important jobs. My best chance was at my alma mater, The Long Island College of Medicine, which had since become state-supported and part of the University of the State of New York, known as SUNY Downstate. It now had a magnificent academic building and a university hospital located across the street from Kings County Hospital. The medical school needed a new Dean and was considering candidates. Chandler Brooks the Chairman of Physiology was Acting Dean and definitely did not want the job. When I contacted Brooks, he was most encouraging and promised to help me in every way in his power. My old buddy Julius Stolfi was medical director of the University Hospital and volunteered to help me. So I put my hat in the ring and submitted my CV, plus the names of several Deans who knew me and were probably disposed to a favorable recommendation. Kellow was now well established at Jefferson, had little to offer, but was looking for me. I put out feelers for a new medical school in Louisiana and even some other more dubious opportunities. I did not go so far as answering ads in the science and education journals, nor did I hire an agent. The later endeavors are seldom productive, but I suppose it was mostly my ego that prevented me from descending to the level of begging for a job.

I waited, but no phone calls or letters came to offer me a means of escape. The situation at Hahnemann meanwhile grew worse with each passing day. Most of the better chairmen were also looking for other positions. Guilio Barbero, the Chair of Pediatrics and a world-class researcher and scientist whom I'd recruited with great difficulty, announced his resignation. He was made Chairman of Pediatrics at the University of Missouri School of Medicine, a new state-supported institution, at a much higher salary and department budget. At Jefferson, Kellow snatched Jewell L. Osterholm, our Chief of Neurosurgery who was gaining a national reputation for his work on spinal cord injury. These were the most prominent of the growing exit crowd.

Other faculty who took matters too seriously became ill and unduly depressed. There were increased requests for sick leaves and sabbaticals. Van Buren O. Hammett, the Chairman of the Department of Psychiatry, had a very severe heart attack that most believed was precipitated by his intense arguments with Shober over the CDT program. The amount of antacids consumed by the faculty and staff during this period would have made an interesting study. Student agitation and demands became excessive. It took all of Bennett's skill and patience to prevent a general uprising. Each day the poison pen letters grew more insidious and aggravating. The Philadelphia newspapers took turns publishing lurid, detailed articles of the goings-on at Hahnemann. A very damaging article appeared in the November 1973 *Philadelphia* magazine entitled, "What's Festering at Hahnemann" with the subtitle, "Behind the sterile hospital façade, the germs of controversy keep spreading."

Who was talking and informing the media? It had to be a faculty member or administrator, but even with my access to most staff, neither I nor anyone else ever found out. I had my suspicions, of course, but in the absence of definitive proof I had to keep any suppositions to myself. I was indeed happy that I did not know because, if I did, it was my duty to report it to Shober and the Board. Now that I'd made my decision to leave Hahnemann, I became bolder and more open in my opposition to Shober's practices. At the next meeting of the Academic Committee of the Board, I made clear, unmistakable complaints about Shober's disregard of the faculty bylaws and his desire to bypass the precautions that had been instituted to safeguard the admissions process to medical school. I no longer recall the exact composition of the committee, but I distinctly recall one member, Charles Hollis, for his immediate and emotional unfavorable response to my statements. Hollis was a retired head of otolaryngology and an alumnus. Why he was on the Board was unknown. Certainly he was not an alumni representative because his fellow alumni had quarreled with him and ousted him from the local group. He'd been on the committee that had finally rubber stamped Shober and was a member of the First Troop of Philadelphia—two items that probably made him a confidant of Shober who was hungry for any kind of professional support. Other members of the committee seemed to have some sympathy for my statements, but there was no clearly favorable comment. It was obvious that the matter would be allowed to fade away without any definite action. I'm sure Hollis ran to Shober and informed him that I must be one of the perpetrators of the growing faculty and staff opposition.

Not unexpectedly, the next morning I received an urgent message to visit Shober's office. I was ushered in without ceremony. Grim faced, Shober was sitting behind his desk. Donald T. Brophy, a fairly recent member of the Board, sat to one side of him. There was no formal greeting that certainly was due a senior member of the faculty of twenty years, the last five of which were spent as Dean. Shober came right to the point, "Mr. Brophy is a member of a Board Committee which oversees the performance of the executive officers of the corporation. He has some serious information for you."

Brophy looked somewhat uncomfortable. At least he had a college education and some graduate work and might be expected to have some respect for scholarly achievement. With some hesitation he said, "Mr. Shober and the Board recognize your good accomplishments, but apparently you have views contrary to those of the president of the corporation. It is untenable that the president can function without the full, uncompromised support of every faculty and staff person in his effort to rescue the institution from its financial and academic failures. The Board is asking you to step down as Dean. You may return to your department as a full professor, provided that you no longer utter any statement or action that is contrary to the policies of the corporation. There will be a reduction in salary, which will be consistent with the rank and years of service to the institution. We hope you will find it possible to stay at Hahnemann and continue your teaching and scientific work."

I managed an ironic smile and looked them both in the eye. "I agree with you that the situation has become impossible. I must thank both of you for making it possible for me to leave the institution, to which I have devoted my life, with a degree of honor. I was about to resign anyhow, deserting my faculty and students. You have solved any qualms of conscience I might have in leaving a sinking ship to its unkind fate. I shall vacate the Dean's office tomorrow and return to my department. After I have completed my research and teaching obligations, which should be by the end of the semester, the institution will be rid of me completely."

They seemed somewhat surprised at my reaction but said nothing. I bowed my head to each of them, turned on my heel, and left the room.

Returning to my office in a somewhat dazed condition, I could think only of the final thought of Anna Karenina in the famous novel of the same name by Leo Tolstoy. As she was about to commit suicide by jumping in front of an approaching train, with its puffing steam, her sole reflection was, "So this is how it all ends." But my situation wasn't over yet.

An ever active secretarial rumor machine began its work immediately. Within the hour, the entire faculty and staff knew that their Dean had been fired. An emergency faculty meeting was called for four o'clock that day. The bylaws called for a wait of ten days after a petition signed by ten members, but they had a petition signed by over 100 and wanted immediate action. Shober was urgently requested to attend the meeting.

The meeting was held in the newly constructed college building's Geary Auditorium that held 630 persons comfortably.

Ordinarily only sixty to seventy-five faculty attended regular faculty meetings held in a lecture hall that accommodated about 100 people so that the impression of lack of interest by poor attendance would be minimized. To my surprise, at least 300 faculty came to the Geary, and it did not look at all empty. This turnout was extraordinary because we had a total faculty of 400, of whom at least quarters were in distant affiliate hospitals. The atmosphere was tense and urgent, which was extraordinary for an academic faculty. Looking over the assembled group more carefully, I noted that all the basic science people were there, which was not unusual, but the good representation of clinical professors was uncommon. Many were from the psychiatry department, whom I surmised were there because of their resentment of the CDT program. Even some eminent surgeons were present, which was amazing considering that I had never known them to attend a faculty meeting before.

This is going to be an interesting meeting, I said to myself, not sure whether it actually was about me or Shober's indiscretions and mismanagements. The chairman of the meeting, a distinguished senior faculty member, soon solved any misconceptions with the brief announcement that the special meeting was called to get an explanation of why the Dean had been fired. It was going to be an open meeting, and Shober had agreed to answer any question.

The President came in alone without any supporting Board of Trustee member. He had a rather jaunty step and confident smile. Striding up to the stage, he assumed a central position and made an inquiring gesture to the Chairman. I don't remember the exact words, but the Chairman turned to Shober and stated, "Mr. President, we the faculty and staff are extremely dissatisfied with your performance. We are going to convey our displeasure to the Board of Trustees and, if appropriate action is not taken, we will take what steps are necessary. In particular, your abrupt and unconsidered action of dismissing the Dean, who by all measures has performed splendidly under adverse circumstances, is of deep concern to all members of the faculty and staff. Can you explain your action in this matter?"

Shober was visibly shaken by the menacing, angry attitude of the group, but he asserted his authority.

"Ladies and gentlemen, Dr. DiPalma is a kindly and knowledgeable academic dean who has done a credible job. However, DiPalma is in an executive position and must answer to the President. His views and attitudes are not in line with the forward progress that the Board and I have planned for the institution. His academic position as Professor of Pharmacology is not in question, and he will return to his teaching and research duties which he performs so well."

As he finished his statement, the entire audience rose to its feet in unison as if it were a military movement. This gesture made an abrupt noise—not quite the shot of a cannon, but more like a heavy crate dropped on the floor. This was followed by a moment of silence. Then again in perfect unison, every person in the auditorium uttered a single word.

A simple and effective "NO" was exclaimed as if it were a clap of thunder. Shober was stunned. His jaw dropped. He looked around as if to seek a ready exit.

To tell the truth, I was astounded at this demonstration. Having some experience with student confrontations, I surmised that an extraordinary amount of effort and planning must have gone into this one, certainly unusual in an academic faculty. I wondered if professional student agitators coached them.

Whatever else he was, Shober was no shrinking violet. Under ordinary circumstances he probably would tell the assembled group to go fly a kite. He was the President and had the support of the Board, and he was going to do what he wanted. The CDT program's disastrous failure and the devastating publicity engendered by the poison pen letters, combined with the exit of several key faculty and the worsening financial position, gave him pause, however. He knew that without the support of the faculty and staff, he could not succeed. While the Board might support him, it was a weak lot and would collapse when the situation worsened.

"Well! I didn't know that Dr. DiPalma was so popular," he said with a smile. "Perhaps I've misjudged the situation. I'm going to reinstate him with the understanding that he will support me in my efforts to make Hahnemann one of the best medical schools in the nation." With that statement the audience applauded loudly and long and then gradually sat down. For the first time since he had taken over at Hahnemann, Shober received applause for something he did right.

Shober walked out with a stride of confidence and the meeting soon broke up. Many of the faculty came up to me to congratulate me and pledge their continued support. For me emotionally, this had been my finest hour. To have such enthusiastic support from the faculty is every Dean's wish but seldom achieved in the real world of academia.

After a night's sleep and some sober reflection, I was not so sure that I had ended up ahead of the game. If no protest had been made and the dismissal held, the reasonable probability was that I would have quit academic life and returned to the practice of medicine. I still had a good fifteen years left to exploit my already proven ability to be a good and successful physician. Financially, it was certain that I would end up much ahead of any academic position that I might be able to secure. I was indeed now more trapped than before because, if I decided to quit Hahnemann, I would be deserting a loyal faculty. So it was with considerable reluctance that I accepted an invitation the next day to have lunch with Shober. I knew only too well what this was going to mean. Shober would try and win my confidence and use my influence to get faculty and alumni support for various money-raising schemes.

At the luncheon he explained that he was not a vindictive man. I didn't know what this meant in reference to me. Did he suspect that I was behind the poison pen letters? I was sure that he'd made a thorough investigation and had hired a private investigator. If there was a distinct link to me, it would have been found. I concluded that he had a mild case of paranoia and was trying to explain that he did not take revenge on his enemies.

Then he brought up the subject of admissions to medical school. He again insisted on a political list and favoring of candidates who might result in substantial gain to the institution. I patiently tried to explain to him what could and could not be done. I finally agreed to handle personally the difficult cases and attempt to find means of eventually helping them gain admission. I had in mind getting the graduate school to admit a small number of these candidates as non-matriculated students so that they could take courses alongside the regular students. This would let them and the faculty find out if they could do medical school level work.

Shober next confided that he had two projects that could use my support and help. One was helping Wilbur Oaks, now Chairman of Medicine, get financing for a project aimed at producing more family physicians for rural communities, especially the Wilkes-Barre area of Pennsylvania. The other was to help acquire space and financing for a Cancer Institute to be headed by Izadore Brodsky, the Division Director of Hematology and Oncology in the Department of Medicine. Both projects were first line, and I was happy to agree to do my best to get them off the ground. In fact, I had already been at work with both individuals in planning and exploring possibilities. Shober and I parted with a friendly handshake and promised to lunch together at least once weekly in the future. I returned to my office relieved, but I knew down deep that my troubles were only starting and that I must spend more time and effort putting out fires. Shober would not change. He had a talent for the creation of crises and calamities.

Nothing had changed. Hahnemann was still an under-financed medical school and hospital trying to compete for the academic and healthcare dollar in an atmosphere of extreme competition in a city with too many first-class facilities. Trying to ride high on the national wave of increased support for medical education and research was precarious. Would Shober be able to raise money for the badly needed new hospital and for expansion of the research effort?

Despite all the troubles of the Deaning business, I managed to continue to lecture and maintain my textbook and other writing. A number of interesting opportunities came my way. The Walter Read Army Institute of Research (WRAIR) was doing advanced research on the chemotherapy of malaria, which became an important military problem because of the Vietnam War. Our soldiers were subject to infection with falciparum malaria which had become resistant to the main effective drug, chloroquine. New agents needed to be developed to be effective against this strain of malaria. I was asked to become a member of a consultant panel that reviewed the progress being made and make suggestions to facilitate the work. I accepted with pleasure and had a very instructive experience attending the several all day meetings each year. The honorarium was small, but travel and motel expenses were paid. My wife got to visit all the museums and other attractions in Washington. I doubt that I contributed very much, but the program itself did develop a number of effective drugs, such as mefloquine and halofantrine that proved useful in subsequent years. The very successful control of malarial infection during the Vietnam War was one of the laudable operations seldom mentioned by the media. The research work done by the WRAIR group and the lessons learned saved many lives and continues to do so even today.

One of the spin-offs of my work with WRAIR was my meeting and becoming friends with a young Army Officer, Stephen DeFelice, who was doing his tour of duty required of every physician in those years. Because his post-graduate training included experience in the drug industry and drug development, he had been able to secure a post at WRAIR instead of the usual physician's duty with an operative unit in the field. DeFelice had a distinct Italian temperament with a keen sense for good food, fine wine, and luscious women. He was a lover of opera and knew most of the singers and arias. While attending medical school, he'd sharpened his talent by being an opera critic for the local papers.

DeFelice was not a natural researcher, but he had an inquisitive turn of mind. His instincts led him in the direction of finding uses for agents that others found interesting but not therapeutically useful. While doing a fellowship in endocrinology early in his career, he found that carnitine (a non-protein amino acid that the body synthesizes) was helpful in alleviating the symptoms of hyperthyroidism. This led to a lifelong interest in developing carnitine for other uses. While he was at WRAIR, he met a Major

Vick who was a physiologist working with a heart-lung preparation that could be adjusted to mimic heart failure. Sure enough, Vick and DeFelice found that carnitine seemed to strengthen the failing heart-lung preparation.

After his tour of duty in the Army, DeFelice started his own firm for consulting and drug development. He was able to convince an Italian drug company, Sigma Tau, to study carnitine further for clinical use, and it eventually marketed it in Italy and Europe for ischemic heart disease of various kinds. It has a fairly wide sale in these countries, and the acetyl and phenyl derivatives are marketed for various central nervous system diseases. Since carnitine was a well-known chemical entity, it could not be patented; hence, any developer of the drug would be foolish to invest large sums of money to prove its clinical usefulness. In the U.S., carnitine began to be sold in health food stores as a dietary supplement. There is little evidence that supplemental carnitine is useful for the average person. Carnitine is present in all animal and plant food. A large amount of this amino acid is in red meat, the source from which it indeed gets its name. (The Latin word for meat is *carne*.) Carnitine deficiency is known to occur in only one animal species, the common meal worm. If its diet is deficient in carnitine, the meal worm grows enormously fat and literally drowns in its own oil. Carnitine is essential for transport of fatty acids across the mitochondrial membrane. A deficiency of carnitine will result in fat accumulation inside the cell inhibiting many other types of essential metabolisms.

While DeFelice used me as a consultant in other drug programs, my real interest was in experimental laboratory and clinical research. My animal investigation of the acute effects of carnitine on the cardiovascular system, done with graduate student Dave Ritchie and my old colleague Bob McMichaels, showed that it did indeed have a tonic effect that increased cardiac output. This was possibly due to the vasodilation, but it also probably caused a release of adrenaline, that might explain its cardiotonic actions. It was unlikely that such acute effects were induced by the metabolic actions of carnitine. Rather, these cardiovacular effects were the result of the large pharmacological doses employed. In any case, the cardiovasular effects of carnitine have not proven to be useful. Carnitine would have died as a useful drug in this country had it not been for the persistence of DeFelice.

New legislation established an Orphan Drug Program under the control of the FDA. DeFelice took advantage of this program, and Sigma Tau was able to develop carnitine economically for primary carnitine deficiency, a rare genetic defect. The public would benefit by having a treatment for a rare disorder; the company would gain seven years of exclusivity that might allow it to find a more profitable use for the drug. Secondary carnitine deficiency occurs in a number of diseases, but is not always helped by carnitine administration. Some evidence indicates that premature babies and infants who fail to thrive may benefit from carnitine. The one form of secondary carnitine deficiency that is helped with some consistency is that which occurs with end-stage renal disease where dialysis must be used. The dialysis depletes the body of carnitine, and the individual suffers muscle aches, fatigue, and weakness. Here carnitine is given intravenously after each dialysis therapy.

I have given the details of carnitine's development into a successful drug because I've been able to follow it first hand from its original inception. It is also illustrative of the many difficulties encountered in the attempt to develop a useful therapeutic agent. Chances of finding an entirely new and useful therapeutic entity, even with the best of preparation and resources, are extremely small. Those who dedicate themselves to the search and development of new agents, however, have just as much adventure and moments of despair and exaltation as those who explore new seas and lands or those who hunt for gold and diamonds.

Despite the travails of the Deanship, my scientific work, writing, and teaching duties, I was still able to devote a good deal of my time to my family. The five girls were quite a bundle. They had reached the age when most conflicts and depression occur. Four of them were in college at the same time. I was grateful that my wife and I had scrounged for years to put aside money for their education.

Maria had continued with her music lessons in the flute, piano, and especially voice. She had been fortunate enough to be accepted as a voice student by Madame Gregory, a famous opera singer who had taught several Metropolitan opera stars, among them Anna Moffo. After attending Temple University for two years for a liberal arts education, Maria decided to devote herself to a singing career. With Madame Gregory's help, she was able to enter the famous Curtis Institute of Music. The high point of Maria's musical education was a recital at Swarthmore College. I invited many of my friends and colleagues to hear Schubert's "The Shepherd on the Rock," which was performed with verve and passion. Mary and I were much impressed and were convinced that Maria was headed for a brilliant operatic career. However, this did not eventuate. Instead, Maria found her real talents resided in teaching and administration. At this writing she is Chairman of the Department of Music at Simpson College in Indianolo, Iowa. She is also on the Board of the Des Moines Metro Opera and exceptional group that has bought opera appreciation to the Midwest. I relate the following episode to demonstrate how parents get into compromising positions in the effort to push along their children's careers. Shober had a grandiose idea of raising money and generating publicity by holding a Bob Hope Gala. It was to be held at the Academy of Music in Philadelphia and be preceded by a dinner in Bob Hope's honor. By the time the plan was fully developed, Duke Ellington and his band and Hope's famous cohort Dorothy Lamour were also invited. The public may believe that personalities like Hope contribute their time and effort to a charitable affair free-of-charge, except for travel and insurance expenses. Better guess again. Hope demanded $30,000 plus expenses for a one-night stand. And a good deal of arm twisting was needed to get him to attend the dinner at which he reluctantly said a few words. The other performers had to be paid. Then there was a rental fee for the Academy and other expenses.

Big Daddy thought immediately of his talented operatic voice daughter, Maria. Here was a chance to put her on the stage at the Academy of Music with no less a personality than Bob Hope. I approached Shober with the idea, and he was agreeable. He arranged for Maria to be introduced by Hope and sing an aria. She chose the famous aria from "La Boheme" and sang it quite well. Publicity pictures were taken with Bob Hope. I doubt that it did much for Maria's career, but it put me in a position of owing Shober more allegiance.

As an aside, the affair did not raise any money despite the facts that the house was sold out and additional donations came in from faculty and friends of Hahnemann. We learned that such galas seldom raise any cash except when the star attraction gives his time and talent for free, but that is seldom the case. Performers have to make a living and must take advantage of their usually brief period of popularity.

Our number two daughter, Dorothea or Dori, had an entirely different personality from Maria. She was less self-reliant, more of a loner, inclined to have phobias, and lacked a sense of spontaneity. She did well in high school but was a slow learner. Mary insisted that she take piano lessons, which she did reluctantly. After a few years, she decided to give them up because she could not stand the prominent veins on her elderly teacher's hands. She actually had a short fifth finger, which is a significant impediment to attaining superior performance in either the piano or violin. Large well-formed hands are a vital advantage for both instruments. But Dori had a competitive urge to outperform Maria and extraordinary persistence. A couple of years later, she requested piano lessons again, which we were pleased to supply. She did relatively well and was a lead performer at the local high school.

She also became interested in the violin so I bought her a cheap instrument that she could practice on her own. The sounds of incessant scales and routine pieces were a constant irritation, even though she was relegated to a remote room. The cheap violin was constantly getting out of tune, and I was elected to bring it in for repair. This was a source of amusement among the medical students who spread the rumor that the Dean was a member of the Mafia and carried a machine gun in a violin case. To add insult to injury, I decided to bring the violin to a local violin shop next to the school on 15th Street. Two brothers who were violin repairers for the Philadelphia Orchestra owned the shop. Stupid me, I laid the cheap violins on the counter and quietly asked if anything could be done to improve its stability. The elder brother took one look at the poor instrument, raised his head to eye level, and exploded, "Take that piece of crap out of here." Thus the great Professor and Dean, who in his day had terrified thousands of medical students and saved countless lives, was aptly humbled. One might expect that the violin story would end here. Such was not the case. The extent that parents go to advance their offspring's welfare is endless.

Much to my surprise, Dori was accepted at Swarthmore College. This was unfortunate as both Dori and her parents found out later. At the time, however, we were all quite pleased because we knew that Swarthmore was an excellent college. She took the liberal arts major with a considerable sprinkling of science to please me. She unfortunately turned out to be a slow learner and soon fell behind in her studies. A chemistry course floored her, and she was asked to drop out. (Swarthmore doesn't flunk students.) We were called in and informed of Dori's failure to perform. The counselor advised taking a year's leave of absence and then returning to Swarthmore and taking a different major, one more suitable to her ability. Both Mary and I laid it in to Dori as if she had blown away her opportunity. There were hard feelings on both sides, and relations were strained for a long time. I advised Dori to seek another college where the standards of academic excellence and the competition were not so great. Stubborn Dori insisted on going back to Swarthmore, which she did after a rest period, and enrolling in the newly developed music program.

The violin now enters the scene again. Dori insisted that this was to be her major instrument. Poor old Dad now visited all the better violin shops in Philadelphia (except the one near Hahnemann) and finally bought a fairly decent violin at a reasonable price. Dori sawed away and polished her treasure with great diligence. I was glad that she was away at Swarthmore where I would not have to listen to endless hours of practice. She was doing quite well in her studies, except that she found out that she couldn't practice the violin at late hours even if she went down in the basement of her dormitory. The next semester the music building was completed and she was able to enjoy a practice room with piano to exercise her violin. Now an unkind fate stepped in and changed the course of events. One night while she went to the bathroom someone stole her precious violin. Despite a police investigation and my own detective work of visiting every nearby pawnshop, the violin was never found. A heart-to-heart talk with Dori convinced her, with great reluctance, that she should concentrate on the piano. I was not about to buy another violin, and in a practical way, pianos are considerably more difficult to steal than violins.

Dori found herself on the piano and convinced herself that she had a chance to become a professional pianist. Mary and I were quite impressed with her musical talent, but we felt that she would not be competitive with the quantity of musical talent who at an early age had already made Julliard or Curtis. On her graduation from Swarthmore, we advised Dori to go on to advanced study in music and get a masters or even a doctoral degree. She would thus qualify for a teaching career in music.

Not for Dori. She was determined to become a performing musician not withstanding her late entry into the field, her small hands, and even smaller pinkie. She engaged the services of a Madame Messena, a renown pianist and a member of the Curtis faculty, and steadfastly stuck to piano practice at least eight hours daily. She also managed to enroll in a summer course conducted by the renowned Madame Boulange for promising pianists at Fontainbleau in France. No one encouraged her to persist in her endeavor. Rather the reverse. Finally Mary and I told her that if she insisted on this course, she would have to support herself. Not in the least dismayed, Dori moved out and rented a modest apartment in the city. She got various jobs, such as a clerk in the music section of Wanamakers, a bank teller, but mostly as a waitress because she could work odd hours and part-time, which enabled her to concentrate on her music. Our last attempt to help her was to buy a fairly decent grand piano that she wanted to purchase from a friend who'd decided that a musical career was not for him. Living very modestly, she persisted for the next ten years investing the flower of her youth in music. She dressed very plainly, no make-up, wearing steel-rim glasses. We found that it was difficult to have social contact with her because she rarely called us. After long lapses, I would make a point of taking her out to lunch.

Madame Messena finally passed on. Her parting message to Dori was, "Go into computer technology. It's a growing field." After a series of piano teachers including one all the way out in Wilkes-Barre, Dori settled down slightly. We decided that it might be now appropriate to urge her to pursue some serious higher education. With the promise that we would support both her board and living expenses, she finally agreed to enroll in Temple University's music program. She wanted to major in the piano but after an audition was recommended for general music theory. It took her three and a half years to get her Master's degree, an accomplishment that many students achieve in one or at the most two. This was due in part to her insistence on studying and practicing the piano simultaneously.

Somehow she managed to get an audition with Robert Good, an eminent pianist. He felt that she had promise but not enough for him to take her on, so he relegated her to one of his better students. Dori spent one day a week in New York with a teacher who she felt could advance her technique and interpretation. Happily her persistence and dedication paid off, and Dori finally obtained teaching positions at two small schools and developed a retinue of students. She also has performed commendably in several recitals. Mary and I were so pleased that we bought a very fine Steinway piano so that we could enjoy her playing.

Joan, our number three daughter, dark-haired and dark-eyed, seemed from the first to demonstrate a characteristic Italian temperament. Happy and outgoing, she early on demonstrated empathy for fellow man. She could listen to the troubles and trials of others with concerned interest and come up with comforting, hopeful suggestions. Everyone liked Joan, and she seemed to fit into any situation. She was a good student and had as much, perhaps more, appreciation of the humanities than the sciences. She was the only one of our girls who, on the exposure to hands-on laboratory work, seemed to grasp the true nature of the experiment. Good with her hands, she easily mastered difficult procedures much to the amazement of older technicians. No slouch in music, she managed to achieve a comfortable mastery of both piano and cello. The latter instrument suited her personality for, unlike the violin's strident, fiery voice or the piano's dramatic overtones, the cello is calm and soothing. It complements other instruments but can emerge in appropriate nuances to express its own opinions.

Joan chose to go to Barnard College, then a women's school separate from its parent institution, Columbia University. I like to think that she chose Barnard because I went to Columbia, but I'm sure that the reason was because she was enamoured with New York City. She decided to be a pre-med and took many of the same courses I took years before, sitting in the same grimy wooden chairs in chemistry courses at the Havermeyer Building. Fortunately she was a good if not brilliant student and had a good time even though the course work was heavy. Playing in the Columbia University Orchestra was a great thrill and being able to see Broadway shows was neat. Of all my girls, Joan seemed to enjoy college the most, knew what she wanted to do, and fused into the social life smoothly and without conflict. No doubt there were romantic interludes, but she remained unencumbered.

Her main goal of getting into medical school dominated her mind and spirit. Her peers knew that her father was the Dean of a medical school and subjected her to much kidding about her chances. She took this joshing with good humor, but she decided not to attend Hahnemann because it might be surmised that her father had helped her get in and would see to it that she passed all her courses. Noble soul, she chose Jefferson Medical College and ignored the obvious fact that I did more to favor her entrance to that school than I had for her acceptance to Hahnemann. She actually had good enough qualifications to gain entrance to either school or even to the University of Pennsylvania or any other top medical school. In fact, I was somewhat pleased that she did not attend Hahnemann because, in my ticklish dealings with Shober, I had no wish to have the question of nepotism enter the picture. My dealings with the admissions process had to be pure, especially when it concerned my own daughter.

Medical school tuition fortunately had not reached the astronomical proportions that it attained recently. Still $4,600 a year, exclusive of books and room and board, was tough to manage at the time, especially since we had three other girls in college. The first year Joan lived at home and commuted. Then she managed to find a relatively cheap fraternity type residence near the school. Adapting remarkably well to medical school life, she was easily in the upper third of her class. The four years passed quickly as her determination to specialize in pediatrics was confirmed. She graduated with honors in this subject, and I was pleased to be permitted to march in the academic procession and sit on the stage when she received her diploma. Such is the pride of a parent. At least one of my daughters had achieved an advanced degree.

Joan returned to her beloved Big Apple when she chose a residency in pediatrics at Montefiori Hospital in the Bronx. She spent four rewarding years and took an extra year in adolescent pediatrics. The work was hard because the hospital served a populous area of underprivileged children. She saw every type of children's pathology, and had excellent instruction because all the physician staff were faculty of the Albert Einstein School of Medicine. Although now fully qualified to take her Boards in Pediatrics, she decided to go on further to qualify for the specialty of Pediatric Gastroenterology. This time she allowed me to help. Guilio Barbero, who had been at Hahnemann as Professor and Chair of Pediatrics, had moved on to the University of Missouri at Columbus where he established a fine Department of Pediatrics with an excellent training program in gastroenterology. He was also an outstanding expert in cystic fibrosis. Joan condescended to apply for a fellowship there, and happily Barbero took her on. Luckily she resonated very well with the program and Barbero. She had empathy for children and mothers, which is the essence of a fine pediatrician. Endoscopy, one of the main tools of modern gastroenterology, came naturally to her. Barbero was anxious to keep her on, but she did not like the Midwest and small towns. She had some big city in mind.

It happened that Georgetown Medical School had an opening in its Pediatrics Department. I knew John Rose, the former Dean of this school, and I encouraged Joan to apply. The Department head happened to be an Italian who liked Joan and practically hired her on the spot. She liked the idea of living in Washington, D.C. I liked it too because it was not too far from Philadelphia to visit frequently. From the start, she seemed to fit in well and made rapid advances in academics and practice. A new Board in Pediatric Gastroenterology was established and Joan took the exam and passed, thus becoming fully qualified not only in pediatrics but also in the subspecialty of gastroenterology.

All our girls were only a year or so apart, so they fit well with each other. Yet Yvonne, Voni for short, the number four child, seemed to be set apart in a more childish group. She struggled to compete on every level with her older sisters. She was naturally beat down and developed the habit of a crying spell at each frustration. From the beginning, she showed great intelligence and a strong tendency towards artistic expression. She was of fair complexion with blond hair and blue eyes. Perhaps the best looking of all the girls, she was blessed with a well-proportioned body. She was good in math and physics and, perhaps under the influence of Aunt Elsie, Mary's sister, decided to major in these subjects at college.

Her teachers encouraged her to apply to the best colleges such as Princeton and Yale that had traditionally not taken women. The movement towards liberalism and equality for women had taken hold by the time Voni reached college age, and she naturally took advantage of opportunities not before available. She was accepted at Johns Hopkins, not a bad second choice. So the proud parents moved their daughter to Baltimore to the assigned freshmen co-ed dormitories. She soon discovered stiff competition in physics but managed to do fairly well in all her courses. In her second year, she was able to find a group of girls who managed a small house where they could live more freely and comfortably than in the crowded, restrictive dormitory rooms. Voni decided that physics was not for her and changed her major to art, not a particularly strong subject at Hopkins. By taking courses at nearby Goucher College, which had more appropriate staff and facilities, she managed to round out her education. By utilizing her summers instead of taking a vacation, she was able to earn her bachelor's degree in three years. To complement her experience and education, she decided on an extensive trip abroad. Mary and I were supportive of this adventure, and so she departed for the art centers of France and Italy.

My sister Aurora had given Voni the name and location of relatives on my mother's side who lived in Vico Equenze, so when she finally arrived in southern Italy she looked them up. They were delighted to see a long lost piasano. Michele and Francesco Attanasio were the sons of Joseph Attanasio, who was the son of my mother's brother. Francesco, the younger of the two, was already married. Michele was a bachelor. Both were talented artists— Francesco more in painting, Michele decidedly a sculptor who worked in marble in the tradition of Michelangelo. Yvonne was drawn to Michele from the first meeting and he to her, although neither spoke a word of the other's language. In a period of two weeks, Yvonne learned enough Italian to get along, but linguistic skill came more slowly to Michele. The romance blossomed nicely, and Yvonne spent the rest of her time in Vico Equense.

At about that time, it happened that I had a meeting to attend in France. We arranged to meet Yvonne and Michele in Fontainbleau where it happened fortuitously that Dorothea was studying the piano. All of us had a grand meeting and were impressed with Michele's manner and deportment. He had brought along a number of prints and photos of his work, and it was obvious that he had talent and great promise. Michele asked Yvonne to marry him, but she was not sure because it would mean that she would have to live in Italy. Michele had a good teaching job in the state education system and connections to get commissions that would all be lost if he moved to America. We naturally wished Yvonne to stay in America but did not raise any objections. We simply told Yvonne that if she was not absolutely sure, she should come back to the United States, get a job, and find out for herself what she wanted to do. Well, she did just that by getting herself a teaching job at Johns Hopkins in the Art Department. At the close of the semester, her mind was made up. She left the American shore for a permanent life in Italy.

Voni and Michele were married in a quiet ceremony in Vico Equence. Once again, Mary and I were not able to attend the ceremony because of my urgent duties at the medical school. This was a disappointment, as I had visions of grand ceremonies in Wayne where we had a large enough house and property to manage such an occasion. Michele was able to transfer to a suitable teaching job in Florence, so they moved to a small apartment on the Via Longarno right on the Arno River near the famous Ponte Vecchio bridge. We visited them soon after and were impressed with the charm and life style of the Florentines. They were able to acquire a studio, and both were soon occupied with their respective art interests.

Our youngest daughter Mary-Jo, although a beautiful and delightful child, gave us the greatest concern. She was delayed in her toilet training and was slow to pick up little bits of learning, such as colors and the alphabet. In the early grades in school she did badly despite much coaching at home from Mary. She had more than the usual interest in the opposite sex, even as early as second grade. I have related the incident of the train accident when she was four years old. This may have contributed to her emotional instability, but it became obvious as she grew older that her level of mentation was inferior. She definitely had dyslexia, but her difficulties were deep-seated. She managed to skim along till her early teens when she became acutely psychotic. How frightening this is to parents, even those like ourselves who were exposed to all kinds of illnesses.

My good friend and former student, Wilbur Oaks, was of inestimable help. Even though Mary-Jo was extremely agitated, he managed to have her admitted to a private room on the medical floor of the hospital where she could have a private room. Mary could have a cot in the room to stay with her during her most difficult periods. Herman Belmont, a child psychiatrist, was agreeable to care for her and proved to be a very competent and caring therapist. It took about ten days for her to get over the agitated stage before it was possible to admit her to the ambulatory ward on the psychiatry floor where she could interact with other patients and receive more intensive psychotherapy. After several weeks of inpatient therapy, she was discharged to home care. She was fortunately able to attend a day mental hospital that the Psychiatry Hospital ran in a hotel located near Hahnemann. I was therefore able to take her in every day with a minimum disturbance to my own work schedule. Mary and I naturally extended ourselves to provide Mary-Jo with a healthy, cheerful, and educational daily experience. It was slow, tedious work but most worthwhile because it avoided the only possible alternative, the dreaded private or state mental hospital from which there is seldom satisfactory recovery.

Over time and with the expert help of P.E. Adams, who adjusted the medication, and Herm Belmont's psychotherapy, Mary-Jo experienced enough improvement to consider continuing her education. Jules Abrams, who ran the psychology program, was very helpful in analysis of Mary-Jo's intellectual status. He finally concluded that she might do well at the Hilltop School, a small private school run by a Mrs. Fischer and her husband that specialized in high school education of poor learners with psychiatric problems. The classes were small and the teaching individualized. Mary-Jo made a difficult but satisfactory adjustment to this school. She continued to learn. At home we devoted much time and effort to enhance her fundamental knowledge of English, simple math, and practical everyday things like cooking, cleaning, and hygiene. Progress was slow and great patience was needed, and Mary's dedicated efforts far exceeded mine. On days off, we took her on short trips to museums, the shore, and amusement parks to expose her to as many normal experiences as possible. She continued to have an abnormal interest and curiosity about sex. Her eyes would follow every male who even remotely crossed her path. We recalled that even when she was in second grade, she wanted to date boys. This extraordinary sex drive seemed to be amplified by her mental illness. While she was at Hilltop, she had many dates. Those we knew about were all with boys who were in just as serious a mental state as she was. None of these minor romances lasted more than a few weeks.

After four years at Hilltop, she received her high school diploma, although Mrs. Fisher assured us that she was functionally illiterate. It was evident that she could receive no further benefit from a staying at this school. Consultation with Jules Abrams indicated that the Ellis School might result in improvement. Located near Newtown Square not far from Wayne, this school had a long and favorable history for the care of disturbed children of high school age. Mary and I enrolled Mary-Jo in Ellis. At first, the novelty of being in a more mature and larger group seemed to have a salutary effect. After a few months, it became obvious that Ellis had a problem with a lack of discipline, and we surmised that many of the inmates had a drug problem as their main defect. We decided to take her out of Ellis because we feared she might acquire a drug habit from her peers.

Mary-Jo was now nearly twenty, and our hope was that she would learn some trade or profession that would make it possible for her to earn a living and care for herself. After extensive consultation with her, her physician, and psychologist, it was decided that childcare might be the most suitable career choice. We were skeptical about this, but it was Mary-Jo's first choice. Jules Abrams was again most helpful. He not only suggested Harcum Junior College, but he also aided in the application process. She was fortunately accepted, and I was pleased to move her into a dormitory room that she shared with another girl. Mary-Jo liked Harcum because she was away from home and could indulge in an expanded social life. The girls attended parties at fraternities at the various area colleges and had numerous social events on campus.

How she managed to pass courses in hygiene, child psychology, and English was beyond my comprehension. Harcum apparently must have had a very liberal marking standard.

Problems arose when she did not get along with her roommate. There were many other problems, and finally we were called in and asked to take Mary-Jo home from the dorm. But Harcum was conveniently located only a few miles from Wayne, so Mary could drive her to classes each day. The following year Mary-Jo was able to live in a single room in a small house on campus. She enjoyed being separated from parental influence, and her relationship to other people improved. She continued to have a very strong attraction to the opposite sex. She somehow developed an attachment to a young man who lived only a few houses from us. We never found out if she even had one date with him. It is doubtful that the young lad even realized that Mary-Jo had a crush on him. She and a girlfriend at Harcum conspired a scheme that was supposed to gain the young man's sympathy and affection for Mary-Jo. The plot consisted of a suicide attempt by Mary-Jo that would gain her admission to Bryn Mawr Hospital. The girlfriend, who had a passing acquaintance with the object of Mary-Jo's infatuation, would then call him up and inform him of the dramatic event caused by his failure to return her flirtations. The conspirators assumed that the lad would then feel sorry and visit the hospital, and this might then blossom into a genuine romance. To any mature mind, the plot was naive and ridiculous. But to the conspirators it was no more implausible than the Romeo and Juliet story. Mary-Jo did supposedly take a whole bottle of Tylenol (acetaminophen) tablets and was duly admitted to the hospital. The object of her affection was duly informed and, as might be expected, he properly avoided any involvement. Mary-Jo made a remarkably fast recovery and proceeded to other pursuits of elusive males.

Mary-Jo eventually received her diploma from Harcum. Although she did not appreciably improve her mental capacity, she did gain in maturity and ability to interact with people. She was now anxious to go to work, earn her own living, and gain complete independence from her parents. So the job hunting began.

Childcare jobs were available, but none paid a living wage. Mary-Jo soon discovered that that she was completely unsuited for this line of work. She was directed towards nursing homes and luckily she found one in Rosemont that would give her a trial. By coincidence, one of the head nurses had worked at Hahnemann Hospital and knew me. She took Mary-Jo under her wing and was of infinite help in getting her started. Mary-Jo did turn out to have a special empathy for patients. In time she managed to develop enough skills to qualify as a nurse's assistant. She earned enough to afford her own apartment, and that considerable burden was lifted from our shoulders. This by no means ended the saga of Mary-Jo, and the amorous adventures continued. However, this is enough for these memoirs.

I have included this synopsis of my children's careers as they occurred during the time of my most active Deaning duties. Have no doubts—children and their perambulations have an enormous influence on a parent's attitudes, mentation, and involvement with work and interactions with peers. I can appreciate the Catholic Church's insistence on celibacy for priests so that they can devote their entire being to their chosen work. I will not go so far as to recommend celibacy for Deans of Medical Schools, but certainly the position is as demanding as that of a parish priest or bishop.

CHAPTER VIII

More Deaning Business

1973-1976

"Very few want to run a medical school but nearly all want it to be operated in a manner which favors their particular specialty, no matter how unfair that may be."

Rupert Black, M.D.

The year 1973 stands out in my mind as the peak year of Hahnemann's slow but accelerating growth. I had occupied the Dean's office for nearly five years and was fifty-seven, the age some savants consider to be the height of greatest mental powers in a man's life. Shober had been in office a mere two years. Contrary to all the dire predictions of a certain and deadly collapse, Hahnemann was in better shape than at any other time in its history. This was the result of increased support by the federal and state governments and the rapidly increasing rate of healthcare delivery, which could be bled for moneys to support medical education. Years of support for basic and clinical medical research were now beginning to make possible the cure of many diseases thought to be hopeless in the past. New medical specialties were developed, such as nuclear medicine, which had been unheard of in the past. Diagnostic technology represented by the computerized tomography (the CAT scan) made an incredible advance in diagnostic radiology. This was paralleled in many other fields that took advantage of technology developed in part by the defense industry during World War II.

Almost overnight, healthcare became a major industry, eating up almost 10 percent of the gross national product. All previous estimates of the number of physicians needed by the nation proved to be seriously on the low side. Existing medical schools naturally began to increase their enrollments, especially since the federal and state governments were offering capitation grants, so much for each student enrolled. It was also possible to increase tuition because of the great demand for medical school placement. States that had no medical schools now felt the need to establish not one but two or three schools within their borders. In a few years, the total number of new schools grew from 90 to 125. The total number of annual qualified medical school applicants increased from about 26,000 to 51,000. About half of this pool succeeded in gaining admission. There was an analogous increase in osteopathic students and enrollment of Americans in foreign medical schools. This increase was due in part to an amazing increase in the number of women applicants, from 5 to 17 per cent.

Hahnemann was right there at the feeding trough. Shober immediately demanded that we increase our enrollment to 250. I had the unhappy task of appeasing the eager president with a more modest number. The Liaison Committee of the AMA and AAMC was coming to inspect us because of Shober's indiscretions, and we would be lucky if they didn't put us on probation. Using the standard technology of academic administrators, I appointed an ad hoc committee of what I supposed were conservative and moderate professors. To my surprise, they were enthusiastic to increase the enrollment to 250. In a tuition-run school like Hahnemann, the faculty soon realizes that salaries and tenure depend in the real sense on the bottom line of tuition income. Sudden increased income from doubling the number of students would make demands for salary increases, expansion of department space and facilities, and increase in personnel not only feasible but mandatory.

After much preparation and documentation, the Liaison Committee arrived and put a serious damper on our ambitions. They reluctantly allowed us to increase enrollment to 160 from the 130 we already had. They also gave us only three years of approval, which was an indication that if we did not improve, we might be in danger of being put on probation. This modest enrollment increase brought in a meager amount of new dollars that allowed hardly any expansion of existing departments. The growing economic inflation eroded the value of the dollar meanwhile. Despite these dire circumstances, there was a great air of optimism in the medical profession stemming from the favorable attitude of politicians who never failed to promise that the United States would have the best medical care system in the world. Money did flow from Congress for buildings, research, and education. Medicare and Medicaid allowed people to be treated for diseases that previously were neglected. Resident house staffs increased dramatically, and the average University Hospital of about 500 beds acquired as many as 300 resident doctors in training—better than one doctor for every two patients. All this bounty allowed medical centers to expand the number and size of new projects.

No neophyte to the value of publicity, Shober took advantage of all the ongoing programs to toot his own horn. In January 1973 he came out with a brochure entitled "Hahnemann Today" that stated in glowing terms the institution's accomplishments and the promise of great future developments. The cover was handsomely illustrated with an architect's drawing of the projected new hospital to be built on the corner of Vine and Broad Streets. Intended for the alumni and friends of Hahnemann, the brochure was designed to gain sympathy and, hopefully, substantial money gifts for the institution. In Shober's own words in the foreword, "Let's have the new publication truly tell the story of where Hahnemann stands today as one of Philadelphia's and the nation's leading Medical institutions." Beneath Shober's bold signature was a picture of him and Billy Likoff before a model of the new medical complex. Likoff deserved this honor because, as the new head of the Cardiovascular Institute, he had negotiated a gift of land to Hahnemann that was worth about $2 million in exchange for certain rights and space in the new hospital for cardiovascular diseases. The brochure also included the usual photos and blurbs of graduation ceremonies, dedication of Geary Auditorium, alumni dinner, a meeting of a volunteer group, a weekend faculty retreat, and the customary pictures of new trustees and new faculty members.

A California alumnus wrote to Shober and pointed out that his photograph appeared ten times and he was mentioned nine times in the text—all in a twenty-five page brochure. The letter ended with the advice that, since Shober had no expertise in any of the matters mentioned, he should come on less strongly. I didn't think much of this criticism, as I had four photos and a couple of mentions myself. The poison pen letters had created such a hostile atmosphere for Shober that anything he did was criticized. He actually was not as bad as subsequent presidents. Alumni don't understand that presidents have to enlarge themselves before the public and their Boards of Trustees. They need to create an aura to justify their increases in salary and the perks they develop in the pretence of good showmanship.

As I reread this brochure a quarter-century after its publication and know the events that have since transpired, I must conclude that 1973 represented a year of greatness for Hahnemann, which had gradually accrued because of the planning and good work of Charlie Brown, Cameron, Kellow, Paxson, and the faculty and staff they appointed and supported. I could give little or no credit to the Board of Trustees with the exception of a few members, which I shall deal with later.

Practically all the meritorious things that happened at Hahnemann came from below. A Board should be strong enough to have an agenda of excellence and see to it that it was carried out. The Hahnemann Board's only contribution was to insist on a positive bottom line at the end of the fiscal year. I suppose most Boards are this way, but it seemed to be especially true at Hahnemann. An institution devoted to education, scientific inquiry, and charitable healthcare should not have to earn its own way by tuition and charges for taking care of the sick. The Philadelphia community could support one good medical school, or perhaps even two, but there were six draining every possible source. Deans of the six

JOSEPH R. DIPALMA, M.D.

medical schools met regularly to discuss means and strategies to extract more support from federal and local governments. I cannot remember an instance when the schools did not cooperate with each other in this enterprise. Indeed the wealthiest schools, Penn and Jefferson, had lobbyists in Harrisburg and were generous in allowing the other schools to use the information that these gentlemen gleaned from legislators. The Deans soon found out that the osteopathic school had the greatest influence in Harrisburg. In any meeting, their representatives were ushered in before any of the other schools and were certainly treated more civilly. It was suspected, but never proven, that they curried favor with the legislators by admitting candidates who were recommended by certain influential representatives and senators. This friendly, cooperative atmosphere did not exist with regard to any other matters. Competition for paying patients, the most qualified students, and the favors of influential and wealthy patrons was lively and often bitter. On stealing one of our better faculty, Kellow chided me with the old saying, "All's fair in love and war." I promptly managed to attract one of Jefferson's faculty to Hahnemann.

In the game of competition, Shober almost immediately gained the enmity of the other CEO's. He was openly aggressive and made no attempt to disguise his intentions. State legislators paid little heed to him because most of them came from modest origins and hated the Main Line bravura of someone born with a silver spoon in his mouth. He was more successful in Washington. How this came about is a good story.

Shober continued to use Holmes as his main confidant and advisor while Moyer and Holmes continued to be deadly enemies. Moyer had his own agenda to get rid of both Holmes and Shober. Meanwhile, Cameron who had been Moyer's main support was out of the picture. Moyer had also made an enemy of Charles Wolferth, who was now Chairman of the Department of Surgery. Wilbur Oaks, Acting Chairman of the Department of Medicine, also was leaning towards getting rid of Moyer because he knew down deep that Moyer would not support his bid to be chairman. These powerful people all had some influence on Shober and convinced him that Moyer was in effect stabbing Shober in the back. Quick to pounce on a conceived enemy, Shober decided suddenly to fire Moyer from his CEO position as Vice President for Academic Affairs. The entire faculty was happy with this move, and it almost made Shober popular. I had some mixed feelings at the development because I could spend more time in intellectual pursuits under Moyer. Without doubt, Moyer got a raw deal. Whether he deserved it or not is a tough call.

Moyer characteristically did not take it lying down. He soon had a lengthy document prepared that lauded his efforts and gave the facts of the administrative improvements he'd instituted. On paper, Moyer looked superb according to Moyer. A faculty movement on his behalf might have saved him, but he could not generate a whisper of support. He sent his document to every member of the Board of Trustees. I doubt if any of them read it. By this time, they were all Shober's boys. Moyer next got himself one of the best law firms and demanded a hearing before the Board with these lawyers present. Shober in return hired Herbert Fogel, one of the most successful trial lawyers in Philadelphia. All I remember about this meeting with the Board was that it was short and loud and that Moyer apparently lost his plea for reinstatement and went on to sue the institution. There was a very long deposition during which I was quizzed continuously from 9 a.m. to 4 p.m. without a rest period or even lunch. I don't know to this day whether I did well for Moyer or for Hahnemann.

The suit never came to trial and was settled out of court. Moyer got his lawyer's bill paid, two years' salary and fringe benefits, plus an office and a secretary. They gave him an office remote from students and faculty in the Bellet building. In return, he was to drop the lawsuit and refrain from all attacks of any kind on Hahnemann. It was pretty much a paid two-year vacation. Moyer eventually found himself a very good full-time job as educational director of the Connamaugh Hospitals in western Pennsylvania. I felt badly about the whole episode because Moyer had done a splendid job of building up the Department of Medicine and greatly improving the quality and reputation of the entire school by his efforts in Continuing Education. He deserved to be allowed to function at Hahnemann and receive an honorable retirement.

Moyer's demotion made it possible for Wilbur Oaks to become Chairman of Medicine. Oaks was young, energetic, and practical. Few physicians ever develop a passion for patient contact to match the fervor that Oaks devoted to practice. His open manner and native friendliness won him the largest practice in internal medicine. He soon learned how to organize for maximum efficiency. No researcher, he had few publications to his credit and consequently few people knew him outside the institution. His creative talent lay elsewhere. He took advantage of the times to conceive the idea of starting a physician's assistant program. This would fit in with the general concept that competent assistants could relieve the physicians' shortage without creating an excess of expensive over-trained doctors. Oaks' enthusiastic support got the Physicians Assistant Program started at Hahnemann. He brought on another young physician, Dave Major, to be in charge of it and made it his personal goal to raise money to get the program under way.

The Wilkes-Barre Program was another project also primarily organized by Oaks and the Department of Medicine. It was supported by the federal government and was directed at supplying primary care physicians to areas of the country that were poorly served by the profession. Wilkes-Barre and the surrounding rural area were considered deprived of the best medical care because of a scarcity of physicians. Wilkes-Barre was in a severe depression because of the sharp decline in the demand for coal after World War II. Mining had been the main industry, and the area was slow to develop other sources of income. Physicians like to be where there is wealth and busy medical centers with the latest technology and advanced medical practice. They shun areas where the work is hard, the pay small, and the intellectual and cultural environment mediocre. Oaks proposed to solve this problem by having an enriched family medical educational program especially designed to favor practice in rural areas. Students applicants would be favored if they lived and grew up in a medically deprived area. Other favorable points were if they came from a small local college, had done community social work, and were sure that the thing they wanted most in life was to be a family physician. To make it sweeter for top-notch applicants to apply for the program, Oaks insisted on an accelerated education in which a candidate could complete college and medical school in six years instead of the usual eight. Daniel Flood was the area's Representative to Congress at that time. He was an old time politician who had served numerous terms. Flood was very powerful because he was Chairman of the House Appropriations Committee. He took full advantage of his position to gain monetary support for Wilkes-Barre. Of course, he was in full support of a program that would gain entrance opportunities into medical school for local students.

When Oaks got to know Flood quite well, Shober smelled a bonanza and lost no time in cultivating Flood. Shober visited Flood in his Washington office and used every trick to humor and flatter the old man. At the Bob Hope money-raising affair, Flood was the honored guest. An Honorary Doctor of Laws for Flood embellished graduation ceremonies. Any candidate whom Flood recommended for medical school got first line treatment. Most of the applicants Flood recommended were fortunately quite good and probably would have gotten into medical school on their own. Those that the Admissions Committee found impossible to admit were usually referred to me to find some remedial method so that, on the next application, they might stand a better chance. Shober gradually worked himself into a pattern of visiting Flood in Washington practically every week. It paid off. The Wilkes-Barre Program, a two-way television link to the Wilkes General Hospital, and cancer research all got significant boosts from this connection. The Wilkes program brought in about $9 million over six years. The NIH Cancer people were more resistant to political pressure. We didn't get a cancer center and had to be satisfied with much smaller offerings. The big payoff was a $14.5 million rider on a much larger Congressional social program for hospital construction money. The appropriation was to facilitate medical education for underprivileged persons. There is no doubt that this nice bit of change helped to float the municipal bond that made possible the

JOSEPH R. DIPALMA, M.D.

building of the hospital. The Wilkes-Barre Program (also known as the Hahnemann-Wilkes Program) enhanced the medical school's reputation because it was one of the few well-designed and financed programs to increase the number of primary care physicians in rural areas.

From the Dean's viewpoint it was one big headache because it greatly complicated the normal operation of admissions, instruction, affiliations, student affairs, and faculty relations. Many well-established principals had to be bent to accommodate the more liberal policies that enabled the program to function. A whole staff of teachers and administrators had to be installed that was not easily welcomed by the existing personnel. I was lucky in selecting Fred Pairent, a biochemist who had shown leanings towards education, as director of the program. Wilkes College appointed its own person with its share of the grant. Pairent turned out to be a very capable and practical administrator. I found that I could trust him in numerous other tasks that are endless in the Dean's office. From my viewpoint, the ability to do more beneficial things for the students and to facilitate education was the best spin-off of the program. As Dean, I had no discretionary fund and the ability to use some scarce resources was most welcome. Nothing comes without a price. I had to make a lengthy trip to Wilkes-Barre many times, which killed a day quite effectively. There were also irate faculty members who thought the program was bad until they were appeased by being given a piece of the pie. The same people who were critical of the program for its governmental-political connections played internal politics themselves. Morality is subject to bias towards self even in the best of organizations.

Who benefited from the Wilkes-Barre program? Was it worth spending so much tax money to populate an economically depressed rural area with doctors? To tell truth, I didn't think so at the time. At least half of the students enrolled in the program changed their minds midcourse, abandoned their solemn promise to dedicate their lives to family practice, and chose instead to become specialists in orthopedics, ophthalmology, and anesthesiology. The students who reneged on their promise gained at least a less expensive and less competitive path to specialization. We made our best effort to prevent this but soon found that it was not possible legally to force a student to stick to his or her promise to restrict the career to family medicine and even more important to practice in an under-serviced community either urban or rural.

Nearly twenty-five years later, I'm pleased to report that in a small but important way the program still continues and is much appreciated by several rural medical centers, especially the Guthrie Clinic in Sayre, Pennsylvania.

As tuition progressively rose, the need for student financial aid grew in importance and complexity. Upon the recommendation of Bachich, I brought on an officer just for this purpose. Barry M. Horwitz proved to be very able in this difficult field. Fortunately, banks considered medical students fairly good risks, and it was possible to borrow long-term money. No school had enough scholarships to finance even a small percentage of its students. At this time in my Deanship, it was not uncommon for students to acquire debts of $20,000 to $30,000 by the time they graduated. This compares to $100,000 to $150,000 today when the annual tuition has risen to $20,000 to $25,000. Yet applicants still consider it a good bargain in view of the financial gain the average physician earns over a lifetime. If an additional five years of post-graduate training at a relatively low salary is added, however, the young physician finds himself or herself at the age of thirty with an enormous debt and accrued interest that, despite the potential of a good income, is very difficult to pay off. The custom now is to marry early, so the additional burden of a family enters the budget as well. The percentage of women entering medicine today is at least 40 per cent. This may mean that medicine is a less attractive opportunity for men, but I really don't think so. Medicine and its opportunities have become more attractive for women, and in the era of emancipation of the fair sex, they are aggressively taking the opportunity to study medicine. More power to them. It's also fair to say that, in the majority of cases, they make excellent scientists and physicians. In any case, the school never suffered from a paucity of applicants—certainly not during Shober's tenure. His antics seemed to attract those who feared that they might not get into any school. There was no Jewish quota, and we had an excellent minority program. We had also constructed a student residence and purchased the Windsor apartment building to provide better housing than was previously available.

At about this time, we received a windfall that was just what Shober needed to bolster the cash position for the proposed new hospital. Out of the blue, I received a letter from an attorney in Austin, Texas. He identified himself as the executor of the estate of William Stiles, a 1920 graduate of Hahnemann, who had recently died. The lawyer included a copy of a hand-written letter from Stiles stating that all the stocks and bonds possessed by Stiles at the time of his death should be given to Hahnemann Medical School. There were no specific directions about how the money was to be used. The lawyer said that he would shortly turn over to Hahnemann Medical College stocks valued at considerably over a $1 million.

I confess that my immediate thought was to find a way to sequester this bonanza for some meritorious academic or scientific purpose. Hahnemann certainly needed more scholarship money. My advisors, who included some trusted members of the Board, however, recommended against any such enterprise. I reluctantly yielded the letter to Shober who hastily took full charge of the matter. The Stiles money, which eventually amounted to about $1.6 million, was a major element in bringing to reality the plans for the new hospital. Whether or not Stiles would have been pleased with this use of his money, we will never know. Someone in the administration must have had some qualms of conscience, and the student residence building that had already been built with government money was with little ceremony named the Stiles Building. At the least, this might indicate to the uninformed that a grateful alumnus helped his medical school by providing a residence for the students. A will, which definitely stated the mission to which the Stiles money was intended, might have preserved it for academic purposes. Yet it is also common knowledge that an ingenious administration can manage to use donated funds for purposes of its own choice. Unless there is strict independent monitoring, unscrupulous accounting manipulations can mask diversion of funds.

This brings to mind the universal misconception that in a medical school-hospital combination like Hahnemann and most leading medical centers, the hospital subsidizes the medical school. The public impression is that the healthcare side diverts moneys intended to provide healthcare to areas of education and research. The exact reverse is the actual situation. To give a few examples: moneys from tuition and government sources in the greater part to finance salaries of full-time clinicians, library maintenance, classrooms and auditoriums, and even research and service laboratories. At Hahnemann 40 percent of the salary of the President came from the academic side, although he spent 90 percent of his time dealing with hospital and health delivery problems. Isadore Krekstein, a member of the Board and a professional accountant, explained on an occasion that accounting is more art than science. In his own words, "Where you put an item in the assets or debit column is a judgment call based more on need than actuality. A skillful accountant can make a statement look good, and it usually takes another independent accountant to correct the statement to a version closer to the truth."

Over the years of my Deanship, I was amused by the annual public statements put out by the different presidents under whom I served. Like most medical schools, Hahnemann was always in a near-bankruptcy state, yet the statements always seemed to reflect a positive balance. The degree of aggrandizement was conditional on the honesty of the Board and the integrity of the chief financial officer. Shober would have liked to issue more glowing statements but was kept in check by Kreckstein and McArthur, the chief financial officer. Ironically, after Shober, a far less honest Board permitted greatly inflated statements that indicated that Hahnemann had an endowment of over $100 million, certainly a great figment of the imagination. Hahnemann was actually in worse financial condition because later presidents spent far more money than they brought in. Compared to his successors, Shober was a piker. Conservatives, including myself, who properly discouraged vain ventures, surrounded Shober.

Shober called me to his office one day, and I could see as I entered his chamber that he was in an expansive mood.

"Joe," he expounded, "We have just concluded a conference with our lawyers and the Feds. They have agreed that they owe us $600,000 in back Medicare payments. We should get the money soon. Why don't you hire some more faculty, get some new equipment, and make some long desired improvements before this money gets assigned to some other less desirable project?"

Frankly I was shocked at his generosity tendered towards the academic side. I thanked him and indicated that I would soon get back to him with some proposals. Having been brought up with the dictum that you never spend money that you don't already have in hand, I was reluctant to plunge into debt without more assurance of the validity of the anticipated funds. Back in my own domain, I consulted with my financial people who promptly informed me that there was only a slim chance that the Feds would ever actually release this money. As it was, the budget of the medical school was already in shortage, and I certainly could have used the money. I reluctantly sat on my hands—and fortunately so, because we never did realize this bonanza. I never did find out, but it would not be surprising if the money was spent on some suddenly urgent project.

Shober did raise more money than any previous president, but he always managed to spend it faster than it came in. Kreckstein and McArthur usually kept him in check. It was ironic that a relatively small extravagance—apartment on the top floor of the Windsor building—gave him more trouble than other, far more significant and unwise investments. All chief executives of big institutions have perks, and Shober was no worse in this regard. He was so open and flamboyant about everything he did that his many critics found it easy to characterize him as excessive. Despite the barebones budget, lack of any endowment, and always near bankruptcy, Shober managed to float a tax-free municipal bond for $39.5 million to build the new hospital. The old hospital would be maintained to house some of the beds and undergo gradual renovation. Because it was a time of high interest rates and a stagnant stock market, the bonds sold like hot cakes. I bought some myself, which paid almost 9 percent. A few years later, when Hahnemann was on the verge of collapse, I sold them at a small profit.

Construction of the new hospital went along quite well despite the customary foibles of contractors with their extra charges and overruns. Fortunately Charlie Paxson was put in charge, and his Quaker qualities enabled a settlement of most problems with some semblance of sanity. When the hospital was eventually finished, its gleaming corridors and handsome, impressive new equipment exhilarated the spirits of the clinical faculty. Unpopular, even despised Wharty Shober had to receive credit for materializing the handsome twenty-two-story structure. Realistically, as events rolled on in the healthcare business, the new hospital provided the means of survival in the developing era of increased competitiveness between institutions.

During the 1970s the commercialization of medicine took hold in earnest. As I look back now, I comprehend what was transpiring. But at the time, the change was so gradual that few of us thought that much was different. Yes, customs were changed and medical school applicants no longer studied medicine to become missionaries; few physicians did volunteer work. For-profit hospitals began to appear, and the introduction of Medicare and Medicaid made available vast sums of money for the sharks to feed upon. Twenty years of medical research funding by NIH had produced much technical development, which translated to expensive machines and procedures that greatly expanded therapy. One device alone, Computerized Axial Tomography, more commonly known as a CAT Scan, revolutionized the whole field of diagnostic visualization of bodily structures. It cost about $1 million, so it was apparent that very few hospitals could afford the device. The Hospital of the University of Pennsylvania had the first one in Philadelphia. Marvin Haskins, the Chairman of Diagnostic Radiology at Hahnemann, was clamoring for one. When word reached the President, Shober smelled profit because the charge for a CAT Scan would be at least $1,000 as compared to a mere fifty dollars for ordinary x-rays. He immediately called a meeting of the executive committee and asked that we buy a CAT Scan machine even though we could not afford it. Without any hesitation and no debate, we all agreed that Hahnemann needed this moneymaking machine. We knew that Jefferson was already planning to acquire one and Temple would also get one soon. We thus ended up having the second such a machine in Philadelphia, but not for long.

None of us could anticipate the remarkable array of diagnostic and therapeutic equipment that was to become available in future decades. Specialization in fields that did not exist before became the way to go. Despite valiant efforts of the American Board of Medical Specialties, new boards and subspecialties multiplied by tens and twenties. The average period of post-graduate training went from three to five years, and it became not unusual for some to train for seven or eight years to achieve proficiency in their main board subject and a subspecialty.

Meanwhile everyone was admiring the success of the group practice set up in California by the Kaiser Industry and known as the Kaiser-Permanente. Started at the beginning of World War II to provide healthcare for Kaiser Industries' workers and their families, it was an ideal model of its kind. Better and more extensive healthcare, provided on an insurance basis, could be delivered on a private-practice pay-as-you go basis. The advantages were obvious to all. Enthusiasm, however, must be tempered by the fact that it was non-profit and backed by a very large, affluent corporation. Most importantly, the members were all relatively young (average age forty to forty-five) and thus not subject to the expensive diseases of old age. Prior to the Kaiser plan, there was a similar organizational set up in New York City known as Health Insurance Plan (or HIP) that was restricted to Civil Service workers. Loud outcries were heard from private practitioners who claimed that this was the start of governmental takeover of healthcare. Initially, very few physicians would subscribe to being HIP physicians because of the lower fee structure. Unlike the Kaiser plan, HIP had a much larger population of elderly patients. Yet it must be admitted that HIP was just as successful as the Kaiser plan. It still exists today and is open to the general population.

During this era, I was a busy practitioner with my own office and private practice. There were relatively few group practices at that time, and most physicians enjoyed the autonomy of a solo operation. Like my colleagues, I was against all health insurance plans, especially government ones. People should set aside money to take care of their health. Those who could not afford it were charity cases to be taken care of in city hospitals and clinics. It must be emphasized that physicians who served in these hospital and clinics received no pay. It was considered an honor and a privilege to do this service. As one who interned at no pay in one of the largest city hospitals, Kings County in Brooklyn, I was well indoctrinated in this concept. The system worked successfully, and in most instances charity patients received better care than those who could pay for more luxurious accommodations. Much is meritorious about the open ward that increases the efficiency of observing and servicing patients' needs. It would not work today, of course. Now we need the privacy of a single, or at the worse a double room, which has its own toilet facilities. But the patient has to have monitors and a telephone, television entertainment, and some signaling device to call the nurse. Astronomical charges of up to $2,000 a day for routine services are not unusual. The result is that no one can afford to be in the hospital more than a day or two. Operations that required at least five days of hospitalization are now same-day procedures. Only one day is allowed for a normal childbirth (in some states changed to two days by legislation).

In the mid-1970s, the changes were impressed upon us because the Hahnemann hospital, built in 1929 and considered then the best of its kind, was decidedly obsolete. Jefferson had built a truly magnificent hospital, and to Shober's credit, he drove relentlessly towards the planning and financing the new Hahnemann hospital and renovation of the old one.

As Senior Vice President and Dean, I was much involved in the changes in healthcare delivery. I didn't like this because it cut deeply in to my research and other intellectual activities. But I was conscientious enough to devote more energy to practical matters than most of my colleagues. Perhaps because I had been in private practice myself, I had some feeling for patient care problems. I learned the most from the Regional Medical Program. Deans of the other Philadelphia medical schools were glad to let me attend the numerous tedious meetings as their representative. This federally financed program was designed to bring the fruits of years of medical research to the general population. The main consultant and instigator was the famous cardiac surgeon Michael DeBakey who, together with his colleagues, decided that the ideal solution was to regionalize expert services with respect to the main killer diseases: heart, cancer, and stroke. Grants were made to encourage selected hospitals and medical centers to construct and operate special emergency units to diagnose and treat heart disease. Special radiation and cancer chemotherapy therapy units were also encouraged. Little was actually done for stroke, as the therapy was not very advanced at that time.

Smart hospital administrators jumped on the bandwagon with alacrity. It was easy to perceive the advantage for attracting business when you had the best intensive cardiac care unit in the community! As might be expected, the more affluent hospitals, especially those with a resident staff, stood to gain the most by regionalization. Many bitter fights followed as the big boys tried by one means or another, often very political, to gain an advantage in technology and equipment. As a matter of course, the Regional Medical Program in time failed to control the monster it had created. There is no argument, however, that the program did accomplish its original purpose of bringing more and better medical care to the general population. This was the period of fantastic increases of technology and the ability to increase control over diseases previously unresponsive to therapy.

The enormous increase in Medicare and Medicaid costs forced the government to try some new method of control. This took the form of local organizations patterned after the Regional Medical Program, with the exception that local community representatives were major controllers. Besides appropriate members of hospitals, clinics, medical and health societies, medical schools and colleges, this also included representative members of unions and other groups, political or otherwise, who were concerned with the distribution of healthcare. It was called The Health Systems Agency, financed by the federal government, but based on volunteer work of local organizations and cooperating with local and state health departments. The agency was slow to get started, but once the political implications sunk in, it gained impetus.

In the Philadelphia area, the agency got its start by the cooperative efforts of the Departments of Community Medicine of the medical schools. I'm pleased to relate that Dean Roberts, our chairman at Hahnemann, was the most active, enthusiastic participant. As occurred earlier with the Regional Medical Program, the medical schools Deans were happy to let me represent them so they could avoid numerous meetings. It was very instructive for me, and I became quite expert in the administrative side of medical care delivery. It also allowed me to become acquainted with some of the more important political figures in Philadelphia. One was W. Thacher Longstreth, the City Councilman and mayoral candidate, who quite impressed me with his intelligence and honesty. But he was a rare politician. Most of the others ground their own axes. I also came to know most of the major hospital administrators in the area.

After tedious maneuvering, a major controversy developed. Should the agency be composed of Philadelphia and the four surrounding counties (Delaware, Montgomery, Chester, and Bucks), or should there be separate agencies, one for the suburbs and one for Philadelphia? It was apparent to all health services in the area that a large proportion of Philadelphians used suburban hospitals. And there was a large flow to Philadelphia from the outside counties. A combined agency of five counties made the most sense to most members of the organizational group. There was strong opposition, however, from the more politically minded members. Mayor Frank Rizzo was imperatively in favor of a separate agency for Philadelphia.

It just so happened that the Mayor was a patient in Hahnemann Hospital at the time the county decision was to be made. He had fractured his leg in a rather ridiculous accident: He was retreating from an explosive fire in a gas tank when he bumped into one of his former policemen. Because of my position at Hahnemann, I had a plausible reason to visit him, so I was elected to try to convince him that a combined agency was desirable. The encounter was pleasant enough in the beginning. When he found out I was a physician, he ripped back the sheets to show me his surgical scar as it were a mark of bravery, a wound earned in hearty battle. But when I revealed the true purpose of my visit, his face darkened and he angrily stated, "Those damned suburbanites. They're always stealing from Philadelphia! No, definitely not, Philadelphia must have its own agency. That's the only way they will get the most from the Feds." So ended the conversation. One did not dare reason with His Honor. Despite all the opposition, the combined five county agency was eventually formed.

Few realized at the time, and certainly thereafter, the great importance of the agency to the welfare and future of Hahnemann. Since I was the only Dean who took active responsibility and also because of Dean Roberts' work, Hahnemann looked pretty good with respect to the other Philadelphia medical schools. It was also a splendid opportunity to meet with community people, union members, and politicians. I began to have a personal relationship with all the local hospital administrators. One of the most impressive and able hospital chiefs was Dick Breckbiel who headed Abington Hospital. Had he not died prematurely, I might have been able to arrange an affiliation with this fine hospital. Yet a twist of fate was to come about that even I did not anticipate.

Gerry Seigler, an able, young administrative type, became head of the agency. I never did find out his educational and career history that led to his being in the health field. I did know that he'd been a Catholic priest and was married to a former nun. His reserved manner and knowledge of Latin gave some hint of his background. His ability to deal with the complex problems of the agency was impressive. It so happened that when the agency was about to be disbanded some four years later and all the employees had to find new jobs, Hahnemann needed a replacement CEO for the Hospital. I was still Dean at the time, and Dick Breckbiel urged me to push hard to get Seigler the job. I made a special effort to see Charles K. Cox, Chairman of the Board of Trustees, and give as good a recommendation as I could manage. Cox was non-committal, but a few weeks later Seigler did get the job. I doubt that my recommendation was a key decision factor, but it probably did no damage. In my opinion, Seigler was a very good administrator especially in an academic institution. Unfortunately, Seigler's skills and personality were not equal to the "dog eat dog" atmosphere that was rapidly developing in the healthcare industry. Seigler became depressed, hit the bottle too heavily, and eventually moved on two years later.

I cannot say that, in the few years that Health Systems Agency actively functioned, it had a profound effect in changing the way healthcare was delivered. It did create a great many experts who knew where the resources were and who understood the potential of various possible organizational patterns. The growing for-profit healthcare industry snapped up many of these experts. Some of the new talent went back to the federal government to concoct new plans that were an attempt to constrain the rapid growth of healthcare services. In the mad rush to exploit the vast sums of money, which the federal government health and insurance plans generate, the sharks care little about how the bonanza came about. The Regional Medical Program and the Health Systems Agency are seldom mentioned today as if they were ancient history of little consequence to modern affairs. Yet they represent the very essence of the logic that dominates our present healthcare system.

Regionalization of services and a systems method of delivery of services (HMOs, for example) are the backbone of the organizational structure today. The magic "Managed Medical Care" of today is the outgrowth of the interaction that transpired when the physicians, government people, businessmen, community activists, and politicians met and discussed a common problem and had the desire to find a solution satisfactory to the majority.

I relate all these problems and developments involving healthcare delivery because it strongly involves the functions of the medical school Dean and his administration. Academic prerogatives are secondary to keeping the hospital beds full and the clinics busy. Boards are so worried about financial solvency that many educationally oriented medical centers establish a senior position such as Vice President of Health Affairs, which in most cases is equal in stature or superior to that of the Dean or even a Provost. This Catch 22 situation is the main cause of the short lives of Deans. Either he must get the hell out, or else get himself promoted to the health affairs position or the Presidency. In my case, I survived only because Shober handily got rid of Moyer and Holmes before he himself was axed. Shober correctly realized that both these characters desperately wanted to get rid of him and become the President themselves. I had no aspirations to be President and wanted to get out. The only reason I did not was because I was unable to secure a more satisfactory position considering my personal circumstances.

CHAPTER IX

The President's Demise and

Its Consequences

1977-1978

"Such is the vagary of fortune that it is possible to be successful in your work and still be unhonored and conversely be a failure and be glorified."

Rupert Black, M.D.

By 1977, my tenth year as Dean and Senior Vice President, I was beginning to feel the weight of my sixty-one years. Shober was in his sixth year as President. He had complete control of the Board and was getting along quite well with at least some portion of the faculty. Students and alumni still hated him, but the poison pen letters had stopped. His family donated $15,000 to Hahnemann with the understanding that Lecture Room B would be named Shober Hall after a forebearer who had done some distinguished medical work during the Revolutionary War. A modest bronze plaque was hung high so that it could not be easily reached. A simple dedication ceremony followed. Very few people attended, and Board Chairman Krekstein made a brief speech. The next day the plaque was gone—apparently ripped from the wall by a vandal. Everyone suspected that some students may have done the deed, but there never was any confirmation. Although I never developed any substantial liking for Shober, this affair appeared disgraceful to me and I was veritably sorry for Shober and members of his family. As it turned out, this event foreshadowed the end of Shober's career at Hahnemann.

Disease, death, or finances defeats many a would-be leader. In Shober's case, it definitely was finances. Despite glowing financial reports, the true story was that the hospital was losing money, and the amount owed the banks was way out of proportion to what could be expected to be earned. Vendors' debts were far beyond ninety days and in quite a few cases as much as a year. A $2 million loan—minimum—was absolutely essential to tide the institution over the next critical period. This was actually not an unusual event for Hahnemann or, to be fair, for most other hospitals. The difference at this juncture was that the banks had become wary of Shober's eccentricities. Even Krekstein who generally had a very good reputation could do nothing to restore the banks' confidence. It simply became a case of getting rid of Shober if Hahnemann stood a chance of getting a loan. Even though most were Shober cronies, the Board did what it had to do (to protect its own liability). The Board called in Shober and his lawyer and made a deal. Shober was to get three years salary, and in return for resigning and getting out of the organization, he had to guarantee not to sue the institution. Thus ended the Shober saga. No portrait graces any wall or hall. His name and actions were expunged from any document that might reach public view.

At the time, everyone was overjoyed at this turn of events. All felt that we had hit bottom and now, with the demise of Shober, things must begin to improve. It did not turn out that way. Kreckstein was old, sick, and dejected, and he soon resigned. The rest of the Board was nothing but a bunch of rats abandoning a sinking ship. Had I the ambition and the drive, I probably could have stepped in as a chief officer and rallied the faculty in a movement to save the institution. My inexperience with the financial world and lack of any considerable personal resources, however, argued against such a venture. I must also admit that I had no guts for a CEO responsibility. Being a Dean was enough for me, and I felt that any potential I might have was already spent. After consultation with senior faculty, I called in Bill Likoff and told him that he was the only man who could save the institution at this juncture.

Likoff was in his middle sixties and not in what might be interpreted as vigorous health. He had a history of a severe myocardial infarction at the age of forty-five that had left him with a compromised heart. In spite of this, he had continued an active private practice and a teaching and modest research program. He was very active in the national cardiology societies. Locally, the Cardiovascular Institute was his baby and indeed now carried his name. Most of the prominent business and financial people in Philadelphia had been or were Likoff's patients. Mark Rubinstein, an affluent business tycoon and one of the stronger members of the Hahnemann Board, was a very close friend.

Without question, Likoff carried the kind of presence and influence that might enable Hahnemann to recover its bearings. His wife Ethyl, to whom he was much attached, had died just a few years earlier of pulmonary cancer after a prolonged period of suffering. This had devastated him. He had given up a beautiful home and lived alone in the Hotel Barclay. Likoff would lose financially because any salary Hahnemann paid him would be far less than he could earn in private practice. He could attempt to maintain some practice, of course. But once he became identified with a full-time executive position, patients would inevitably desert him for other physicians who could devote more time to their ailments. It was obvious also that he could realistically expect a term of office of only five years, probably less. Despite all these misgivings, Likoff took the job. I don't know the details, but I am quite sure he got a three-year contract. Everyone breathed a sigh of relief.

Likoff did manage to put the institution on a more stable financial path but at a terrible price. He knew a certain Mr. Gallagher, the president of a newly formed Valley Bank. Yes, Gallagher's bank would lend Hahnemann $2 million but only on certain terms. The clinical faculty must put up their practice incomes and the other faculty their homes or other reliable income as collateral for the loan. Gallagher and his henchman Kelly eventually were to become Chairman and Co-chairman of the Board respectively.

As might be expected, there were many faculty meetings and fractionation into groups, each with a sure solution. In the end, those clinicians whose financial stake was most endangered came through with the required collateral. Not many basic science professors put up their houses as collateral, but one or two did. I must be included among those who put nothing on the line. My opinion, then as now, was that it would be better to declare bankruptcy and put the institution at the mercy of the state, the city, and the public. The bankers were playing business hardball and using their favorite devices to gain control of the institution to protect the investment they already had. (Hahnemann owed the banks about $11 million at that time.) If the institution declared bankruptcy, the banks would probably only recover a small portion of this amount.

Likoff went about the tricky business of finding a suitable Chairman of the Board. He asked everyone's help but received little because this was an unpaid job that carried very little prestige. Only the banks, insurance companies, food vendors, and other suppliers were interested in forcing one of their executives into doing this responsible community work. So it developed that the business community finally beguiled Charles K. Cox who was retiring after a credible career as Vice Chairman of the INA Corporation. He was a large man with a business like presence and a diffident manner. He gave little indication that he was really interested in the job and was only doing it because it was his duty to round out his vocation and fulfill some obligations to his business cronies. He was definitely not a friendly type, and I confess that I got along much better with Shober than with Cox, but perhaps there are other reasons for this that I need to explain.

When Shober lost his bid to get rid of me, he made an agreement to get along with me as long as I didn't fight his objectives. Besides the usual routine meetings, we had lunch together quite frequently. More importantly, I managed to become friendly with some members of the Board. The most important one with respect to my dealings was Maurice Fox, a most interesting character. Of average height, he was inclined to be amply rotund. From his jovial face and merry manner, I sensed immediately that here was a person who enjoyed life in the fullest degree. It was rumored that his father left him a fortune of some $6 million that he had gambled away, but he managed to gain most of it back through some shady deals in trucking and other business ventures. I never did find out how he got on the Board, but I would guess that he sold Shober a bill of goods in some kind of enterprise. Why he took a shine to me, I never clearly comprehended. I sensed that he admired the loyal support that the faculty gave me when Shober moved to fire me. Fox phoned me one day out of the blue and invited me to lunch at the Sheraton Hotel in Fort Washington, a considerable distance from Hahnemann, where it would be quite unlikely that any busybodies'd observe us. The meeting had an air of mystery that intrigued me. He came right to the point.

"Joe, I know that you and the faculty are out to get rid of Shober."

I naturally thought to myself, here is one of Shober's stooges trying to brainwash me. I did not say anything but listened nattetively to his next statement.

"Understand that I'm completely faithful to Shober, and I'm convinced that he is trying to do his best for Hahnemann," Fox said. "However, I'm willing to keep you informed as to what goes on in the executive sessions of the Board and to take your side and that of the faculty whenever I can."

I was frankly surprised at his generosity, and I smelled a rat. Perhaps he wanted to get someone into medical school, so I asked to him, "Why are you being so helpful? There is little I can do for you, and the faculty is not in a position to do you any favors."

"Well," he replied, "I have a great admiration for scholarly, educated people. You know that I belong to the Franklin Institute and greatly enjoy their programs. I have respect for you. As Dean of a Medical School, you are a unique person as there are only 100 schools in the country. That assures that you must have unusual talent and ability to have achieved such a rare position."

I thought to myself, flattery will get you nowhere, Maury. Instead I replied, "It's nice that you think of Deans as unusually talented people. However, most critics think otherwise. To them, a Dean is a person who has been a failure at the practice of medicine, who can't do research, and who doesn't know how to teach, so there is nothing for him to do so they make him a Dean."

He smiled at this and asked if there was anything he could immediately do.

"Yes," I replied, "You could become a member of the Academic Affairs of the Board of Trustees. I present at this subcommittee and need supporters to get across some urgent needs of selected academic programs."

Fox agreed and, true to his word, was an excellent ally for the academic side. As a matter of fact, the Chairman of the Committee was Bowen C. Dees, President of the Franklin Institute and a very academic person. Prior to his position at the Franklin Institute, he was President of the University of Arizona. He understood and appreciated academic prerogatives and was a very convincing spokesman for the academic side. During his tenure, and with additional help from Fox, I was able to propose and get action on a number of projects that would otherwise fall on deaf ears. My main objective was to get final state approval of university status so that we could change the name from Hahnemann Medical School and Hospital to Hahnemann University of the Health Sciences. To me, the inclusion of the term "hospital" degraded the primary purpose of the institution from education and research to one that was mainly service. We were the only medical school in the country that included the word "hospital" in its title. The hospital would actually gain the most from university status because it could then be known as the Hahnemann University Hospital, which definitely established it as a notch above the average excellent community hospital.

The top twenty medical schools in this country are university based—for example, Harvard, Yale, Hopkins, and University of

Pennsylvania (the latter being the first medical school established in the United States). If there was a hospital, it was usually separate with an individual board, although there might be interlocking members with the board of the university. In contrast, the great majority of medical schools at the time of the Flexner Report (1910) were part of a physician practice group with or without a hospital. There was only one controlling board for both the educational and practice group. In many cases, the students were nothing more than captive labor and a source of additional income. Flexner's great reformation strongly recommended that all medical schools be university based. His educational requirements both in the humanities and the sciences definitely mandated a university facility and capacity. This pronouncement caused many schools to close. Some survived, among them Jefferson Medical College, Hahnemann Medical College and Hospital, and The Women's Medical College of Pennsylvania all located within the City of Philadelphia. Their hospitals were all on campus under a single board and all non-profit and charitable. They were only able to survive because grateful patients left their money to the hospital. Medical education gained from this because the hospital was the main teaching laboratory and classroom. Thus the hospital-medical school combination has subsisted to this day whether or not the medical school was university based.

My alma mater, The Long Island College of Medicine in Brooklyn, started as a medical school-hospital combination in the last century. The Long Island College Hospital separated from the medical school in 1930, however, with a separate board and finances. The medical school continued to control its physician staffing and practice standards. Simply, no physician could be a hospital staff member unless he also had an appointment in the medical school. This insured that his qualifications were first-rate and that he was available for education and research. This arrangement worked quite well until America's medical education system became predominantly staffed by full-time physicians in all the clinical departments. Full-time meant that these physicians were to devote the majority of their working hours to teaching and research. Their salaries were fixed by contract and did not depend on what practice income they could develop. When the full-time system first started in the 1940s and 1950s, salaries paid to the full-time clinicians were usually considerably less than the same individual could make in private practice. Some compensation for this difference was the pension and insurance benefits and less working hours, plus other perks that the full-time staff was supposed to enjoy. As time went by and the number of full-time physicians increased, the medical school or the university found it expedient to establish a practice plan for their academic physicians so that they could earn the major portion of their salaries. Under these conditions, the full-time people instinctively desired to make as much if not more income than physicians in private practice. The traditional antagonism between the two groups of physicians was intensified. The result was that the economical, harmonious volunteer physician staff disappeared from the educational scene for the most part. They definitely were not going to do for free the work for which their full-time confreres were receiving generous pay. Today this situation has intensified because both sets of physicians are reimbursed by health maintenance organizations (HMOs) that make no distinction between the two groups. Also HMOs do not pay for any treatments or procedures that are considered research oriented. Thus even more distress enters into the life of the full-time physician.

One should not forget the great advantages of a hospital that's the integral part of a medical school has over an equivalent community hospital. Not the least is the ability to get government financing to educate residents and post-doctoral fellows. As a result of a medical school affiliation, hospitals have hundreds of residents, which makes possible many types of special treatments and surgeries that require several cooperating specialists. Great technical advances like cardiac surgery and renal dialysis were originally developed in medical school hospitals. Excellence attracts excellence, and the presence of distinguished professors attracts the best of the crop of medical school graduates. Completion of a residency at a top teaching hospital practically assures a notable career. The availability of a large medical library, laboratories, conference rooms, and scheduled learning exercises also are features not accessible in the average community hospital. The presence of medical students and an abundance of allied health personnel, as well, make for an esprit de corps that heightens the competitive edge.

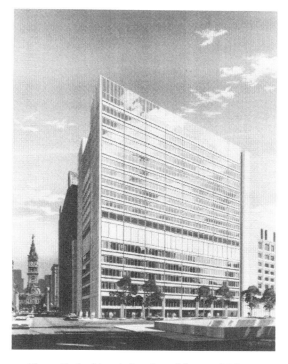

Figure 5. Architect's drawing of the new Hahnemann Hospital completed in 1978. Capable of housing 600 patients together with the old hospital and equipped with the most modern equipment the new structure of 21 stories provides a superb health care facility for Philadelphia and the adjacent suburbs. President Shober deserves the credit for having the foresight and determination to foster the construction of this building so important to the future of Hahnemann.

The commercialism now rampant in medicine has tended to destroy the academic quality of even the finest teaching centers. Full-time clinical professors must earn their salaries, do research, pay for the space they occupy, and in most cases earn enough to pay for secretarial and nursing services. This forces a clinical professor to see at least four patients an hour and order tests and procedures that may not actually be needed. Research is done because the center needs the overhead money to finance the competitive structure it has acquired. Genuine teaching—which means actual contact with students—is neglected because it does not bring in the kind of money that accrues from practice and high status research. Gone is the leisure time to investigate new and innovative directions. Early retirement is mandatory for a modest producer (one who doesn't bring in enough money for his or her rank).

I have described today's commercial state of affairs to contrast my relationship that was characteristic of the 1970s. First of all, faculty governance was very democratic. The Academic Affairs Council consisted of all the Department Heads, and four elected faculty made all academic decisions. The standing committees of the Council controlled such matters as admissions, curriculum, appointments, promotions, and the formation and deletion of departments. There were standing committees for each of these functions, and a committee in consultation with the Dean elected members. Affairs beyond the scope of these committees were solved by the Dean's appointment of ad hoc committees with the approval of the Council. An Executive Faculty and a General Faculty met in joint session twice a year. These meetings were quite dull and mainly of informative value but could get quite active, as in the Shober Era. As Dean and Senior Vice President, I ran the Academic Affairs Council quite successfully until the late 1970s. Under Likoff as President, I became weaker because most of the clinical faculty were Likoff's friends and colleagues and found it easy to bypass the Dean to get what they wanted directly from the President. Much as I liked and admired Bill Likoff, it was evident that he was an incompetent administrator. It was unfortunate, in a way, that he was a brilliant physician because he carried his professional experience into his administrative functions. He treated everyone as a patient and every situation as a disease. The treatment was medical, not business-like. He was a prime example of why hard-nosed business people say that most physicians make poor business decisions.

Nevertheless, he was the savior of the institution and must get credit for the achievement of university status. He was far more acceptable to the accrediting bodies and the State Board of Education, and after fifteen years of tedious documentation and formation of credible schools and educational goals, Bondi and I were finally fulfilled. I think we both felt that we had achieved an honor much like winning an Oscar. To celebrate achieving university status, a nice ceremony was held which everyone enjoyed because they realized that Hahnemann, with origins predominantly in homeopathy, was now a medical university, fully accredited, and competitive with the best in the field.

Although university status meant a great deal to a few dedicated faculty and to me, it seemed to be of little significance to the majority of clinical staff. The students could not have cared less. Most painful of all, Cox and the rest of the Board were completely ignorant of its significance, much less its commercial value. Few, including myself, anticipated that some fifteen years later, an imaginative, ambitious executive individual would capitalize on the university status to merge a string of hospitals into one organization under the umbrella of medical and health sciences education by making dexterous, strategic changes that favored a profitable bottom line. (More later about this venture which turned out to be disastrous.)

Even in retrospect, while I feel that I devoted my entire capacity to the Deaning business, I made a dedicated effort to maintain my intellectual activities. At this interlude, I had been Dean for about ten strenuous years, and my age had advanced to the early sixties. I was about thirty pounds overweight and smoked and drank too much. The insidious process of atherosclerotic disease was creeping up on me. Now in view of my subsequent health history, I suspect that I was ascribing those vague chest pains to any reasonable cause other than coronary artery disease. Physicians are not immune to self-denial. They are, in fact, all the more prone to it because of their more extensive knowledge of alternate causes suggestive of chest pain.

McGraw-Hill, publisher of my big pharmacology book, decided that wasn't selling too well. The publisher believed that a smaller, more pertinent volume, suited to the "Core Curriculums" then the rage, was needed. I went along with this wish, and we were able to publish a decent text by using as authors only the existing members of the Pharmacology Department and abstracting the bulk of the material in the big book. Dick Sample did a credible job of editing while the rest of us divided various chapters into the fields of our expertise and revised, shortened, and updated the material. It fortunately turned out to be a minor success and went on to several editions. I might point out here that such an exercise greatly improves the teaching prowess of the faculty.

I managed to maintain a laboratory fully outfitted for cardiovascular research although the equipment was becoming obsolete. Bob McMichaels had risen to the rank of instructor, and I no longer had to find money to pay his salary from grants. We continued to collaborate, and I feel that we were doing some fairly credible work. As grants from NIH became more difficult to get, however, we had to face the fact that we were no longer competitive. To support the laboratory with supplies, animals, and minor equipment, I took on consultations for drug companies and some legal testimony in litigations involving drug toxicities. With rare exceptions, I always asked that the checks be made out to Hahnemann Medical College and Hospital, and I deposited the money in a Pharmacology Research Fund that I controlled. In this manner, I was able to generate $8,000 to $10,000 a year to support our research. Other faculty did this, I'm sure even taking money from hard earned practice funds. There were undoubtedly faculty who did outside work but diverted the funds into their own pockets. This was not allowed, of course, but it was virtually impossible to police this racket. Like other institutions, policies and procedures were written but never actually enforced.

These activities served to keep me abreast of general trends in medical research. This was the era of the rapid expansion in molecular biology, however, and there was no way—with my heavy administrative load—that I could even begin to comprehend all the new science and technology. I tried desperately at least to learn the new language and concepts, and to some extent I succeeded. The reality of the situation was brought home to me when I gave a lecture on membrane structure and functions to an evening class of graduate students. The students justly complained that my presentation was out-of-date and not consonant with the newer information then available. This disturbed me greatly, and I determined to institute corrective measures. I still had charge of a graduate student or two, fortunately. Dave Ritchie was just starting his graduate work, and I was able to put him to work on artificial membranes made from soap bubbles. These are capable of simulating a real cell membrane and actually can generate an action potential under appropriate circumstances. For reasons that I cannot recall, we studied effects of helium on the membrane. The work was fairly productive, but I doubt that it had any practical value. Ritchie wrote his thesis on this subject, but I made sure he had the opportunity to do other types of research that would be of more utility in his later life. Although this work helped me to understand some newer nuances, rapid advances of technology made possible revolutionary developments in membrane physiology that oldsters like myself couldn't even dream about. That the living membrane of the cell had specific channels for all the major ions (sodium, potassium, and calcium), in addition to having particular receptors for many different hormones and other control substances, was a monumental advance that made possible explanation of membrane functions that had been only conjectural. Looking around at colleagues my own age, I could perceive that even the most sharp were deficient in their comprehension of the advancing technology. Perhaps because I read a lot and wrote articles and edited a textbook, I felt that I had at least some modicum of understanding of the new knowledge. It became obvious to me that my colleagues and I were no longer able really to comprehend the articles in first class journals like *Science, Nature,* and *The Journal of Clinical Investigation.*

Large universities meanwhile were producing great volumes of talented PhDs and post-doctoral fellows who were expert in the new technologies. Industry and the more fortunate academic institutions greatly elevated the general level of scientific competition for grants and the ability to do cutting edge research by snapping up these young experts.

I was not completely devoid of professional and intellectual opportunities, however. I faithfully attended the weekly Grand Rounds sponsored by the medicine department. This reflected my old, persistent love of the practice of medicine. It satisfied my interest in keeping au courant in the latest and advanced clinical thinking. Through an odd connection, I was invited to join the editorial consulting staff of *Facts and Comparisons* (*F&C*) a large, very excellent compendium of prescription drugs. This volume started by a pharmacist in St. Louis, MO, was intended to aid physicians in the selection and use of the best-marketed drugs. Actually it was very popular only with pharmacists. Physicians, who received the *Physicians Desk Reference* (*PDR*) free of charge courtesy of the drug companies, did not even know *F&C* existed. It was quite obvious that the producers of this fine volume wanted some prominent M.D.s to appear on the title page in order to make more sales to practitioners of medicine. It was a loose-leaf arrangement with monthly additions and deletions. While the *PDR* discussed only trade name drugs, *F&C* also covered all generic preparations. It was therefore a more useful prescribing book. The staff of *F&C* was congenial, talented, and energetic. Bernie Olin, the chief editor, had a good sense of humor and a deep perspective of drug usage as concerns the practicing pharmacist. Mr. Kastrup, then in his seventies, had originated *F&C*. He was an interesting character who came to all the meetings even though he was retired and insisted that the original concepts be rigidly maintained. All were trained in pharmacy, and some had the advanced degree of Pharm.D. The other physicians who, like myself, had been brought on the consulting editorial staff were Louis Lasagne and Thomas Whitsett, both experts in Clinical Pharmacology and related matters. Once a year the administrative staff and consulting editors met for two or three days to go over editorial matters and new plans for the manual. New projects were explored. These meetings started in St Louis, and I have fond memories of the fine dinners at the Cafe Bergerac. In later years, as *F&C* became more prosperous, the meetings moved to Hawaii and the Caribbean. Wives were now included, and the meetings became lavish affairs. Much good work was accomplished, but I must admit that I probably would not have vacationed in such affluent places if left to myself. Mary enjoyed the trips immensely and eagerly looked forward to them each year. Thanks to my work with *F&C*, we got to visit all the main islands of Hawaii and most of the lovely Caribbean vacation spots. We enjoyed the best hotels and the finest meals.

I continued to attend the yearly meeting of the consulting pharmacologists at the Walter Reed Army Institute of Research (WRAIR) where research continued in the therapy of malaria and other tropical diseases as well as on possible antidotes for radiation toxicity. The work on malaria was fascinating, and WRAIR's contributions to the advances in knowledge and control of this devastating disease must stand as one of the greatest achievements of government directed research. My role was very minor, and I certainly learned more than I bestowed. Much technology was developed: for example, how to grow the parasite in vitro and the development of valuable animal models. New chemotherapeutic agents were produced, some of which are now in clinical use for drug resistant falciparum malaria. Malaria still remains as the major killer disease worldwide and accounts for over a million deaths each year in tropical belt countries. Drug companies are hardly stimulated to develop drugs for this disease because they see little chance of profit in treating a disease that is endemic only in poverty-stricken countries. To be frank, the United States government has devoted resources to fighting malaria only because it has the obligation to protect its soldiers in war theaters where malaria is endemic.

My attendance at the yearly national Dean's meeting of the American Association of Medical Colleges had a useful spin-off. I became acquainted with John Rose, the very able Dean of the Georgetown University School of Medicine. Like me, he had an early interest in physiology and continued to do research and teaching despite his Deaning position. He also was interested in family medicine and was editor of *American Family Physician*, the official journal of the American Academy of Family Practice. He knew of my interest in Clinical Pharmacology, and one fine day he asked if I would be interested in running a series of monthly articles on this subject in the journal. I was to write at least three or four of the annual series while the rest would come from outside authors procured and edited first by myself. I agreed without hesitation despite my already heavy load of administrative and other duties. Writing had actually been my worse subject in college but it became one of best the things I now did and enjoyed the most. It suited my interest in advancing the new field of Clinical Pharmacology, and I also felt that it would be good advertisement for Hahnemann. Little did I imagine at the time that I would continue this series for twenty more years. The series still continues under the editorship of Richard W. Sloan, a Family Medicine Practitioner and Clinical Pharmacologist at the York Hospital in Pennsylvania. I'm pleased to think that this series of articles came from Hahnemann, a former homeopathic school, and did much to establish the institution for the ability to join in the accepted clinical science of the day and even to be a leader in some areas. In the 1970s this was the ethical and gentile way to advertise the scientific and clinical prowess of the institution. Today the competitive method of tooting your horn is to purchase a full-page advertisement in the local newspaper, accompanied by radio and television spot items in prime time. This incidentally is extremely expensive, especially as compared to the former method where the author received no recompense from the institution for his efforts other than a half-hearted pat on the back. Of course, it must be admitted that the author was also advertising himself, and this was undoubtedly a paramount consideration.

Despite these seemingly meritorious ventures I had the premonition that I was slipping into a state of obsolescence. Yes, I'd had enough of the deaning business. It was time to retreat to the laboratory.

CHAPTER X

Decline and Fall of the Dean

1979-1982

"Know that when they paint your portrait that soon they mean to get rid of you."

Rupert Black, M.D.

The appointment of Bill Likoff as President was obviously of great benefit to the institution. It was also the beginning of my decline. Likoff was insecure in his position and sought to cover his deficiencies by bringing in professionals who could devise new, effective approaches to management. After an exhaustive search by headhunters, Paul Gazzerro, an MBA, was discovered and installed as CEO, second in command to Likoff. I was presumably third in command, as Holmes had left soon after Shober's demise. Lew Mills, who assumed Holmes' position of Vice President of Health Affairs, was benign and kept out of academic matters. Number three in this situation meant nothing, however. Gazzerro completely ignored me. Meanwhile the faculty, all good friends of Likoff, bypassed me and went straight to the president with their plans, complaints, and ambitions. Likoff passed the problems on to Gazzerro for solution without consultation with me. Naturally, Gazzerro gave them high priority. Please the President is always the road to success.

A short stocky fellow with an alert assertive manner, Gazzerro conveyed an aura of authority. He had made his mark at the Medical School of Vanderbilt University where he was able to engineer the operation of several large grants. He apparently demonstrated singular dexterity and resourcefulness. There were successes and failures over time. As a result, some faculty members were very pleased, and others who were on the short end were very critical.

Vanderbilt, a very well endowed university, had a medical school that was easily in the first quartile while Hahnemann was definitely in the bottom quartile. Its thin budget and sparse staff could not offer Gazzero the facilities and opportunities of his former post. Undaunted, Gazzero plunged ahead with grandiose plans to reconstruct the institution.

Likoff made valiant efforts to recruit substantial new members of the Board and get rid of the deadwood. He was helped by his acquaintance with the important members of the business community, a good many of whom had occasion to use him as an expert cardiology medical consultant. Several new additions were made, none of whom could be considered a major philanthropist or even an expert in any pertinent field. Eventually, Likoff got Mark Rubinstein, an influential businessman, on the Board. The Board was too big (thirty-five members), and too much deadwood remained. The ability of a President to get things done depends on a sympathetic and supporting Board. Likoff did not have one. Cox, the Chairman, and Donald T. Brophy, the Vice Chairman, had only one aim in mind—to maintain a satisfactory financial status. There were no plans for expansion, no ambitions to excel, no pure desire to improve the academic status. The faculty anticipated a salary increase, but this was just wishful thinking. Students, staff, and professors all had a great fervor for new projects nevertheless.

A valiant effort to raise more money from the alumni was started. If anyone could raise funds from the graduates of the institution, it should have been Likoff. A superb clinician, a doctor's doctor, and the most popular instructor of clinical medicine with a national reputation, he was universally loved and admired. Although there was some response, no substantial funds eventuated. Alumni of medical schools seldom contribute large sums. Physicians do have good incomes; some surgeons and specialists become millionaires, but truly large fortunes arise from industry, real estate, and investments. Those rare alumni who are so endowed do not make their medical school their major beneficiary. Rather they give to the undergraduate college where there are sweet memories compared to the torture of the onerous study of medicine and science.

The glorious 1980s were a period of the greatest growth and expansion of medical services and science. Faculty and staff who felt the Shober Era had compromised them, as well as those who had flourished, now saw the chance to advance their personal interests. An environment of plotting and intrigue soon developed. Gone was the orderly democratic process of discussion in properly appointed committees and presentation for consideration in Academic Affairs Council. Rather, entrepreneurs made a direct thrust to the President and the Board. Important matters were already decided by the time they reached Academic Affairs Council.

During the Shober Era, the faculty had gained the right to have two elected members to the Board. In addition, there were two elected alumni members who were generally sympathetic to academic perogatives. Thus there was an unusual ability for members other than executives to get acquainted with and to influence Board Members to support certain projects. The Dean, with no direct access to the Board, just gave a monthly report that was not read. He could talk to the President who didn't listen. Under these circumstances, the Board thought of the Dean as a species of office boy who took care of student problems and some pesky academic matters.

Two particular faculty members took advantage of the situation to get themselves elected to the Board. Evangelas T. Angelakos from the basic sciences and Sheldon Bender from the clinical sciences achieved this distinction. Both had the institution's best interests at heart (if it fit in with their personal agenda). Angelakos was the Chairman of Physiology. Recruited in 1967 by Bondi and myself after a difficult search, he turned out to be a very able researcher, a good teacher, and a clever department head. His sterling academic record could have predicted this: an M.D. from Harvard, a Ph.D. from Boston University, about fifty first-rate publications, ample NIH grants, and superb recommendations. He certainly was qualified and his subsequent performance was commendable. At this time in his career as he approached age fifty, his personal ambitions turned towards administration with an eye on the deanship or presidency. He wisely took a business course at Harvard especially designed for deans. Naturally fluent in math, Angelakos became expert in the analysis of budgets. Impressed with this calm, well-spoken scholar who knew the lingo of businessmen, the Board made him secretary to his delight. This position gave him access to documents and personnel that made possible acquisition of valuable data, as well as the ability to discuss it with various members of the Board. Combined with ingenious politics with prominent members of the faculty, Angelakos was able to develop ample support. His co-conspirator was Chernick, Chairman of Pharmacology, who let on to me some sparse details of Angelakos's machinations.

Sheldon Bender was a popular cardiologist of the part-time volunteer clinical staff. He represented a rugged type who defended the rights and entitlements of his group against the full-time medical staff. He fancied himself a researcher in arteriosclerosis particularly as it affected the coronary arteries, but he was not a lab type. Whether or not he had ambitions to become a Chairman is uncertain, but he valued his academic professorial title. I felt that he was a practical type who could converse reasonably with the Board members and protect the rights of the practicing physicians who were valuable teachers and contributors to the institution.

There were several other ambitious, aggressive groups who were anxious to protect and extend their piece of the pie. Brodsky and his oncology cluster wanted to be an institute rivaling the cardiovascular institute. Without argument, Brodsky had raised much money and his program was superior in both research and clinical performance. Sylvan M. Tobin, his brother-in-law, was on the Board and was able to protect Brodsky's interests. My impression was that Tobin was a sterling character who acted entirely within the confines of what was reasonable and proper. Luther Brady, head of Therapeutic Radiology and Nuclear Medicine, was also a main actor. His research program was good, his clinical work superior. Nearly everyone who came in contact with Brady found him to be abrasive. Paradoxically, he was sweet with patients and charming at social events. Internationally known in oncology circles, he did a great deal of traveling. I liked Brady, but the only bone of contention was that he overspent his grants year after year. His influence on the Board was not too great. Arnold Berman, the head of Orthopedics, was the savviest, most politically astute of all the contenders. He had made some real estate investments that reputedly made him a millionaire many times over. He seemed to know seamy characters that operated within city government politics. His influence on the Board was considerable since he had taken care of quite a few backs, hips, knees, and ankles of Board members. "Reds" Bagnell, ex-football player and now prominent businessman, was in his pocket. Berman wanted his own institute and desired to control affiliate hospitals so that some lucrative surgery could be channeled his way. There was no end to Berman's ambitions, and subsequent history confirmed this. Naturally there were more contenders for power, but Surgery was not one of them. Since Charles Wolferth had left, there was a decline in this department that seemed to be chronic. Teruo Matsumoto, a Holmes protégé, was Chairman. He was a superb surgeon who did some praiseworthy research. His popularity was attenuated by a short stature but even more by poor speech. He spoke rapidly with a marked Japanese accent. He was the only chairman who consulted me regularly on how he might improve his department. I did what I could for him, which wasn't much.

I still had some friends on the Board, but they were of the benign type who never made waves. Donald T. Brophy, a long time member of the Board, was well acquainted with me. He was very businesslike and straight-laced as becomes a senior officer of Rohm and Hass, the great chemical firm in Philadelphia. One did not dare to make a direct approach to Brophy to advance a worthy project. Thus I was in a weak position at this time to control any situation.

While I still had considerable support among the general faculty, there was a disturbing movement towards tenure and more involvement of the general faculty in decision-making and governance issues. Naturally there was the underlying interest in salary raises and fringe benefits. Hahnemann did not have tenure, and all efforts to establish it in the past had failed. I was not opposed to tenure, but I had a clearer view of its impracticality in a school so poorly endowed and always on the edge of financial failure. My personal experience over thirty years at Hahnemann was that very few faculty were fired or treated unjustly. The salary structure was comparable to that of the University of Pennsylvania School of Medicine. Department Chairmen tended to be paid more than the average, and perhaps this was one of the reasons that the faculty did chide the Dean for running a "Chairman's Club." Some faculty were members of the American Association of University Professors (AAUP), while the rest imagined that it's good to be protected by a union. They wanted a Senate elected and run by the faculty, with the power to make recommendations that had to be heard. The Board, of course, never understands why the Dean cannot suppress such activities that are a nuisance. I had to go along with the faculty and appointed an ad hoc committee to study the matter and come up with a proposal that could be considered by College council and then the Board. There was sparse talent that could engineer a plausible study and proposal. The best I could find to head the committee was Melvin Benarde, Associate Professor of Community Medicine. Benarde was a microbiologist by training, but somehow he had gotten into things like germ warfare and the environmental contamination affecting human welfare. He had written several books, one of them achieving *The New York Times'* bestseller list. Benarde plunged into the assignment with enormous enthusiasm He made plans completely leftist and inconsistent with the majority of what was essentially a conservative faculty. He was outspoken, and irritated his colleagues No amount of advice seemed to help, and the committee's report was laughed off the stage. Benarde's career at Hahnemann was damaged by this episode, and certainly my own reputation was damaged. Some actually thought that I was Machiavellian enough to have appointed Benarde to kill the project. The truth is that there was no real interest in a faculty

Senate except by a small militant group. When it came to do serious work, none came forward to put his head on the block. In a few weeks the senate idea died away, and the faculty turned its attention to other matters. There was no tenure until many Deans and years later—ironically, when most universities were dropping the concept of tenure.

Likoff blossomed into his position and obviously enjoyed the responsibility and drama of running a large medical center. His personal life also thrived. He courted a female medical resident nearly forty years his junior, married her, bought a house in the city and another at the shore, acquired a Jaguar, and lived the bon vie. I even observed, as did others, that he sneaked in some cigarette smoking. With his past medical history of vascular disease and his age, it was inevitable that some deterioration would occur. He began to have symptoms of Parkinson's Disease Nevertheless he hung on functioning fairly well despite his disability.

In my own case I was beginning to experience chest pains that were suggestive of coronary heart disease. I was finally hospitalized and a cardiac catheterization showed a 75 percent closure of my anterior descendants' coronary artery. I refused a by-pass operation. At the time, it was believed that with single vessel disease, medical therapy did as well as a surgical approach. Now many years later, I'm sure it was the right decision. The loss of thirty pounds, a change in diet, abstinence from alcohol and tobacco, and a change in lifestyle was an effective treatment. This regime unfortunately is hardly consistent with the rigors of the Deanship. I was sixty-four years old and ready to move on. Besides, the Board felt that it was time for a change, and Angelakos felt that it was the strategic time to move himself into the Deanship. Chernick, who was grateful for my many favors towards him, managed a campaign to have my portrait painted. It was handsomely done, and I was most pleased and grateful for this commendation. It has hung in the library all these years and is a constant reminder that I was appreciated in my time.

The year was 1980. Retirement age had traditionally been sixty-five. Now it was, at least theoretically, any age when you could still stand up and function. This movement came on because of the failing financial status of Social Security. New regulations were passed that allowed retirement at seventy, after which you could work and earn as much as you liked without penalty of your Social Security income. As result, the retirement age practically became seventy, and many worked after that if they were able. With Likoff's help, I managed to hang on as Dean for two more years.

The Board felt that I should retire in June 1981 when I would be sixty-five. I pointed out to Likoff that it would take at least a year to find a suitable replacement, and he would have to work with a replacement Dean, which might be cumbersome. Likoff agreed and apparently convinced the Board to let me stay on another year. Because of the new laws with respect to retirement age, I could have insisted on being maintained. This was entirely inappropriate. First of all, I wanted to step down as Dean. I did want to work a few more years in teaching and research, and the Board was entirely agreeable to this.

Little did Likoff anticipate that the Board would not renew his Presidential contract in 1982. Instead, he was pushed upstairs to be Chancellor. Undoubtedly his Parkinson's Disease which had now become more symptomatic influenced the Board's decision. Deeply hurt and bitter because he had sacrificed much to take on the Presidency, he continued to support Hahnemann, at least on the surface. Poor health and the breakup of his second marriage speeded his decline. He returned to full-time practice and never was much of an influence on the future course of politics and finances of the institution.

As might be anticipated, the final two years of my deanship were "Lame Duck" squared. As I have pointed out in these memoirs, a Dean's popularity depends entirely upon what moneys and opportunities for the faculty he can procure. The pickings were now scarce. State and federal governments had come to the conclusion that there were too many physicians who became specialists and caused an inflation of healthcare. About twenty new medical schools scooped up the NIH funds that would have gone to the weaker older schools. Five medical schools in one city whose population was diminishing was extreme competition for already scarce funds. Programs like the Wilkes-Hahnemann, which had brought generous funds to the Dean's Office, were now phasing out. Tuition raises did not parallel the inflationary rises in salaries and maintenance expenses. Students were demanding more services and the minority program required infusions to keep it alive. New technologies for office management required expensive equipment and the consumption of enormous quantities of paper. Copiers, fax machines, and computers all had to be installed and maintained. Gone was the simple typewriter that limited copies to two or three with carbon paper and lasted twenty years. Somehow an old pinchpenny Dean did not look germane in the midst of the humming new machines.

In the final years of an executive's reign, his trusted and faithful staff begins to fade. Recognizing the handwriting on the wall, they seek to find other opportunities that promise advances not likely in their present position. Bachich, my capable financial officer, managed to get more integrated in the central financial operation, but he knew that ultimately he would have to go outside for real gain. He finally became financial officer of a moderate size university and has done very well. This forced me to secure another finance person. Amy D. Waldor, a very competent young lady, performed a competent job but was short on the confidence and aggressiveness necessary to combat the financial wolves of the hospital. Bob Walker, my trusted manager and systems expert, successively tied himself more to the central business administration and anticipated the time when I would no longer be in power. He didn't get along with my secretary, and a quasi-armed truce endured. Hugh Bennett, the Associate Dean, stuck to the bitter end. He took care of all student services, the clinical curriculum, and such pesky things as graduation. Meanwhile, he taught a good deal of clinical medicine and had a fair size practice. Most students liked him, and he deservedly won the Golden Apple Award five times. He stuck it out with me loyally to the end, for which I will be ever grateful. If there was any hero in the Dean's Office, Bennett was the real candidate.

I began to pursue more scholarly pursuits, knowing full well that soon I must step down and sequester myself in the Pharmacology Department. The easy way to go was to start a more active research program. Laboratory space was no problem as I had maintained a working active laboratory during all the years that I was Dean. Robert McMichaels, whom I hired as a technician many years before, was a great help to me in this. Justification for the laboratory also lay in the fact that it was the home base of the best minority programs, which were run by McMichaels. They had NIH support, which greatly helped to sanction its existence. I managed to support the purchase of equipment, supplies, and other expenses from a research fund into which I put all earnings that I made in consultations, giving legal testimony, and doing small research projects for industry, so my laboratory was not a drain on departmental resources.

NIH grants in cardiology research had become so competitive that I had little hope of securing enough funds to modernize the equipment. Besides, I wanted to get into more molecular biology research that was expanding rapidly and offered more opportunity for significant discoveries. Over the years I had become friendly with Burton Landau, Associate Professor of Microbiology. He was an expert tissue culturist and had a laboratory for this purpose. He kindly allowed McMichaels and me to work in his laboratory and learn the technology of tissue culture in a practical way. I had a realistic reason for turning to tissue culture as an experimental technology. The animals I had worked with, mainly dogs and cats, had grown prohibitively expensive, and the red tape even to use them was tedious and wasteful of time. Tissue culture was not cheap but had other advantages, the most important being that it was more consonant with the concepts of the day. A vast variety of cells were also available for any experimental purpose.

I must digress to explain how I got into the research, which occupied the declining years of my academic pursuit. Steve DeFelice, the young army officer I'd met years before at the Walter Read Army Institute of Research, was successful in establishing a consulting practice aimed at enabling smaller drug companies to develop and market new drugs. He was unusually talented for this profession because he was trained in both medicine and science, had worked for the drug industry, but most importantly he had a nose for business and sales. As a great lover of opera and Italian culture, he naturally gravitated towards Italy and the Italian drug industry. Fidia, a fairly new and growing Italian drug firm, was making a fortune selling a special preparation of the ganglioside GM_1 for the therapy of various degenerative neurological diseases. There was ample experimental evidence that gangliosides cause regeneration of certain nerve cells in tissue culture and sprouting of cut axons. The clinical work proving efficacy was weak. Despite this, Fidia's preparation of GM_1 Cronosial, was very popular in Italy, Germany, and South America for the therapy of unresponsive neurologic diseases such as peripheral neuritis and other brain disorders. It was an injectible and had to be administered subcutaneously two or three times a week on a chronic basis. Doctors liked it because they could charge a fee for administering it. Patients liked it because injectibles are in their mind are much more effective than oral drugs. Cronosial had practically no side effects, and this also gained patient's acceptance. It was very expensive, but at the time the Italian Government paid for it, which greatly added to its popularity. Fidia had a virtual monopoly on GM_1 because of its patents on the manufacture from calves' brains.

Fidia felt that Cronosial should have a market share in the United States and hired DeFelice to promote the drug with a view to getting the Food and Drug Administration's (FDA) approval. This would not be easy, as the FDA would require exhaustive proof of efficacy and toxicity. Undaunted, DeFelice took on the assignment. He asked me to look over the scientific and clinical data that Fidia had assembled. This gave me a chance to visit the Fidia Plant in Abano Terme, Italy, and talk to the staff of scientists involved with Cronosial. I was impressed with the facilities and the scientists, especially with Francesco Della Valle, the President of the firm. After a thorough study, I came to the conclusion that Cronosial was being used clinically in humans essentially on the basis of laboratory data and theory without any clinical studies that would satisfy the FDA with respect to Cronosial's efficacy. Fortunately, while it had no meaningful clinical effect it had no appreciable toxicity. My hunch was that it probably was a powerful placebo especially as it was expensive and was given by injection.

I decided to see for myself if gangliosides had any activity in intact animals. Madhu Kalia, a young Indian neurophysiologist in the Department of Physiology, was agreeable to working with me in establishing a test animal model. Incidentally, she was a thorn in Angelakos's side because of her aggressiveness and frank criticism of her colleagues. This caused me some concern because I did not wish to antagonize Angelakos. With me she was sweet, and I found her to be most able and resourceful.

We settled on a test of the healing ability of ganglioside in a nerve crush injury in the hind limb of the rat. The crush injury results in a paralysis of the limb, which is capable of natural recovery over a period of ten to fifteen days. We found that indeed ganglioside shortened the period of recovery by a significant number of days as compared to non-treated animals. I was encouraged and recommended to DeFelice that a clinical study be instituted to learn of the therapeutic potential of ganglioside in peripheral neuritis in humans. Peripheral neuritis occurs frequently in diabetics and is seriously crippling. Fidia was enthusiastic and a fairly comprehensive clinical study was performed in a different institution. The results unfortunately were completely negative. As so frequently happens in drug research, what works in a laboratory test fails when put to test in the human.

With the help of a graduate student, Kalia and I went on to study possible benefit of ganglioside in spinal cord crush injury in the rat. This model resembles paraplegia, a common disabling injury in athletic and automobile accidents. We were disappointed to find no perceptible benefit. After this I decided to move on to other pastures.

Not so Fidia. Still making millions in world sales of ganglioside, Fidia could not understand why it did not catch on in the United States. It suspected a low opinion of Italian science and clinical investigation by American scientists. Determined to change this atmosphere, the company conceived a plan to establish an outstanding institute of neurobiological science in the United States. Fidia selected Georgetown University School of Medicine, perhaps because of its Washington D.C. location near the FDA and NIH, and promised an income of at least $50 million over a period of years. Georgetown had to provide extensive laboratory space and administrative know-how. Without this available space, Georgetown decided to close its Dental School, which was in the state of decline. The dental building became the new Neurological Institute, much to the dismay of faculty devoted primarily to teaching. Erminio Costa, a truly outstanding neurophysiologist, became the head and assembled a very able staff. The Institute began to do cutting-edge research. None of this research was even remotely related to gangliosides, and apparently Fidia kept to its promise not to exploit this venture for self-interest. Hahnemann, incidentally, wanted this bonanza and solicited my help. Although I was no longer Dean, I must admit that I too would have liked to bring a $50 million windfall to Hahnemann. Sadly by this time, I had lost my interest in gangliosides and broken my relationship with Fidia. Such is the fickleness of destiny that Georgetown eventually lost heavily on the deal. In a couple of years, Fidia went bankrupt and never completed its commitment. The Institute broke up. Costa returned to NIH, and many scientists and staff were left high and dry.

Thousands of papers have been written on the gangliosides, which remain of great interest because they are involved in Tay-Sachs Disease. Their function in the fetal development of the nervous system is vital. What they do in the adult is mysterious. The only reliable evidence that I could find was that gangliosides serve as part of the cellular membrane receptor mechanism for certain natural peptide structure hormones and control substances. Among these is interferon, a complex peptide agent manufactured by fibroblasts and other tissues, which has anti-viral and anti-cancer cellular activity. At the time, the early 1980s, interferon was in the early stages of development, but it was already known that its efficacy was limited. Only certain types of cancer cells and virus were susceptible, and then there rarely was a complete kill. These facts gave me the idea that gangliosides could perhaps enhance the activity of interferon by increasing its binding to cellular membranes. This was quite a wild idea. Was it worth exploring? I asked Dr. William Carter, a world class authority on interferon and a new member of Brodsky's oncology group. After cogitating a few minutes he replied, "There's about a fifty-fifty chance that you will get a positive result." That was enough for me, and I boldly decided to gamble on this project. Fortuitously, Carter had a share in a company that manufactured interferon from fibroblasts obtained from the foreskin of the human penis. He kindly let me have $3,000 worth of interferon to do the study.

With great anticipation McMichaels and I began work. The first step—to obtain a cell line of a human lung cancer and grow it successively and reliably—was accomplished in a matter of a few weeks. We next established a dose of interferon that was able to cause a 20 percent reduction in growth of the lung cancer cells. Next, the crucial experiment was adding the ganglioside. Disappointment! The ganglioside did absolutely nothing. Baffled, we went back to original work on the gangliosides and found that neuroaminodase, an enzyme that splits off neuroaminic acid from the total molecule, is necessary to cause binding of some substances. So we got some neuroaminodase and added it to the experiment. No soap. Neuroaminodase turned out to be a growth factor for this cell line. This would enhance the growth of the cells masking the inhibitory action of the interferon. Eventually we gave up after learning some hard lessons. In my younger days, I would have tried to publish this negative result, at least to get a publication out of hard work. At this stage in life with more papers to my credit than I needed, I did not bother to try to publish negative results. So we went on to see if we could devise tissue culture methods to study microgravity. We had some contact with the

Space Agency and felt that there might be some chance of getting financial support from this source.

Gangliosides remain a domain of interest and development to many investigators. There is some experimental work, which indicates a possibility of benefit in Parkinson's disease and in spinal injury.

Despite my research endeavors, I made a distinct effort to leave the institution in as good shape as possible for my successor. The early 1980s were a time of vast growth in the delivery of medical services because of increased availability of Medicare and Medicaid moneys. Congress doubled budgets of the National Institutes of Health. Hahnemann needed a young vigorous President who was well qualified and had strong connections in Washington in order to optimize income from this source. I had nothing to do with the search committee for the President, which greatly depressed me because it was evident that whoever was selected would have a great influence on the future. I wanted to be sure that the right person be chosen.

By some twist of fate, the person who had the main influence in the selection of the new President was a former Brooklyn student of mine from the old Long Island Of Medicine. Israel Zwerling had a Ph.D. in psychology before he went to medical school. He was a brilliant student, and it was natural for him to specialize in psychiatry. State and federal governments wished to move mentally ill patients from institutions back to the community. In his professional life, Zwerling was much involved with this maneuver. The discovery of effective drug therapy led society to believe that mental patients who were incapable of taking care of themselves could now be returned to a more normal existence, provided that appropriate services and drug therapy were available in a community setting. At the same time, significant cost savings could be achieved. The National Institute of Mental Health (NIMH) was much involved in this movement, and many large grants were distributed for the study and facilitation of effective community services. In his work at the Albert Einstein College of Medicine, Zwerling was very involved with the NIMH and became friendly with its head, Burton Brown.

Meanwhile, Van Buren Hammett, our distinguished head of the Department of Mental Health Sciences, retired. Zwerling turned up as a nominee to replace him, and I gave my blessing when the selection committee chose him as the top candidate. We had a large and active department, and I was anxious to maintain forward movement. They were primarily of the analytic school, and I was pleased to observe that Zwerling, although more broadly trained, was also of the same calling. Although not as popular as Hammett, he made an effective department head, and that is how some years later he successfully sold Hahnemann to Bertram Brown. Cox, the Board Chairman, asked my opinion of Brown. I must confess that I told him that he was a choice I would have made myself and that I was surprised the Board would select someone who was an intellect, a government official, a psychiatrist, and a consultant to the Rand Corporation.

Bertram Brown was tall and thin, with a sharp face topped by copious dark wavy hair, and a toothy smile. Yet his eyes had that insouciance that indicated he was smarter than you and whatever you were suggesting was old hat. By the time Brown took over Hahnemann, he had already done everything except climb Mount Everest. Trained in psychiatry and pediatrics, he never practiced either profession. He was head of NIMH for over ten years and was involved in moving the mentally ill from chronic care hospitals to community care centers (which did not exist and so created the problem of homeless street people). In his work at NIMH, he made many important contacts with government officials and politicians. He brought along to Hahnemann a fellow government official Gian Carlo Salmoiraghi, who was head of the grants division of NIMH. (More about him later.) Brown was a consultant to industry in many areas but especially with respect to crime and particularly terrorism. In addition to all these great accomplishments, Brown was also a brilliant pianist. I heard him play myself and must admit that he could have been a successful musician.

Brown installed himself at Hahnemann with fanfare worthy of an event such as Napoleon's coronation or the inauguration of George Washington. He conceived the idea of a Constitutional Convention similar to the one that took place in Philadelphia in 1789. On October 24, 1983, delegates (Brown's government cronies and other dignitaries) gathered at the Friends Meeting House at 4th and Arch Streets to discuss in depth the delivery of healthcare and appropriate management systems. In this one-day meeting, specific recommendations and luminous new concepts were to be conceived. Without a strict agenda and serious exhaustive preparation, it was bound to produce nothing but tepid air. And that was exactly what it did, despite the attendance of Arthur Fleming, Elliot Richardson, Josh Lederberg, and other very intelligent, capable people. It did not attract much press and in reality turned out to be nothing more than a demonstration of Brown's contacts rather than a constructive educational creative event. It was also a very expensive undertaking for Hahnemann's sparse budget. Brown was apparently thinking that he had the government's copious treasury behind him. Sadly, the underpaid archivist, Barbara Williams, wrote up the great event in summary without much help from the well-paid participants.

Brown's next extravaganza was a complete remodeling of the nineteen floor into a handsome suite of offices. In his five years as President, Likoff had managed to get along with the quite adequate former Shober suite. I can't say that Brown was completely out of line. The 1970s and 1980s were a period of rapid expansion and the firm establishment of a credit philosophy in money matters. Banks gave out large loans with abandonment and without realistic collateral. Credit cards blossomed, and people began to spend money they didn't have, hoping that a future increase in income would rescue them. The old solid Victorian philosophy of "have the money in your pocket before you spend it" was gone. The healthcare industry was growing rapidly, and medical schools that were hospital-school combinations rushed to take advantage of this bonanza. In Philadelphia with its five medical schools and many fine hospitals, the competition was fierce. Jefferson with its fine new hospital, good business oriented Board, cash reserves, and a cagey Dean and resourceful President did the best. Not counting the University of Pennsylvania, of course.

In some ways Bert Brown was a good choice. He had the vision, he was smart, he was ambitious, and he had important contacts in the healthcare industry and in government. The only detriment was that Brown was a psychiatrist with an extraordinary ego. When you had an interview with Brown you felt that you were undergoing psychoanalyzed by a superior brain. Indeed, his approach to all problems was psychiatry oriented, including favoring the Department of Mental Health Sciences—at best a loss leader as far as income to the institution was concerned. Presumably he could get big grants for this department, but they never did materialize. His personnel decisions were questionable. For example, he insisted on dragging Salmoiraghi away from his secure government job. Salmoiraghi had a valid M.D. degree from an Italian medical school, but since he had no clinical experience in the U.S., he could not get a license to practice medicine in most states, certainly not in Pennsylvania. For reasons only he understood, he had put the stipulation to Brown that a Pennsylvania medical license must be obtained for him in order for him to leave his safe job and come to unstable Hahnemann University. Brown made a solemn promise to get him a Pennsylvania license to practice medicine. His solution was to call me.

"Joe, as a former Dean, you must know the people on the Medical Board of Licenses." Brown said. "Salmoiraghi needs a medical license. See what you can do to get him one." He fluffed off my response that the Medical Board was very strict and above influence peddling. I didn't dare tell him that the chairman of the Medical Board was a Hahnemann alumnus whom I knew quite well. Instead, I diplomatically replied, "I'll see what I can do. Have Salmoiraghi send me his curriculum vitae." His C.V. showed that he did have an authentic medical degree from an Italian medical school. His postgraduate training was entirely restricted to neurophysiology where he had secondary positions to some prominent physiologists and had managed to get his name on some quite good scientific papers. He had immigrated to this country and maneuvered to get a government job at NIH. There was no acceptable clinical training, and it would be impossible for him to qualify for a medical license. He would have to spend at least two years in an approved residency program to stand a chance. Despite this, I tried to help him. As expected. I got a dressing down by the Medical Licensing Board for even suggesting that they make an exception. This failure on my part was the first of a series of events that resulted in a lack of endearment between Brown and myself.

Salmoiraghi was a charming and attractive fellow. With his foreign accent and his European manners, he made friends easily. A big push was being made in research for neurological disorders because, as compared to cancer and cardiovascular diseases, there had been little advance in this area. Competent in neurophysiology and with know-how of getting a grant application through the red tape of NIH, Salmoiraighi became acceptable to most faculty. No doubt he was Brown's man but his appointment as research coordinator made sense and was an advantage to those who wanted to develop neurophysiology and neurology.

Brown had a style of operation peculiar to himself. He loved large conference meetings meant to be idea sessions to find solutions to difficult situations. To this end, he formed the "Alert Group" composed of about twenty major and minor executives. They met each week, early in the morning in the Board Room, without specific agenda or prior preparation. Brown always presided in an informal manner but in complete control of the discussion. He would present a problem and then pick any member at random for discussion and solution. Since the person selected rarely knew the background or what had already been done, their comments were perforce pedestrian. His confreres who knew more details about the particular subject would jump in, and the discussion would often get lively. Brown would listen with a silly smile on his face. After a few minutes, he'd cut the discussion short and modestly let on that he had thought about the subject and pointed out what, in his estimation, would not work and what could be the ideal solution. He called upon me many times, especially when the problem concerned some academic fringe. I would usually give a conservative answer based either on personal experience or what neighboring institutions had done in similar circumstances. I don't know why this approach seemed to irritate Brown. Perhaps his brilliant intellect could not accept the fact that an old solution was probably better than an expensive new strategy. Brown also saw fit to ignore Likoff, who at the time was the Chancellor and organizationally his superior officer.

In all fairness, it must be acknowledged that Brown did bring a new approach to Hahnemann that was more consonant with the burgeoning 1980s. The institution that had struggled to overcome the stigma of homeopathy and had managed, against great odds, to become a respectable university, now began to feel that, with the leadership of a talented former high government official, it could really compete with the big boys. Department chairmen and section heads lined up behind Brown in hopes of getting support for their special projects. He helped those he could, and quite a few thought Brown was a great president. Regardless, all great leaders have their own agendas on the path to greatness. Brown was going to make Hahnemann a leading center for neurological research.

Such an undertaking unfortunately would require seed money ideally of at least several million dollars. With Hahnemann's lack of endowment, and with a Board controlled by bankers who were protecting their loans, there was little hope of local support. Raising money from the Philadelphia area philanthropists was also virtually impossible. Brown had worked with the Kennedy family in establishing its philanthropy in the neurological sciences so everyone thought that Brown would raise outside money for this ambitious project. No such luck. Brown resorted to the same old game: Rob Peter to pay Paul. Use departmental teaching funds to support a new research area.

During my years as Dean, I followed the dictum that a medical school's excellence depends upon having well organized and balanced basic science departments in Anatomy, Physiology, Biochemistry, Microbiology, Pharmacology, and Pathology. These supported the clinical departments of Medicine, Surgery, Pediatrics, Obstetrics and Gynecology, and Psychiatry. There usually were other departments, but those above were considered essential and followed the subjects that were the bulk of material on medical licensing exams. Many important subjects could also have departmental status, such as Radiology, Preventative or Community Medicine, but in less affluent schools were incorporated as divisions or sections of a major department. The by-laws of the institution clearly delineated the rules of appointment of department chairmen and the powers and jurisdiction they might have. Major decisions ultimately fell upon the Academic Affairs Council that had faculty representation and involved all departments in any decision involving one department. The Dean or President could not appoint Department Chairmen or change the structure of departments without due process. Brown wanted to appoint Salmoiraghi as Chairman of the Department of Physiology to appease the latter's desire for the safety of job permanence. I would have never allowed this appointment to go through had I still been Dean. I was still a member of the Academic Affairs Council but without a vote. By some stratagem, Angelakos (Chair of Physiology and faculty board member) accomplished Brown's desire. Thus began a continuing decay of the carefully constructed by-laws of the institution. Departmental structure and operation would never again be the same because now there would be far more emphasis on research and much less on teaching.

Salmoiraghi did have commendable expertise in neurophysiology but was not of the caliber expected in the full professorship category. He had no experience teaching medical students or running an educational department. There is no way he could have been competitive for the position if the appointment had been carried out in the ordained fashion. Angelakos, on the other hand, was very well qualified for the position of Dean. Moreover, it is entirely within the province of the President to appoint an Interim Dean of his choice. I knew that Angelakos was astute enough to know that the appointment of Salmoiraghi would be a catastrophe for the Department of Physiology. Why did he allow it? I asked my buddy Chernick for an explanation. He blandly replied, "Van is terribly ambitious to become the permanent Dean and wants to better his chances". By being Interim Dean, he can dig in his tendrils to insure his continuous tenure. Besides, as Dean he can control what goes on in Physiology. Down deep he thinks Salmoiraghi is no more than a mouse who can be controlled, and Brown can be dispensed with in due time."

Well, it didn't turn out quite as the connivers expected. In a few months Brown got rid of Angelakos by throwing him a bone, the Deanship of the Graduate School, a gift he could not refuse because he was no longer even a Department Chairman and would have to return to his department as an underling to Salmoiraghi! The plan to build an important presence of neurobiology at Hahnemann began in earnest. Using his knowledge from NIMH about up and coming researchers in the field, Salmoiraghi began to recruit by using the money that was originally intended to support the Physiology Department and the Division of Neuroanatomy of the Department of Anatomy.

I did what I could to support the effort to develop neurobiology and the clinical sciences of neurology and psychiatry. Nevertheless, without the support of the President, I could only play a passive role. I had to sit back and watch the destruction of basic science departments for the sake of a gamble that neurological research and therapeutic developments were the great blossoming fields of the future. It wasn't a bad gamble, but the funds for development should have been secured first.

Brown had grandiose ideas for developing the hospital and wanted to secure an aggressive, resourceful hospital director to carry out his plans. A large, cumbersome committee was appointed composed of faculty, physicians, and administrators. Even I was allowed to be an insignificant member. Headhunters probably did the nationwide search. The name of Iqbal Paroo eventually appeared as the lead candidate. Paroo was born in Egypt of a well-to-do family and had an excellent education. Dashing and sporty in his youth, he had a serious motor accident in which he lost a leg. His hospitalization and subsequent fitting of prosthesis made a deep impression on him. Impressed by what could be accomplished by expert medical care, he decided to devote his life to the health field. He migrated to this country and enrolled in Georgia State University where he earned a Bachelor of Business Administration (cum laude) and went on to a Masters in Health Administration. After some clinical residencies, he held a number of jobs in hospital administration and performed in an exemplary fashion. He eventually became CEO of the Meharry Medical School Health System, which was in deep financial straits, and he was able to bring some order to the operation.

On paper, Paroo looked good. In person he was young (thirty-four), thin, tall, dark, and if not handsome at least very good looking. You would not notice a slight limp unless you knew that he had only one leg. He had the authoritative bearing of a leader and the determination and will to succeed. The committee was unanimously for Paroo, and Brown promptly appointed him. Little did he suspect that this was the man who would soon replace him. I was even enthusiastic myself about his appointment.

It soon became apparent that Paroo was a very able operator and completely consonant with the rapidly developing free-spending 1980s. He soon revamped the development department, got rid of deadwood, and made some strategic appointments. He was mindful to consult Brown at every step and to make the chief feel that all these good ideas were his. Brown, an ingrained intellectual type, was happy to relegate all these mundane business type matters to Paroo and began to spend more time and effort in the academic development of the institution. Meanwhile Paroo worked the old double agent game and went about ingratiating himself with key Board members.

There were problems. Angelakos, the former Chairman of Physiology, was Interim Dean and had access to financial information that showed that the institution was spending money too lavishly. Gene Busch, the financial officer, was also well aware of the situation, as were the more conservative Board members. The faculty and staff were becoming disenchanted with both Brown and Paroo. Salmoiraghi was not pulling the NIH rabbits out of the hat that every one expected. Paroo was telling eminent clinicians where they could go if they did not fill the hospital beds. The alumni were told they were disloyal to the institution. Brown's witticisms no longer enchanted the faculty. Something needed to be done. The solution? Bring in a strong Dean who could secure the allegiance of the faculty and alumni, and this, of course, would get rid of Angelakos, a thorn in the side of the free spenders.

The usual large search committee was set up, and headhunters soon found that John R. Beljan, M.D. was the most qualified and desirable candidate. He was the Dean who installed and managed the new Ohio State Medical School in Dayton, entitled Wright State University School of Medicine. A Detroit native, he did his training at the University of Michigan at Ann Arbor. A four-year surgical residency qualified him as a surgeon. His main interest however was Aerospace Medicine, and he spent nearly ten years in the U.S. Air Force Medical Corps serving in a number of important projects in the States and in Europe. One was Project Gemini where he served on the General Support Team. After leaving the military, he became a faculty member of the new medical school at the University of California at Davis where he served as Associate Dean for Medical Education. On paper, Beljan was more than qualified to be a Dean. A Provost or better a Presidency was a more fitting position.

I had a chance to interview Beljan before he took the job. I liked him immediately with his attractive smile and the bearing of aviators whom I admired in my youth. There was no doubt that Beljan knew the deaning business inside out. One reservation that I knew inherently was that he would have to deal with an established, hardened faculty. This would be much different from his experience at Wright State where he had a younger, unsophisticated faculty that he'd hired himself and who owed him allegiance. At Hahnemann he would also have nothing to give away to appease a hungry, ambitious faculty. I knew all this, but I also realized that the likelihood of finding a better candidate than Beljan was remote. Knowing that I was not doing Beljan a favor, I encouraged him to take the job. Hahnemann, I told him, had great potential, was in a great medical city, had very good students, had first-class accreditation, and had a blossoming University of the Medical Sciences. These were true statements. What I did not tell him was that Hahnemann was constantly on the verge of bankruptcy. Knowing that Beljan really wanted to be President, I cunningly suggested that Brown was sooner or later going to shoot himself in the foot.

Beljan took the job, much to my wonder, as I felt that he surely could have done much better with his qualifications. They did give him the additional post of Provost to appease his desire to be the chief officer of the institution. He started with little fanfare but soon used his experience to make fast judgments about faculty. His conduct of affairs was more military than civilian, and it did not take long for the faculty to hate him. To be fair, under different circumstances Beljan might have been a great success. His positions as both Dean and Provost were incompatible. The Dean is the protector of the faculty; the Provost is by nature a hatchet man. Furthermore, the local faculty was not acclimated to a Provost function. My title, Senior Vice President for Academic Affairs and Dean of the Medical School, was more appropriate for the state of affairs at that time. I did the work of a Provost without the imposing title. Regardless, Beljan's weak point was that he lacked diplomacy and instinctive ability in dealing with problems involving eminent faculty and administrators. Although he was usually right, his bluntness earned him lasting enmity from his victims.

An imbroglio that illustrates his lack of finesse arose from the Admissions Committee's refusal to admit the son of a prominent faculty member. The applicant had an acceptable record from an Ivy League School but did poorly in his interview because of an immature attitude. In its wisdom and experience, the Admissions Committee recommended that the applicant spend at least a year in a further cultural or maturing occupation. The faculty member was naturally irate and claimed that the Admissions Committee was discriminating against his son in order to get back at him. Beljan properly took the side of the Committee but handled the matter with a complete lack of tact. Eventually the dispute got to

President Brown who decided to have his buddy Zwerling, the Chairman of Psychiatry, examine the applicant with respect to his immaturity. It was no surprise when Zwerling announced that, in his estimation, the applicant was immature and needed more life experience. At this stage the father was seething mad. He got a group of faculty together, myself included, who had a confrontation with Brown. The end result was that the applicant was eventually admitted. Not only did he become an outstanding student, but he has a brilliant career in Hematology-Oncology at John Hopkins Medical School. Admissions Committees and Deans little realize how many potentially meritorious candidates are denied a career in medicine on the basis of a nebulous defect. In my time as Dean, I handled many of these cases for Cameron and certainly many more for Shober without ruffling any feathers.

The faculty exceedingly disliked Beljan for this episode and others. His fate was settled by a misjudgment so extreme that there could be no recovery. It came about this way: Angelakos, the interim Dean, appointed Ralph Dehoratus as interim Chairman of Medicine when Oaks retired as chairman. Dehoratus was an excellent rheumatologist, a fine teacher, and a competent researcher. He lacked, however, the kind of administrative skills and craftiness indispensable to running the largest, most influential department in the medical school. Spontaneously, an earnest desire to acquire a really exceptional chairman developed among the faculty. A Blue Ribbon Committee was elected. After a nationwide search, it came up with the names of some great looking candidates. Everyone knew instinctively that Hahnemann was unlikely to be able to acquire candidates who had their eye on Harvard, Yale, or Hopkins. Rather they put their faith in Beljan to make an ingenious choice and somehow convince the candidate to come to a less prestigious institution.

Among the final choices of the committee was Victor Herbert, nephew of the well-known violinist of the same name. There was no argument that, on paper, Herbert was an attractive choice. He had trained at the famous Thorndike Laboratory and was internationally known for his seminal work on Vitamin B_{12} and folic acid. He was chief of research in Oncology and Hematology at the Bronx Veterans Hospital. Although he had teaching appointments at several medical schools, he had not had a full-time professorial appointment nor had he any experience in the private practice of medicine. Most people who knew Herbert personally had a problem with the fact that he was eccentric and an odd ball. His work on vitamins had led him to believe, with justification, that the current craze with megavitamin intake was unjustified and definitely harmful. He undertook a vigorous campaign against this and other types of faddism in medical therapy. He even acquired a Law Degree to defend himself against the many enemies he gained as a result of these activities. His books on cultism and faddism had considerable circulation, and he was frequently asked to appear on radio and television programs. While not exactly inappropriate, these endeavors did little to enhance his image of what was expected to be a great clinician, administrator, researcher, and teacher reminiscent of Osler, Soma Weiss, Henry Christian, George Thorn, and others.

For reasons known only to himself, Beljan latched on to Herbert, and it was obvious to everyone that he was going to insist on his appointment. Almost everyone who could reach Beljan's ear warned him that it would be a catastrophic appointment. I made an entreaty myself, practically on bended knee, against appointment. Beljan responded by having me meet Herbert in a privately arranged dinner. I suspect he had already told Herbert that he could have the job. I liked Herbert personally and admired him for the courage he had to fight against the exploiters of vitamins and natural products.

Herbert took the job and as predicted was ineffective in every respect. Fortunately for him, he'd been wise enough to take only a leave of absence from the Bronx Veterans Hospital and was able to return gracefully to his former position. This misadventure gave Brown ample justification to ease out Beljan, which I'm sure he would have done in any case.

Beljan and I got along very well. He gave me some purpose in life by making me Associate Dean for Affiliate Hospitals and Continuing Education. This was a very generous gesture in view of the natural distrust associated with former Deans who desire to retain their former powers. He let me know, of course, that he knew much more than I did about these subjects and favored me with his writings pertaining to these matters. I swallowed my pride and plunged into the serious task of attempting to improve and develop our hospital affiliations and, at the same time, restore our former distinction in Continuing Education.

CHAPTER XI

Concluding Years as Administrator, Researcher, and Teacher

1982-1986

"Rarely do successful scientists achieve important contributions in old age. Occasionally ingenious concepts conceived in their youth can be revived with meritorious results."

Rupert Black, M.D.

I vacated my office on the second floor and moved to the sixth floor to be near my laboratory and the Pharmacology Department. With alacrity, I demanded a competent secretary. After a short search, I convinced Evelyn Cavalaro who was working in the President's Office to come with me. She was a mature woman with excellent secretarial skills who rapidly learned word processing. As I have related, Chernick had no room for me, but my secretary could be located in a small office off the Pharmacology reception space. Through the kindness of Oaks, I was able to borrow an office about twenty-five yards from my secretary. It really was a storage room with no windows and steel cabinets on two walls. William Weiss, Professor of Community Medicine and Environmental Health who had been occupying the room for some years, gleefully informed me how happy he was to escape this isolated, gloomy room. I had done my best work in the attic of the ancient Hoagland Laboratory in Brooklyn, so this was no hardship for me. The room had excellent lighting and was air-conditioned. Moving the furniture from the Dean's Office on the second floor to this room and adding some attractive pictures and a rug made the place quite habitable. As I write this now, I've been in that room for over twenty years!

Beginning in the 1960s and even earlier, the rapid advances in science and the technology of communication made certain that any physician's education would be obsolete in just a very few years. So many new drugs and therapies were becoming available— and were announced to the public by the radio, television, and numerous journals—that patients often knew more than doctors. Organized medicine indeed became disturbed that physicians were being informed by detail men who were agents of drug companies rather than by impartial, more authoritative educators. The increasing extent of specialization and the formation of boards, which had specialty journals and organized scientific and clinical meetings, added to the excellence of the delivery of new information.

Perhaps the greater practical stimulus for Continuing Education had occurred earlier as a result of World War II. Physicians who'd been drafted and spent a number of years in the military, found when they came out of service that their knowledge of the practice of medicine was not at the level of the physicians who'd managed to escape service. Many physicians had been drafted with only a year or two of residency. When they were released, the average well-trained physician had at least three or four years of postgraduate training. As consequence, many decided that additional training in a specialty was the way to go, even though most of them would make quite competent physicians and surgeons with a little brushing up.

Both medical schools and industry jumped into this vacuum of need and hunger for Continuing Education. Several of the leading universities formed programs in continuing medical education. Some actually instituted schools for this purpose, among which the most outstanding was the Graduate Medical School of the University of Pennsylvania. It was organized mostly around the Graduate Hospital of Philadelphia and many of the leading scientists and clinicians of the Medical School of the University of Pennsylvania participated. Julius Comroe, a superb clinician, scientist, and educator headed the venture. For about ten years this school flourished, and many who participated attribute their success to the advanced education they received. In time, however, the supply of physician-veterans who were able to pay tuition through the veterans' benefit program diminished, and the school eventually closed. Short one—or two-day courses, meetings and demonstrations, home study, and correspondence types of learning replaced this formal kind of Continuing Education. Most of this was and is financed by drug and instrument companies who write this expense off as a very efficient kind of advertising. Most medical schools finance their Continuing Education efforts by moneys generated from commercial sources rather than from endowment and tuition. An obvious example is the combination of a vacation to an exotic spot combined with some Continuing Education. An additional inducement was that a physician could get an income tax break on vacation expenses. In many cases, speakers received their stipends from the commercial source. Some states require Continuing Education credit for license renewal, while all insurance companies insist on evidence of Continuing Education as a requirement for issuance of malpractice insurance. Despite these obvious conflicts of interest, Continuing Education is beneficial as long as the audience is aware of the source of finance and can evaluate the particular recommendations of the speaker with reference to a specific product or procedure.

Specialty boards require periodic renewal by examination for clinicians to maintain their qualifications. This requirement is real and cannot be bypassed. Clinicians who wish to remain on top of their specialty must continually strive to maintain their intellectual machinery at least at par. Some physicians and most scientists are very fastidious about maintaining their Continuing Education credits, but many need some enforcement mechanism. This takes the form of educational credits issued by certificate of attendance and guarantee of subject matter by medical schools, universities, and other organized, recognized bodies such as medical and scientific societies. The more established and prestigious courses charge tuition. The less well-oriented ones have to find financing from commercial sources and scarce benevolent agencies. Small fees for issuance of certifying certificates bring in some funding, but this scarcely pays for paper work and record keeping. Deans and provosts refuse to finance Continuing Education, but they want it as an inducement for alumni support, resident, training, occupational therapy for tenured faculty, and a kind of indirect advertisement for the institution. Consequently, anyone who undertakes to operate a Continuing Education program has to row his own boat. Continuing Education therefore has been financed, and will continue to be financed, by commercial interests, which is a serious conflict of interest.

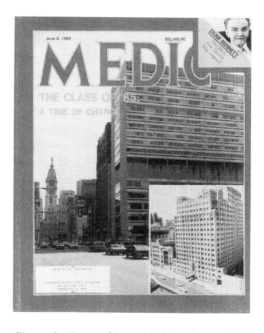

Figure 6. Cover of 1985 Medic. Illustrated on the cover is a comparison of the view of the new and old hospitals on Broad Street. Also shown is a portrait of Hugh Bennett the favorite Associate Dean. The location of the Hahnemann Medical Center in center city in the shadow of City Hall has always been a strong factor in the growth of Hahnemann.

At Hahnemann, Continuing Education was a major project of the Department of Medicine and its chairman, John Moyer. Starting in the late 1950s through the 1960s and 1970s, Moyer conducted a program of lectures, seminars, and volumes of written material in Continuing Education exceeding in scope that of any other medical school. There is no doubt that this effort had a salutary effect on the reputation of Hahnemann Medical College. It also was a considerable source of financial support for the department, and Moyer was able to build up both clerical and professional staffs. At one time Moyer indeed had five secretaries and kept them all busy. Another added value was the ability to establish a growing presence in Clinical Pharmacology, a growing field at the time.

When I took over Continuing Education in June 1982, it was on the books as one of the schools of the University. It was actually nothing more than a minor program consisting of a director, Robert J. Schaefer, and secretary, Faye Zelle. Its offices were on one of the unremodeled floors of the Bellet Building. An ancient typewriter and some filing cabinets were the only equipment. There was no specific budget from the University. Apparently it managed to operate on borrowed funds, which hopefully would be paid back by successful operations. Schaefer was an agile, resourceful procurer of contracts for various projects that could be classed as having educational value. Over the years when Moyer and Oaks were active, he had developed a clientele of drug companies and other commercial outfits that supported Continuing Education as a means of gentile promotion of their products. Admittedly, some of the support was free of strings, and the supported program might be even injurious to their product. But the great majority of support was for the promotion of a specific product or device. Enough money remained, after expenses of running of a program were paid, to cover Schaefer's and the secretary's salaries and office expenses. The University did not charge any rent for the office space and maintenance.

Continuing Education programs were surprisingly expensive to run. An average one-day exercise might cost between $12,000 and $15,000, with the biggest items being hotel and travel expenses and honoraria for the speakers. Local faculty who participated were not paid about half the time, so naturally they were less anxious to participate. Tuition was rarely charged in the hopes of enticing a decent audience. This was the early 1980s. Today expenses have nearly doubled, and drug companies are spending money on direct-to-the-public advertising, which makes financing of Continuing Education more difficult.

Schaefer soon perceived that the University was not about to invest any funds in Continuing Education, so he soon found a much better opportunity in a New York City commercial enterprise. I encouraged him to go because I could not foresee that I could raise the kind of finances that would insure a stable, superior program. Since I had to allocate my major time and effort to the affiliate hospitals, I sought provisional solutions. Bob Walker came to my rescue. He found Virginia Marsh, a Speech Pathology and Hearing staff person, who wanted to change professions. I liked Marsh and felt she could do the job given an even chance. Besides, I could only afford a modest salary. For obvious reasons, Faye Zelle was not pleased because she felt that she could manage the office herself. The two women fortunately got along fairly well after some adjustments, and I was able to run a very modest program. I put on several courses myself, and there were some others that were reasonably good, but inevitably Continuing Education languished under my leadership.

In the 1990s Continuing Education became a loss leader. In the past, it was essentially a method for Medical Centers to show their wares, and it attracted the attention and support of administrators. Now commercially oriented executives find it expedient to spend millions on media advertising directly to the public and reluctantly spend only a few thousand on Continuing Education. It's the competition, they explain. If the medical center across town presents lurid advertisements in the local paper, radio, and television, then we also have to do it.

The most recent advances are the result of computer and communication technology. Two-way television programs can be individually transmitted between institutions. Correspondence courses of all types are available via the wizardry of CD-ROM and the Internet. Prominent Journals like the *New England Journal of Medicine* offer excellent correspondence courses for credit. Even lay magazines like *Scientific American* and other journals offer medical correspondence courses that are accredited. No physician can claim that Continuing Education is unavailable either at no charge or at a modest fee.

Every medical school needs affiliate hospitals to supply clinical education requirements of medical students and resident staff of its major hospital. In Hahnemann's case, the hospital was part of the corporation and consequently was not technically an affiliate hospital, but it actually served as such in a practical sense. In the U.S. and most advanced countries, the university hospital serves as the main service and research facility for the delivery of healthcare and advancing medical technology. Every staff member has a professorial appointment in the medical school. A great many physicians are employed full-time, which means that their salaries are paid by the university through contract arrangement. This defines the amounts that arise from teaching, research, and administrative duties. Ordinarily at least three hundred residents and fellows are in essence highly educated slaves who are paid just a living wage. There are also attending physicians who admit patients and do some teaching and committee work on a volunteer basis. University hospitals usually have five hundred beds or more and facilities for all the specialties. Without argument, the value of a medical school is judged in major part by the quality and excellence of its university hospital. Harvard Medical School with its three university type hospitals, Brigham and Women's, Beth Israel, and Massachusetts General, tops its sister institutions by far. (Yale and Hopkins would not like to hear that.) Yet even Harvard finds it necessary to have additional affiliate hospitals for other specialties such as psychiatry.

Affiliate hospitals are needed because medical educators believe in a one-to-one instructional basis. And they believe that medical students should have a maximum exposure to clinical material as handled by both advanced medical centers and community hospitals. This means that the student should have responsibility for the diagnosis and therapy of patients and not be relegated merely to a third—or fourth-hand observational position. Medical education is primarily of the apprenticeship type, and a plethora of clinical material handled by well-run hospitals and clinics with highly motivated physicians is needed. In the real world, the average medical school needs at least three or four affiliate hospitals in order to provide clinical material and quality instruction. At Hahnemann at least 50 percent of clinical training was done in affiliate hospitals. I suspect that this is the case at most medical schools. There is another imperative reason for this situation. Instruction at affiliates comes cheap compared to the full-time staff at the home-base university hospital. All it costs is prefixed professorial titles and, in some cases, a part-time salary for an instructional director.

Why do affiliate hospitals capitulate to an unfair monetary contract? Sometimes it is just a question of pride and esteem of their institution. Traditionally there is the credo that a hospital that's associated with a medical school is held to a higher standard and thus does superior clinical work. No doubt there is considerable truth to this concept, but the overwhelming factor is the desire to have a resident staff. Specialty boards will not approve a residency program unless there is satisfactory evidence of a substantial educational program. In some instances, particularly in the surgical specialties, the university hospital will rotate its residents through the affiliate hospital. This is mutually beneficial because it allows residents the opportunity for direct exposure to more clinical material than would be available at the home base. On this justification, it was possible to have strong, valuable affiliations with St. Agnes's Hospital in Philadelphia and Crozer Hospital in Chester, PA. In more recent years, as the Surgical Board severely restricted the number of residents any institution might have, there was much less opportunity to work this game. As a result, those hospitals could establish their own residency programs. The affiliation with a medical university was still valuable to them as a recruiting device. Medical students who rotate through a hospital have a chance to see the opportunities of education available and to consider the chances of settling in practice in a bordering community. The hospital can observe the intelligence and work behavior of the students and decide if it wants them for future house staff. There is another important consideration: Medical students, especially in their clinical years, are an important source of referrals. The public naturally feels that a student in direct contact with practicing physicians has the opportunity to observe who is the most skillful and who has the most empathy for the patient. Many physicians enjoy a greater degree of satisfaction in their work if they can share their knowledge and expertise with a younger mind, if only to show that they can still cut the mustard.

In my negotiations to secure an alliance with a particular hospital, I found that many factors were important, such as proximity, similarity of interest in programs, need for dependence on educational programs, and perspectives of the Boards of the respective establishments. In most instances, however, I found after bitter experience that the determining factor in most cases was the number of loyal alumni who held leverage positions in the target institution. Hahnemann was in a particularly bad position with respect to obtaining first-class affiliate hospitals in Philadelphia or its suburbs. Because of its homeopathic origins, at the turn of the century it had only relationships with hospitals that practiced or favored homeopathy. Rarely did its alumni gain important positions in allopathic hospitals. By 1945, when homeopathy was dropped from the curriculum, all the choice places had been snapped up by Jefferson, Penn, and Temple. Women's Medical College was in a similar position as Hahnemann. The Osteopathic School also had to confine itself to osteopathic hospitals. Fortunately in those days, Philadelphia General Hospital (PGH) was the large city hospital run on a charity basis, supported by tax funds, and replete with the best clinical instructional material. It had a grand history dating back to Revolutionary War times and establishment by

Benjamin Franklin. The great William Osler made rounds at PGH, which was known as Old Blockly in his time. Since the hospital and The Medical School of University of Pennsylvania were established at the same time and were adjacent to each other, there was an obvious affiliation. Hahnemann shared the affiliation with the University of Pennsylvania and in it's day it was the best instructional opportunity for students. But that ended when Mayor Frank Rizzo closed the PGH in 1974.

After World War II, many Veterans Hospitals were built close to medical schools wherever there was the geographical possibility. In order to establish some equity of access to government financed clinical material, Philadelphia's five medical schools had to divide the spoils so that each had a reasonably equal share. Hahnemann got a share of PGH, and Woman's Medical College received privileges at the Veterans Hospital. The Veterans Hospital was built adjacent to the University of Pennsylvania, which gave it an immense advantage of access. Hahnemann's share of PGH proved to be tremendously important for the development of a full-time clinical staff and the proper education of medical students. In some ways, Hahnemann's clinical services at PGH were equal to or superior to those of Penn. Consequently when PGH closed, it was a great loss to Hahnemann. As Dean at the time, I had the burden of finding suitable replacement clinical services. Not an easy task when every decent hospital in Philadelphia and its environs was already affiliated with another medical school.

Moyer, the Chairman of Department of Medicine, was of great help because he understood the problem and was willing to devote the time and energy required establishing a stable, efficient relationship with the affiliate hospital. Other departments were also helpful, particularly Psychiatry which was able to establish on its own a fine affiliation with Friends Hospital in Philadelphia. Proceeding with a great degree of optimism, I began to make overtures to suitable hospitals within a twenty-five mile radius. Lankenau and Bryn Mawr Hospitals, both on the Main Line, were great possibilities but were staffed mainly by Jefferson graduates and soon succumbed to the overtures of that institution. I turned my attention to Crozer Chester Hospital, which was some thirty-five miles away. Even though it too was a Jefferson stronghold, that venerable institution did not desire it. Here I had some support. Danny Marino, an old friend, Hahnemann graduate, and member of the "Circolo," was on the staff of the Cardiovascular Department. There were other connections developed over time. One was James Loucks who was hospital director. Although he was an M.D., he had a fine business sense and got along with the hospital board. Another very able person was James Clark, a nephrologist and head of the medical division. An excellent clinician and teacher, he was most helpful in establishing good instructional practices. The big point of affiliation with Crozer was that Hahnemann would supply six surgical residents in a joint program. This proved to be feasible, and this affiliation proved to be the best, second only to Hahnemann Hospital. In fact, some years after I had left office, Crozer Chester became a Clinical Campus with teaching services in all the major specialties.

I next turned my attention to Monmouth Memorial Hospital in Long Branch, New Jersey. This extraordinarily excellent educational hospital had residents in all the major specialties and a full-time Educational Director, William S. Vaun. Fortuitously, he was very dedicated and savvy about the political medical situation in New Jersey. Certainly Monmouth should have been affiliated with the New Jersey College of Medicine, but it preferred to control its own destiny, fortunately for Hahnemann. This independence and fine quality was due to the fact that Monmouth County was a rich community full of retired, wealthy New Yorkers. Another important and favorable reality was the fact that Hahnemann graduates held the Chair of Surgery and several other important positions. With the help of Moyer, Oaks, and others, I was able to bring about a very satisfactory working affiliation that has been appreciated by students and has been permanent. This was accomplished despite all the difficulties that distance and crossing a state line creates.

Another good but distant affiliation was in Sayre, Pennsylvania. This consisted of the Packer Memorial Hospital and the Guthrie

Clinic, plus a research institute. Located near the New York State border, the medical center was at a great distance from any large medical center in Pennsylvania. It related to the closest large city, Binghamton, N.Y. Relatively few students chose a clinical rotation at Sayre because of the distance. Those who did, however, found that it was an admirable instructional experience. Students were housed and fed and treated just like house staff. Because of this fine treatment, the Packer Hospital recruited many very excellent residents. Paul C. Royce did an excellent job as Director of Medical Education.

My greatest accomplishment in my final year as Dean for Affiliations was to finalize an affiliation with the Allentown Hospitals. They had traditionally been with the Medical School of the University of Pennsylvania. Many of their attending physicians were from Penn, but there were also a number of Hahnemann alumni in the area, which helped. After much negotiation and many trips to Allentown, an agreement was reached. The clinching factor was a strong relationship with Brodsky's cancer group. This was an across-the-board affiliation, meaning that students would be rotated in Medicine, Surgery, Obstetrics and Gynecology, and Pediatrics. When Bert Brown heard about this new affiliation with an affluent practice group in a strategic geographical location, he immediately took hold of the situation. He and Iqbal Paroo (then Hahnemann's Hospital CEO) had meetings with the CEO of the Allentown Group and together they made an agreement that looked more like a contract related to healthcare delivery rather than education and research. There was much advertising and ballyhoo. Of course, the event was presented to the Board as one of the important achievements of the President. This did not bother me because I'd long become accustomed to the duty of "making the President look good." But I was disturbed by the increasing obligation of educational objectives to be integrated with, and secondary to, healthcare delivery goals. I did have the satisfaction, at least in the early years, that the affiliations worked quite well and benefited both institutions. All this was accomplished without the exchange of vast sums of hard cash that is obligatory today. In this enlightened era, it is now required to buy hospitals and private practices and have contracts with HMOs in order to keep the hospital beds full. Educational and research objectives are diminished to an inconsequential state. This is the background of the massive financial debacle and health systems bankruptcies of the late 1990s.

CHAPTER XII

Retirement

1986-2000

*"Old age is depressing because it has no future unless you
believe in an afterlife where errors of the first life can be repaired."*

Rupert Black, M.D.

My retirement in June of 1986 was very uneventful. I was
seventy-years-old, and the most impressive feature was going from
a regular salary to Social Security and pension checks. Because of
my frugality and savings habits, I had actually accumulated a
reasonable estate. My last close relative, my sister Aurora, died in
1983 and left a considerable sum to me the sole heir. Interest rates
had been and continued to be excellent. As a consequence, at least
for the next five years, my income was actually better than my
salary had been. All of my daughters were well established with
their own apartments or homes. My wife and I were left with an
enormous empty house. Most of my friends in this situation either
moved to Florida or found an agreeable continual care community
center.

As I write this more than fifteen years after the event, I recall
only one unpleasant incident. Brown was still President at the
time. Although I had already had adequate discussions with Donald
T. Brophy, Chairman of the Board committee on hiring and firing
executives, Brown abruptly called me into his office. I was ushered
in unceremoniously. Sitting behind his big desk, Brown beamed a

toothier smile than usual. His eyes danced as if he was having an orgasm.

"Joe," he airily spit out, "I've decided to get rid of you. I'm keeping Bondi. He is a very useful Dean." The remark was obviously intended to be a rapier thrust right to the heart. Bondi, Dean of the Graduate School, was a few years older than I and well over seventy at the time. Brown was thus telling me that praiseworthy workers were kept on even after any age limit, but I did not belong in that category.

I smiled sweetly and said, "Bert," (He liked being called by his first name.) "As you know, I have already discussed my retirement situation with Brophy. Your present remarks are redundant." With that, I just exited.

Dean Zwerling fortunately felt somewhat more kindly towards me and arranged that I received Emeritus Status, both for my Dean position and my Professorship of Pharmacology. This allowed me certain privileges, but I was also allowed to remain a member of the faculty. I was able to teach, do research, maintain an office, and receive all the academic values allowed a regular faculty member but at no recompense.

The first year after my retirement, Chernick felt he could use me in the teaching of the medical pharmacology course. I was happy to cooperate and acted pretty much as a full-time instructor, lecturing, taking responsibility for a conference group, instructing in the laboratory, and constructing and marking exams. Chernick even managed to pay me a small stipend for this work. I was glad to do it because it helped enormously in my editing and writing, especially of the textbook of pharmacology. Still, I could perceive a certain discomfort both with Chernick and the other professors in the department. What was this aging ex-Dean doing? Competing with younger professors who were struggling to excel and climb the shaky academic ladder?

With the mutual consent of all, I decided to devote my energies just to research, scientific writing, and serving on committees that no one else had any desire to serve on. I was now free to do consulting work and use the income received to support the modest research program that my long-time collaborator Robert McMichaels and I performed. McMichaels had now advanced to rank of Senior Instructor. Besides his teaching duties and technical support, he also ran a minority program for which he was able to secure NIH support. The program was mainly for high school students and ran during the summer months. I was more than pleased to lend my laboratory facilities for this purpose and give any other aid I could manage to this program.

At last free of teaching and administrative duties, I was naïve enough to imagine that I could still be productive in cutting edge research. Regrettably, such was not the case. My field of expertise, cardiovascular physiology, had become very sophisticated and most of the good research was done in humans. My electronic equipment was of the tube type and completely obsolete. Research in cats and dogs was extremely expensive and virtually impossible to justify before the Animal Rights Committee. I was forced to direct my efforts where the experimental material was cheap and easy to obtain. I decided therefore to continue research adaptable to tissue culture. I needed a laminar flow hood, a carbon dioxide incubator, and a suitable microscope just to get started. I could use other equipment, such as a deep freeze, in community-shared facilities. I did not even worry about the large amounts of plastic ware and culture media required. By using an obsolete but still serviceable laminar hood, which microbiology was willing to discard, I estimated that I could get started if I managed to raise at least $7,000. McMichaels was most cooperative and even enthusiastic, and so I began to seek some means of support.

Fortune smiled when an old acquaintance from the orchid society approached me with a drug problem. Ed Waxman owned a small drug company whose main product was a diaper rash ointment called Balmex. It had been on the market for many years and sold quite well, both in the United States and abroad. Although no serious adverse reactions had occurred, the FDA was on a campaign to rid the market of all drugs that had not been proven to be safe and effective, especially those available over the counter without prescription. Balmex contained bismuth subnitrate which, when given by mouth, had caused bismuth and nitrite poisoning. But since Balmex is applied to the skin, absorption is minimal. Another main ingredient of Balmex was Balsam of Peru. This natural organic agent has been used for thousands of years to treat many conditions, especially those affecting the skin. It has an attractive fragrance and is also used in the cosmetic industry. Some individuals are allergic to Balsam of Peru and can have severe reactions on exposure to this substance. Waxman was well acquainted with this potential reaction and took great care to avoid most allergic reactions by putting an especially purified preparation of Balsam of Peru into Balmex, and at a smaller dose.

The FDA wanted a full-scale clinical investigation that would easily cost several hundred thousand dollars and even then might not satisfy the FDA. I told Waxman that he had two choices. He could remove both the bismuth subnitrate and the Balsam of Peru from Balmex and be left with a preparation of zinc oxide, which would probably be effective but not in the least unique. Understandably, Waxman was reluctant to do this. The second option was to find a Washington lawyer experienced in FDA cases. I would be willing to do a simple pilot study on ten cases. These would be randomly assigned to five subjects who would receive Balmex therapy plus standard care and five who would receive a placebo plus standard care. This plan was agreeable to Waxman, and he soon secured a suitable lawyer. Consultation with the FDA, with the lawyer's help, encouraged us to proceed. The FDA insisted that bacterial cultures be made in each case. This greatly increased the cost of the study, and I made little profit from the modest sum that Waxman could afford. I nevertheless put all the money I could into running the study. With the cooperation of Gerry Kaplan, a fine pediatrician, I arranged to use the pediatric ward to study babies with diaper rash.

Fortunately, both Balmex and plain zinc oxide ointments were commonly used for diaper rash so I had no difficulty randomizing patients. The study was finally completed with fully detailed culture studies and toxicity determinations of bismuth and of nitrites. S.N.S. Murthy gave me very valuable aid in the toxicity studies. It showed no difference in the toxicity of the two ointments and a barely statistical therapeutic superiority of Balmex.

Some months later when we presented the study to the FDA, it was not impressed. The FDA statistician said that the small number of patients lent no power to our conclusions. The study nevertheless did show that the company had made a serious effort to assure that the product was safe and effective. Pending additional studies, Waxman was able to keep his product intact for several more years. When he sold the company, however, the new owner was forced by the FDA to remove both the bismuth and the Balsam of Peru from the product. It is still sold as Balmex and seems to have good sales. I suppose that this suggests that the brand name is more important than the ingredients in a drug product. Thus ended my experience with the important problem of diaper rash.

Another potboiler that earned some cash to carry on more erudite research was the problem of baldness. The success of Minoxidil (Rogaine) in growing hair spurred interest in exploitation of other agents. My good friend Steve DeFelice put me on to a European firm that had a competitive product. The main ingredient was hyaluronidase, an enzyme that softens tissues and allows the penetration of fluids and nutrients in the skin when applied locally. The firm felt that its product, really classed more as a cosmetic, would enhance the growth of hair, but there was little scientific evidence. I proposed a pilot study in rabbits that they were willing to finance. After dickering with the Animal Welfare Committee, I bought a dozen Belgian rabbits that had beautiful hair. They were kept in individual cages, fed, and watered daily by McMichaels or myself. A veterinarian inspected them weekly. Their backs were shaved. After four days of rest, the shaved area of each rabbit was divided into a right and left side, allowing each rabbit to serve as its own control. Each rabbit randomly received daily applications of active product to one side and placebo to the other side of the shaved area. The side with the active ingredient was coded so it could be blinded to independent observers. The backs were examined daily and accurately photographed at the beginning, middle, and end of the thirty-day period. The result was just a significant increase in the rate of growth in the treated area. The manufacturers were ecstatic with my scientific report to them, mostly because of the colored photographs. They wanted me to publish and act as a sponsor for their product. I refused because I felt the data was weak and should be repeated. Also, the baldness in men is caused by testosterone and is an entirely different mechanism than normal hair growth in rabbits, which grows in cycles related to season. I did agree to talk to reporters in a publicity campaign to sell the product. My carefully worded explanation probably did little to increase sales. Nevertheless, the hair product has been fairly successful commercially even though it is no competition for Minoxidil and the newer inhibitors of testosterone.

The money earned from these studies allowed McMichaels and me to continue doing research and providing a structure to continue the minority program. McMichaels' NIH grant for minority high school students was of great help because it also provided funds for laboratory essentials. During these years, we also had a summer program for high school science teachers who did research that complemented what we were working on. The institution categorized our work as unsponsored research, and as interest in minority programs waned and the pharmacology department was completely restructured, my laboratory of so many years had to be closed. What lives on are the products of the laboratory in scientific papers, students trained, research fellows inspired, and technical support for other researchers.

From 1963 to 1994, I edited a major medical pharmacology text. During this time I was also a professor, chairman of a department, and Dean. The first two editions of *Basic Pharmacology in Medicine* published in 1976 and 1982 did well because they were brief and fit the then current idea of a core curriculum. Fortunately, I was now retired and could devote more time to editing a text that needed a major revision and updating. There

were several very good competitive texts, including that edited by
Bertram G. Katzung of the University of California at San Francisco,
which was superior. I decided to bring in outside authors and use
our local faculty as section editors. McGraw-Hill, the publisher,
was supportive and we set upon a three-year task to produce a
finished product by the spring of 1989. But many unanticipated
difficulties delayed its appearance until 1990. Although very
credible and even outstanding in some respects, the text failed to
strike a competitive stature among the newer ones. Several schools
adopted it, our students thought it was great, but the sales were
disappointing. It was obvious that if the text were to continue,
some very drastic and innovative improvements were needed.

In 1991 meanwhile, I had to undergo bypass cardiac surgery.
Although I did well, I no longer had the passion required to produce
a superior product. In addition, McGraw-Hill bought out
Pergomon Press, which published Goodman and Gilman's
outstanding pharmacology text. They naturally no longer needed
my text and were anxious to drop it. They politely told me that I
could have the copyright and seek another publisher.

Under these circumstances, I was quite agreeable to abandon a
fourth edition and let the book die a quiet death. To my surprise,
my collaborators DiGregorio, Barbieri, and Ferko were enthusiastic
to continue. I had great misgivings about this and felt that, unless
we could find a publisher and indeed a prominent pharmacologist
as chief editor, a successful outcome could not be assured. I made
a considerable effort to find both without the least success.
DiGregorio had a connection with a small publishing firm, Medical
Surveillance that had some success in publishing pocket medical
books. It would undertake the project of a full-size medical text,
provided that we could prepare a manuscript that was a finished
product complete with figures and completely copyedited. No
color or extensive artwork would be permitted. These restrictions
would preclude our ability to produce a contemporary text that
would be competitive with others in the field. It turned out that
Barbieri had computer and editing skills that could make the project
feasible. Even with these restrictions, my colleagues remained

enthusiastic and urged me to continue as chief editor. I would have willing bowed out, but the flattery to my ego was sufficient to make me believe that I could continue the eminence of my baby. I finally succumbed, provided the other editors would do most of the work. I agreed to write about five chapters in the area of my expertise. I ended up writing nine and doing all the correspondence and tedious paper work required to produce a full sized textbook.

The fourth edition of *Basic Pharmacology in Medicine* came out in the spring of 1994 and caused no perceptible ripple in the textbook market. Despite the many difficulties, in my estimation it was quite a decent text, consonant with the times but still in a classical cast that lacked the avant garde of the competitive texts. Even our department head, who admitted the superior writing in our text, insisted instead on recommending to students a newer text that was replete with colored cartoons. Considering that the total yearly market of medical students is about sixteen thousand and that at least half don't buy any text, there are only eight thousand potential users. That's the first year. The second year, second-hand copies further cut down the market. Considering competition from at least ten other books, the possible medical student market is only about eight hundred. The average medical text sells about three thousand volumes in a three-year period— and this is considered a success. Based on this estimate, the fourth edition was definitely not a success. Yet so convinced were we that we had a good, useful product that we even seriously considered producing a fifth edition to come out in 1998.

Although we set out with mighty ambitions, the whole project was a disaster. This time it was the changing fortunes of the institution and the reorganization of the basic sciences into self-pay status. Locally, the takeover of Hahnemann University by the Medical College of Pennsylvania and the Allegheny Health and Education Foundation (AHERF) put an excessive price on academic endeavors. (More about this in the next chapter.) Modern business philosophy in medical schools is that writing a scholarly book or doing unsponsored research does not bring any funding into the institution and is therefore discouraged. There are sound reasons for this attitude. A vast sum of government money is going to those who are eligible and capable, and modern competitive biological research requires very expensive equipment. Only the most richly endowed institutions can afford to carry on compatible functional research without government or research foundation funds. So the end result is that very few talented faculty are available, or even willing, to write chapters in textbooks. After more than a year of dedicated work, only about 10 percent of the intended chapters were finished, and it was obvious that it was very unlikely that the fifth edition of the book would ever be completed. So with much reluctance and a sense of shame and defeat, I wrote to each author stating the problem and offering to return their chapters so that they could publish elsewhere. So died forever *Basic Pharmacology in Medicine*. Counting the two editions of Drill's *Pharmacology in Medicine*, I had edited six editions of a major medical text over a period of thirty years. Not a bad accomplishment!

Basic Pharmacology in Medicine was only one of my writing experiences during retirement. I continued to submit monthly articles in clinical pharmacology to *The American Family Physician*. This was a continuation of the arrangement I had with John Rose, the editor in the late 1970s. The series continued until 1991, so in all there were about 250 articles, about a third authored by myself with the rest solicited, edited, and sometimes completely revised before being submitted.

Of my later years, I think that the best thing I authored was the review article, "Use of Niacin as a Drug", with my collaborator, the biochemist William S. Thayer. It was published in the 1991 *Annual Review of Nutrition*. Over the past years, I had written articles on the use of vitamins as drugs, on vitamins as anticancer agents, and on the toxicity of vitamins. The editor of the Annuals of Nutrition asked me to do this article, which was flattering because I knew there were probably others who might be more qualified than I. However, I undertook the task but, realizing my weakness in biochemical approaches to the subject, I recruited

Thayer to help me. Without reservations, I considered Thayer's contribution to be the better part of the article, which attempted to clarify the use of niacin in the great cholesterol problem.

I naturally continued to contribute monthly articles on clinical pharmacology to the *American Family Physician (AFP)*. These were a pleasure to write and edit. Eventually, failing health forced me to turn this task over to younger hands. Over 250 articles had been contributed over a period of twenty years. The new editor of *AFP*, Jay Sewik, was most gracious and had a nice editorial written about my contributions. I like to feel that this series had a beneficial advertising spin-off for Hahnemann. I did receive many letters from alumni, most of them complementary.

My work with *Facts and Comparison* was of a different nature. There was little original writing but much review and suggestions for improvement in the organization of material already constructed by in-house writers. As I have mentioned, the yearly meetings of *F&C* were the real attraction because they were usually in a great resort spot, the company was affable, and there was a feeling of productivity. In 1991, I was prepared to go to the February annual meeting when failing health of both myself and my wife caused me to bow out of the group.

No one escapes the ravages of old age. The body and mind degenerate ever more rapidly as the sixth, seventh, and eight decades approach. My dear, wonderful spouse Mary was seventy

in pretty fair shape despite years of combating hypertension. She was always on the obese side, but now her main problem was severe back pain that became so incapacitating she could not even walk. Her fourth and fifth lumbar vertebrae were compressed and her spinal canal had narrowed. The best advice I could get from experts was for conservative therapy. Injection with cortisone did not work. Months of bed rest, then graduated exercise with ample analgesic and anti-inflammatory drugs made life bearable.

Although limited in the amount of walking and activity, at least Mary could function and do useful chores, drive a car, and do shopping.

My own health status was deteriorating. I kept up my pace of activity despite increasing warning signs of chest pain. Finally I awakened one morning with chest pain and a weak pulse. I called my trusty physician, Bill Oaks. Characteristically, he admitted me immediately to the hospital for catheterization. It showed that I had almost a complete block in my anterior descendant's coronary artery. In over nine years from my previous catheterization study, medical therapy had not been able to prevent the further atherosclerotic changes in this vessel. I had avoided surgical intervention then, but now it was obvious that further damage to the myocardium was imminent and a decision to risk surgical repair was needed. At the time (1991), Stanley Brockman was chief of Cardiothoracic Surgery and certainly the best in his field available to me. He recommended bypass surgery using the internal mammary artery and, if necessary, also a venous graft. I was seventy-five-years old. I knew that the surgery probably would not increase my life expectancy, but it might enable me to be more active during my remaining life span. After consulting with my family, I decided to go ahead with the operation.

As I write this eleven years later, I am reasonably sure that the surgical intervention was beneficial overall. But whether or not the operation was worth the risk and the permanent accompanying side effects is another question. Two days post operatively; I suffered the most dreaded complication, a pulmonary embolus. I fortunately recovered, but this prolonged my hospital stay to nearly one month. Most people undergoing the same operation are sent home in five days. I also had atrial fibrillation and several bouts of atrial tachycardia. These arrhythmias are far more common complications of bypass surgery than are reported. In my case, the atrial tachycardia became a permanent defect that has required drug and other interventional therapy. Removing the internal mammary artery decreases the blood supply to the chest wall and in some cases causes symptoms of paraesthesias and even pain, which are annoying. Balance this against the fact that the area of heart muscle supplied by the damaged vessel had not deteriorated over the years, and you have a reasonable estimate of the value of the operation. Was the price worth the benefit? In my case, probably yes. I believe that I preserved more heart function than I might have in the absence of surgical intervention.

Until this event in my health status, I had been working pretty much full-time. Having reached the age of seventy-five, I felt I should slow down. The onerous task of editing the textbook of pharmacology was now over. I decided in addition to give up, as I have mentioned, the writing and editing of the Clinical Pharmacology series in the *American Family Physician*. In addition to my diminishing cardiac status, Mary's serious back problems were not capable of resolution. This forced me to conclude that our traveling days were over, so I gave up the editorship position with *Facts and Comparisons* and any attendance at national meetings. I began to restrict my attendance at Hahnemann to two days a week, to devote myself to taking care of Mary, and to do projects that could be done at home. There were plenty of repairs to do on my 100-year-old house, and my greenhouse needed reorganization. The most intellectual project I began was the writing of these memoirs.

Now as I look back, the most disheartening ravage of old age is depression. The trouble is, the brain does not deteriorate on the average as rapidly as the rest of the body. The result is that you observe other people doing things you could have done better, had you not lost your physical stamina. On my retirement, I decided that I would conduct myself very low-key and not attempt to retain any influence in matters of governance or conduct of the institution. I could not, however, avoid being an experienced observer who thought he saw errors of judgment that would be deleterious for the long run. I saw greed and wild ambition supersede the moderate considerate planning that becomes a university. There was a serious deterioration of democratic ideals in the mad rush to surf the crest of the good times of the late 1980s and1990s. I'm introspective enough to realize, of course, that if I had a similar situation when

I was in power, I might well have acted in the same manner. Was it all "sour grapes?" Not so. A devoted faculty kept Wharty Shober in check. Why could they not moderate the wild executives who followed him? This was all very depressing to me as I observed the destruction of the worthwhile progress Hahnemann had made during the years of my tenure as an executive officer. I vented my despair at the time by writing the following note to myself:

"The horror in the medical school exists not in the weird specimens in the pathology museum, nor in the walk-in refrigerator wherein hang the corpses for the anatomical dissections. Not even does it exist in the operating theater where the blood flows, brains are spooned out, and the wrong organs are removed. Then where is the "Chamber of Horrors?" It resides in the carpeted, luxurious offices of the administrative persona where ambitious, greedy, uncaring administrators have the privilege to make decisions that affect the health and welfare of the public. The medical school and the hospital have lost their charitable character. Delivery of health education, science, and service has become an extremely lucrative business where the almighty dollar reigns, whether the structure is declared for profit or not-for-profit. Aggressive individuals have seized this opportunity for personal gain and profit." Robber Barons" of industry today dominate the healthcare delivery business."

This statement turned out to be uniquely prophetic of the events that most observers hold responsible for the biggest twentieth century debacle in the healthcare industry. On July 21, 1998, Allegheny University (the name Hahnemann inherited as a result of a merger to be discussed in the next chapter) and its nine affiliated hospitals declared bankruptcy that would eventually prove to be a total loss of $1.6 billion. The hospitals were put up for sale. The University, as an integral part of the corporation, was cast into an extremely precarious financial and ethical position. How could such a huge catastrophe happen to a charitable institution that received state and federal funds to carry on its good works? Who was minding the store? Where were the American Association of Medical Colleges and other accrediting bodies? Who had changed the bylaws so that this debacle became feasible? What were the factors of the healthcare industry that predisposed this catastrophe?

All this was extremely depressing to an old man who had seen better times for his institution. It was very disheartening to see my department deteriorate and all of the people whom I'd helped to advance get eliminated. So I have decided to put down on paper how I saw these events as they happened, which in my view caused the horrible setback. I was the silent observer of the saga of near destruction of a modern university health center.

CHAPTER XIII

Bankruptcy and Collapse

1998

"Great and successful men let success go to their heads. There it ferments and gives birth to even greater enterprises."

Rupert Black, M.D.

In the construction of human events there are three main components. The first is the cast of characters with ambitions and motivations. No less important is a situation that can be exploited. All will fail unless the timing and environment are favorable for the event to be accomplished.

First, the characters: Sherif Abdelhak was born into a prosperous family in Cairo on March 14, 1946. A sturdy baby, he grew into a handsome young man. Although short in stature, he was muscular and played football well enough to become team captain. An excellent horseman as well, he might have become a professional jockey. He was a good, if not particularly brilliant, student at the American University of Cairo where he was a student leader. After graduation his direction was confined to industry, with particular reference to becoming an expert purchasing agent. It is a fair supposition that during this phase of his life he became obsessed with the contention that you can buy yourself into fame and fortune. All you have to do is develop purchasing power by any feasible method. Then anything can be bought and operated to your advantage.

By the age of twenty-five, this ambitious Egyptian was employed as a buyer for the cafeteria of the famous Allegheny General Hospital in Pittsburgh, PA. He so impressed the administrators that in less than a year he was promoted to be General Purchasing Agent for the entire hospital. He quickly climbed an additional step by becoming Assistant Director of Nursing. At this juncture he sensed the need to increase his buying power so he acquired a new credential, an MBA from the University of Pittsburgh School of Business. He received his degree in 1981 and was promoted to a full Vice President.

Now the big opportunity presented itself when an unexpected event led to a vacancy in the office of the chief executive. As next in line and only thirty-five, Sherif became interim CEO of Allegheny General Hospital. Despite his best efforts the search committee chose another person for the permanent position. Sherif was bitterly disappointed, quit Allegheny, and landed a job as chief of Canonsburg General Hospital, a good community hospital but certainly no match for Allegheny General. Still ambitious to achieve his goal, he managed not only to perform brilliantly at Canonsburg but also to consult at Allegheny—thus ingratiating himself with the movers behind the scene. The key person at Allegheny was the influential William Penn Snyder, III.

With characteristic shrewdness, Sherif spent the next three years doing a superb ingratiating job on this pillar of Pittsburgh finance. In 1986 Sherif became CEO of Allegheny General Hospital under Board Chairman Synder. From this point on, his career blossomed, and he became known as the guru of CEOs of healthcare providers. As a community hospital, Allegheny General competed successfully with the prestigious Pittsburgh's University Medical Center. Sherif managed this by establishing a credible research institute, buying outstanding medical specialists, and supporting first-class residency programs. He also had the good fortune to ride the crest of the wave of the expanded federal Medicare funding of the late 1980s.

Compared to well-recognized historical types, Sherif resembles Napoleon more than Caesar, Hitler, or a Renaissance type. His resemblance to Napoleon is physical, and one almost expects to see him stick his hand into a well-paunched vest. In ambition, again like Napoleon, there were no limits to feathering one's own nest. Among the notorious immigrants to this country in the last century, Sherif resembles most closely Carlo Ponzi both in the scope of his enterprise and the belief that he has discovered a new, workable moneymaking formula. Ponzi reworked the ancient pyramid scheme by forming a completely fictitious company based on foreign postal card exchange. He promised huge interest rates and attracted numerous investors. Sherif's formula was less fraudulent and considerably more sophisticated but was nevertheless a type of pyramid scheme intended to favor his own income and at the same time be beneficial for the institution. Sherif floated bonds, borrowed from restricted research and educational charity funds, and meanwhile siphoned off funds in the form of interest free loans to buy a house and raised his own salary and pension among other perks. Justification? Why, it's what is commonly practiced in industry.

②

William Penn Snyder, III was tall, handsome, and the scion of one of the wealthiest Pittsburgh families. They owned and managed banks and industries, played on their own golf courses, and were members of the New York Yacht Club. There were also strong ties to Carnegie and Mellon. Snyder III continued the family tradition of supporting Allegheny General Hospital. A member of the Board since 1965, and more recently Chairman of the Board (a position he held for several more decades), he was there to protect the family investment in the twelve-story Snyder Patient Pavilion and the magnificent Snyder Auditorium.

It is hard to judge the mettle of a man who has inherited such position and wealth. Certainly Snyder III was a man of considerable accomplishment. At the time Sherif had made him his pigeon, Snyder III was in his middle sixties and ambitious enough to want to be remembered as one who'd established an outstanding healthcare delivery and management system. He was thus suitable fodder for Sherif's overtures. Besides, the banks that loaned money might make handsome profits with a minimum of risk.

Walter David Cohen, DDS, was a capable, accomplished dental surgeon and recognized expert in periodontics. His father was a very successful dentist who established a lucrative Center City practice in Philadelphia. Following in his father's footsteps, Cohen continued what is considered the best dental practice in the city. Dedicated to academic pursuits, he rose to professorial rank at his alma mater, the University of Pennsylvania. In 1972 he became the Dean, a position he held with dignity and accomplishment, not only advancing academic prerogatives but also raising funds to fulfill faculty wishes. These features of his character (especially the latter) were very attractive to the Medical College of Pennsylvania, the former Women's Medical College. At the bottom rung of the five Philadelphia medical schools, MCP was desperate to find a leader who could advance it to a more prominent position. It urgently needed a new physical plant and funds to hire a more able faculty and staff. It was a natural to court Cohen. He fell for these overtures and became President some five years before Sherif invaded Philadelphia. Cohen was in his early sixties and anxious to crown an already highly successful career with an opus magnus of even greater magnitude. He gave generously of himself and his wealth to this medical institution that continued to believe that their main purpose was to advance the cause of women. His talented wife also dedicated much of her time to the affairs of the school and the hospital.

Iqbal F. Paroo, born in 1951, was some five years younger than Sherif. There is a distinct parallel in the careers of these two men. Both were born in Africa. Paroo in Nairobi, Kenya. Sherif in Cairo, Egypt. Both of the Islamic faith and educated abroad in good schools, they immigrated to America to make their fortunes in the rapidly advancing healthcare system. Tall and debonair, Paroo is the more handsome and likable of the two. The motivation of each is fundamentally the same: to make a fortune out of a business venture. Sherif got into the healthcare field quite by accident by answering an ad and becoming a buyer for the dietetics department of a hospital.

Paroo's story is more touching. He wanted to be an aviator and was already a pilot-in-training for the Kenyan Air Force at the age of seventeen. A freak motor scooter accident led to the amputation of his left leg and a long hospital stay and rehabilitation. He was fascinated by the workings of the hospital and decided to devote his life to hospital administration after talking with a hospital administrator who befriended him. He decided to come to the United States where the best educational programs were available. He enrolled at Georgia State University and took a full course of study while working part-time at a nursing home. After getting his bachelor's degree, he went on to earn a master's degree in health administration in 1974. A series of jobs followed here and abroad and culminated in the Executive Directorship of Hubbard Hospital of Meharry Medical College in Nashville, Tenn. This black college and its hospital were in deep financial trouble. In only one year, Paroo straightened out the hospital's finances and reorganized its administration so that it could function. Despite this brilliant success, Paroo decided that Meharry and its hospital did not offer the future he envisaged. He went on searching for opportunities, including Coral Reef Hospital in Miami and HealthCare International. Only thirty-three years old in 1984, he landed the position of Vice President of Health Affairs and Hospital Executive Director of the Hahnemann University Hospital.

I was on the large, elaborate committee that selected Paroo. Bertram Brown, then President, believed in doing things right and insisted that every faction of the University, even students, be represented on the committee. Paroo's C.V. was most impressive, and his personal appearance outstanding. If Sherif had been a candidate in competition with Paroo, everyone would have picked Paroo. I had only one reservation. He'd had eight different challenges in ten years and had not stuck with any of them. Would he last at Hahnemann? Was this opportunity big enough for him?

As it turned out, he did stay—unfortunately long enough to almost destroy the institution. Brown was a relatively weak, inept president, and it did not take Paroo long to stab him in the back. Paroo ingratiated himself with all-powerful Board President, Joseph

Gallagher. Brown was fired, and Paroo was appointed interim CEO. A hastily appointed search committee selected Paroo as the best candidate for the top job. At age thirty-nine, in April 1990, Paroo was installed as the twenty-fifth President of Hahnemann University. It did not take him long to assert himself. Trusting no one, he fired everyone who did not declare absolute allegiance to him. If a person was too efficient, in fact, he was suspect. Paroo's worse mistake was firing Gene Busch, a competent, conservative financial officer who had helped save the Institution in its previous financial difficulties. Busch would not let Paroo manipulate the budget, so Paroo got rid of him. Soon the annual budget reflected a profit line and—most astounding—an endowment of $25 million. The by-laws were suitably altered to suit Paroo's style, and the democratic quality of the governance changed towards dictatorship. He liked to travel the high road. Advertising brochures, signage, or any public relations event had to be first-class. Always in financial difficulties, Hahnemann, was used to more modest style. This new extravaganza alarmed some faculty, but on the whole most faculty and staff were pleased with this new refreshing attitude. A master plan was soon developed that was aimed at greatly improving the quality of the medical school and hospital.

One must not be too critical of Paroo. He was simply keeping up with the times. Not many could have done better under the circumstances. He was superb at building up a board and controlling it to do his bidding. He failed, however, to recruit able faculty and staff. During his tenure, there never was a strong Dean or a really capable Chairman of the Department of Medicine, personnel vital to the professional success of a medical center. Paroo's ego was too big. He thought he could do it all himself.

Leonard Ross Ph.D. was Dean of the Medical College of Pennsylvania in the 1980s. Ross ascended to this position from the Chairmanship of Anatomy. Born in New York City in 1927, he had the usual excellent primary education afforded in that era. His undergraduate and graduate degrees were earned at New York

University followed by an Assistant Professorship at the Medical College of Alabama and an Associate Professorship at Cornell University School of Medicine. A visiting professorship at Cambridge rounded out his career, and in 1973 he assumed the Chair of the Anatomy Department at the Medical College of Pennsylvania.

Ross was not a great anatomist in the traditional sense, but he was a very good scientist and his publications attest to it. Few students raved about his teaching abilities, and his faculty was not overly enthusiastic about his leadership. He knew how to gain favor in high places and was very fastidious in his personal conduct. Decidedly ambitious, he understood how to exploit a situation that might favor him. When Sherif entered the scene at the Medical College of Pennsylvania, it was astounding how well these two characters saw eye to eye on each problem. About the same height and demeanor, cocking their heads together, waving their arms, they looked like a pair of penguins hob-nobbing and flapping their flippers. Ross had his own agenda, however: He was going to make the Medical College of Pennsylvania one of the best research medical centers in the country.

6

Daniel Kaye, M.D. was the most assertive and disliked of all the characters in this saga. Kaye was born in 1931 in New York City and received his early education there. He got his bachelor's degree at Yale. Returning to his native city, he achieved his medical degree at the New York University College of Medicine. He was an outstanding student who showed interest and ability in research. Microbiology fascinated him perhaps because of the blossoming field of antibiotics. His post graduate work in internal medicine was done at the famous New York Hospital of Cornell University School of Medicine. He went on to specialize in the field of Infectious Diseases and distinguished himself by both basic and clinical research. This enabled him to become a member of the prestigious American Society of Clinical Investigation, an achievement of which he was justly proud. At Cornell Medical School he worked his way up the ranks to become Associate

Professor of Internal Medicine. In 1969 he came to Philadelphia to head the Department of Medicine at the Medical College of Pennsylvania.

There is no argument that Kaye was an extremely capable, progressive department chairman. He held everyone to the very high standards, which he himself followed. His unfortunate style of expression and conduct was, to say the least, brutal. Aggressive behavior was characteristic, which earned him the hatred of most who had to work with him. Needless to say, this type of personality suited Sherif in his grandiose plans to dominate the entire health services of eastern Pennsylvania.

Obviously, there were many more characters in this large disaster that were key to certain events. Sherif's financial officer, for example, had to go along with some very shaky financial manipulations. Another key character was hired to make deals to buy practices. There were faculty members who indeed perceived financial gain for themselves and eagerly threw their support to the enterprise. In this summary, I will deal only with the principal responsible players. Most important, no shrewd executive goes about his manipulations without legal advice. Sherif was smart enough to have persons with legal sagacity at his side to bolster his intentions.

Next component, the exploitable situation: In the late 1980s, the last vestiges of charitable healthcare were practically eliminated. No more free clinics; most cities had closed their city hospitals or else converted them to the pay-for-care basis. Medicare, Medicaid, and medical insurance were intended to finance all medical care from birth to death. Medical schools and other health related establishments were increased in number and capacity so that physicians, nurses, and other health workers were in adequate supply. Enormous amounts of money were expended yearly on healthcare, estimated at that time to be about 11 percent of the gross national product. Yet about a third of the population had no health insurance, and this was a great embarrassment to planners and politicians who had promised the best of healthcare to all.

Nearly forty years of government and industry grant support of biological and medical research to the tune of many billions of dollars, meanwhile, had produced enormous advances in the diagnosis and treatment of disease. Disorders that had received only custodial care could now be treated. Diagnostic machines such as Computerized Axial Tomagraphy (CAT scan) and Magnetic Resonance Imaging (MRI) picture the internal structure of the body in detail—never before considered possible. Miniaturization of instruments, such as the endoscope, as well as computers, miniature cameras, and television enabled surgeons to perform internal operations through a tiny incision. Such advances reduce hospital stay and increase safety, and thus can be argued to reduce cost. Because of the cost of instrumentation and highly trained personnel, however, they end up costing more. There is increased demand and utilization, especially of elective procedures. Diagnostic laboratory tests involving genetic analysis also became available. While very useful, this is also very expensive. Gene therapy may be possible for still incurable diseases like cystic fibrosis. Transplantation of the heart, liver, and kidney are widely practiced and limited only by the availability of replacement organs.

Here is the dilemma: The ability to deliver medical services that increase well being and prolong life is limited only by finances. The United States, admittedly the richest country in the world, manages to deliver more medical services to its citizens than most other modern world powers. Yet it finds it necessary to ration medical services because otherwise the cost would cripple the national economy. In the late 1980s, the amount spent on healthcare (11 percent of the national gross product.) was considered to be excessive, and legislators took steps to ration the delivery of healthcare. Several devices were applied. The most successful were regulations that limited the length of hospital stay. The average number of days spent in the hospital decreased from about twelve in the 1980s to about five-and-a-half in the late 1990s. Medicare led the way in establishing methodology, which controlled finances.

Diagnostic Related Groups (DRG's) were published which covered practically all common diseases, their variations and complications—along with a price list dictating what amount of money could be charged for each entity. An uncomplicated appendectomy was might involve a hospital stay of at least a week in the past. Now only one or two days were allowed.

Established health insurance companies like Blue Cross resisted these regulations in the beginning. The government, however, encouraged the establishment of Health Maintenance Organizations by letting them handle Medicare clients on a contingency basis. Simply put, an HMO receives an annual sum for each Medicare patient enrolled, regardless of whether or not the patient has any medical problem requiring the expenditure of funds during the year. Medicare patients are obviously elderly, and the incidence of disease is high. It is expedient and profitable for an HMO to keep the patient healthy and avoid expensive treatments. Physicians are rewarded if they cut the diagnosis and treatment to the bare minimum. Cheaper generic drugs are preferred

DRGs have worked well but have fallen far short of containing healthcare costs. The HMOs more recently force competition between hospitals and medical groups by having contractual arrangements with the lowest bidder. Even further, this allows HMOs to make arbitrary decisions about what they will pay for. All this leads to frustration and bitterness by physicians and patients who are the victims of the system. In countries with national socialized health plans, the situation is actually worse although it may appear better because everybody is covered for minimum healthcare. Willy-nilly, the conclusion is that no matter how the system operates, only that amount of healthcare can be delivered which is affordable. One method or another must ration healthcare.

So how can big money be made? It happens that during periods of expansion, the rationing is forgotten until the cup runs over. The period from the late 1980s into the middle 1990s was one of great growth in healthcare financing. As has been explained, the astounding development of technology and science made possible unprecedented therapy and control of disease.

How to take advantage of this situation? Sherif knew the answer. The situation in Pittsburgh was no different from any other large urban medical center. Average routine medical care was the domain of the community hospitals. While they handled the bulk of medical care, they had no access to lucrative high-end diagnosis and therapy. Catheterization, cardiac surgery, advanced cancer chemotherapy, transplantation of organs, and the prestigious University of Pittsburgh Medical School Hospital and its clinics monopolized advanced technology of all types. Allegheny General Hospital, certainly a first-class community hospital, could not compete against a staff of full time professors, scientists, a research aura, and more important high class slave labor in the form of over four hundred M.D. residents and fellows. No less important was the ability of the University to raise seed money for new projects of prospective importance to the hospital. Add to this political influence with state and federal governments and a loyal alumni group ready to support and assure referral pathways.

Sherif achieved his long time ambition becoming Chief Executive Officer of Allegheny General in 1986 under Board Chairman William Penn Snyder III. His plan to gain supremacy had long been cooking in his brain. The Allegheny Health, Education and Research Foundation (AHERF) would serve as a substitute University, i,e., a storefront to run operations in a legitimate but none the less cutting thin-ice fashion. AHERF could raise funds for research and education, present a front of community service to the public, enjoy the profits of the non-profit hospital, and thus have the same advantages of a university hospital in a practical way. It worked for two reasons. Snyder put his own money and reputation on the line with the banks. Health business was good, and Sherif knew how to exploit the situation. Allegheny General made extraordinary profits, and the surplus was pumped into AHERF. Staff physicians and the Board were overjoyed. For the first time, Allegheny General was competing successfully against its old enemy, the Pittsburgh University Hospital and Health System. In only two years, Sherif became the guru of CEOs of healthcare systems. Admirers came from far and wide to study his methods.

The third component in this overall picture was the environment of healthcare in Philadelphia. Like all great men, Sherif not only let success go to his head, but he also let it ferment there. If he could achieve such wonders in Pittsburgh, why not invade the eastern part of the state? The gimmick with AHERF had worked so well in the west, why would it not work in the east? All he had to do was acquire a number of fine academic and community hospitals and run them in an efficient health plan. Indeed, the situation in Philadelphia was ripe for such a venture. Five medical school hospitals, an osteopathic medical school, and at least six very fine community hospitals served a prosperous industrial area of some four million people.

Sherif put out feelers. Of the five medical schools, The University of Pennsylvania was definitely not interested because it had its own plans for expansion. Jefferson University Medical Center was also not attracted to Sherif because it was well endowed and successfully competing for its share of the market. Temple University Medical School was state-subsidized and did not feel the financial pressure to run a profitable clinical program. That left two that were always in financial difficulties and anxious to merge with any agency that had the means for development and expansion— Hahnemann University (HU) and The Medical College of Pennsylvania (MCP).

HU was in every way superior to MCP. Strategically located in Center City at the 15th Street exit of the Schuylkill Expressway, HU was the most assessable medical center to the affluent western suburbs. MCP was located in East Falls, which was more remote from Center City. HU also had a relatively new Medical School Building and a brand new modern twenty-story hospital. Compared to MCP's old, inadequate hospital and non-existent medical school buildings, HU was palatial. Aside from these differences, both medical schools would be classed in the fourth quartile of the over125 medical schools in the nation. Both well over one hundred years old, they carried a stigma of segregation. HU started as a homeopathic school and remained so until the early 1940s. MCP was originally a female medical school exclusively.

Both medical schools managed to survive the Flexner Report of 1910 by conforming minimally to the requirements of state and federal agencies. Despite the low standing among the cadre of medical schools, both institutions rendered high quality education, excellent scientific research, and first-class clinical services comparable to the best. No mediocre, non-conforming medical schools are allowed to exist in the United States. The control is simple and very accurate. No one can get a license to practice medicine in any state of the Union without a diploma from an approved school. The real problem is that medical schools without state support or connected with an affluent university are operated on a marginal budget and are always in financial difficulties. They also tend to have weak Boards fearful of being financially committed and hence eager to unload the money burden to someone else.

Sherif knew all this and was an expert in dangling bait with generous perks for the main negotiators. Both institutions were approached. Which one was first did not matter at the time. The crucial factors were who the negotiators were and whether they could get Board approval. Faculty and staff approval were actually important also, but hardly a decisive factor. The big dealers for HU were Iqbal Paroo, Dean Harry Wolman, and the Board Chairman, Joseph A. Gallagher. As CE0, Paroo had the most to gain or lose and so was the key actor. Could he slice a deal that was advantageous to the institution, but at the same time lucrative and one that left him in a superior leadership position? Actually HU was not in severe financial stress at the time, but there was a strong desire to expand and grow with the accelerating health system.

Although Sherif and Paroo were kindred souls, the proposed merger of AHERF and HU did not go well. There were the usual financial projections and arguments about who was to do what. The bottom line, however, was who was to run the show. Paroo was not about to let Sherif become President of the University and Chief CEO because that would relegate him to a subordinate position, so the merger deal did not eventuate. A public statement was issued stating that, while the concept of a merger was a very good idea, it did not seem appropriate at this time.

Sherif lost little time in negotiating with MCP where he found much more malleable flesh. Cohen, the President of MCP, saw an opportunity to leap his institution ahead of its rivals. Tired at being at the bottom of the pile, he was anxious to get his hands on new, abundant finances. He had no aspirations to become CEO and would be happy to be pushed upward to a Chancellorship. After all, he had a substantial private practice to maintain, and the medical school was just one of his side ventures. Dean Ross was ecstatic with the prospect of being able to fire old non-productive faculty and hire some new stars. Kaye, the Chairman of the Department of Medicine, was certain that he could install and successfully run a whole health system for the City of Philadelphia. The faculty at large was not too enthusiastic, especially when they found out that Sherif was trying to slip a female friend through the Admissions Committee. Most of them, however, anticipated better salaries and new facilities and were willing to make what sacrifices were necessary. Everyone wanted a new medical school building that they could call their own. So with little fanfare in 1988, Sherif bought himself a medical school and its hospital lock, stock, and barrel. Oh, how many people have dreamed of buying their own medical school and hospital! It was like winning the lottery. What was Sherif going to do with this bonanza?

In his customary operating fashion, Sherif sought out the most aggressive persons, gave them promotions, generous salary raises, and other perks. He demanded in return absolute allegiance to him, creating a henchmen-type Mafia style operation. In a general faculty and staff meeting, he laid down the law in no uncertain terms. Anyone who dared to ask a question or make a comment was immediately shut down and knew that he or she was likely to be fired soon. In brief, he instituted a mode of operation that demanded full-time clinicians to earn their salaries by seeing enough patients to cover their own income, office, nurse, and secretarial expenses. Basic science professors had to earn most of their salaries from grants. There was nothing wrong with this mode of operation. It indeed was standard practice at large prestigious universities. They could attract the type of people who could easily perform under such conditions because they had the facilities, reputation, governmental and political contacts, referral pathways, and a credible history of successful performance. For MCP, a small medical college with inadequate facilities and funding and very modest record of performance, the sudden institution of such drastic changes would be ridiculous without the influx of large amounts of money. Sherif said he had it, and the changes in policy went ahead. New by-laws were written. Old timers who could make trouble were bought out with generous exit packages. Very soon everyone was in line and pleased with Sherif.

Another faction of faculty and staff was highly motivated with the advent of a new, credible medical school building. There was no room to build at MCP's Henry Avenue campus, but a suitable building was found in a nearby neighborhood. The Lutheran Church, which had built its headquarters on Queen Lane, now wanted to move to the Midwest. The building had adequate acreage but was almost a mile away from the hospital, which would make it difficult to integrate education and science functions with clinical services. Sherif managed to float a $40 million bond that enabled the remodeling of the long three-story structure into an attractive, small academic style building. The larger lecture hall accommodated at best 150 students. There were few or no laboratories for medical students, and the library area was too small. Although, handsome in many respects, such as an attractive lobby, the building was inadequate for the expansion that Sherif and his henchmen contemplated. Nevertheless, it satisfied the ego of the main executive operatives, and they soon made it the base of their operation.

No time was wasted in planning meetings. Sherif knew exactly what he wanted to accomplish. Leonard Ross was put in complete, absolute charge of educational and scientific operations. He was to institute standards of conduct that matched the best that were recommended by the American Association of Medical Colleges and practiced by the top ten medical schools in the country. Daniel Kaye was installed as chief operative of clinical services, both outpatient and hospital. It was up to him to set rules of full-time versus volunteer physicians. He was furthermore to develop a system of healthcare delivery that would insure referrals to the medical school hospital for advanced care. The whole operation was to be integrated with that of Allegheny Hospital and AHERF. All financial operations, including billing, were to be managed from Pittsburgh. Walter Cohen was made Chancellor, while Sherif took complete charge of running the medical school and hospital.

For the first two years, enthusiasm and hopes ran high as money poured in, new people were hired, and old professors were encouraged to retire. AHERF was able to stimulate research by giving out grants, especially in diseases of old age and cancer therapy. They naturally favored MCP professors, and this certainly made some faculty who had trouble getting NIH grants happy. The completion of the physical plant on Queen Lane boosted morale. Attempts to increase the clinical practice were less successful.

The Philadelphia health market was more competitive and complicated as compared to that in Pittsburgh. In the midst of a serious project to reduce the length of hospital stay; Philadelphia and its suburbs had an excess of well over three thousand beds. Sherif was having trouble filling the beds of the Medical School Hospital. So was every other hospital. Yet Sherif was so confident that his methods would succeed that in 1991, only three years after his invasion of the Philadelphia market, he bought out St. Christopher's Hospital for Children and Rolling Hill Hospital in Philadelphia and Warminster Hospital in Bucks County. The last two were typical financially troubled community hospitals. And it's well known that children's hospitals lose money and must be subsidized. Times were still pretty good for funding of healthcare, and somehow Sherif was able to put on an appearance of success. There was no doubt that MCP was growing in stature, both locally and nationally. Other Philadelphia medical schools were beginning to regard with awe this growing monster in their midst.

Sherif was not alone in his concept of health systems. In the lush early 1990s, the University of Pennsylvania Health System (UPHS), Jefferson University Health System (JUHS), and Temple University Health System (TUHS) began to emerge. Under the

vigorous leadership of Dr. William H. Kelley, UPHS began to buy
doctors' practices, establish satellite clinics, and consolidate its
affiliate hospitals. It also plunged into high tech genetic research
in hopes of becoming the first and the best in the therapy of disease
on a molecular basis. JUHS took a more practical, expedient line.
Using its loyal alumni base and affiliate hospitals, it formed a health
system of Main Line area hospitals, including Lankenau, Bryn Mawr,
and Paoli. It also consolidated its traditional South Philadelphia
catchment area. TUHS stuck with the poor community of North
Philadelphia and tried to expand its business to the northeast and
adjacent suburbs. Practices were bought and affiliation with
Abington Hospital negotiated.

Well aware of what was going on, Sherif realized that MCP
and its hospital alone could not compete with giants UPHS and
JUHS. Feelers began to be projected to Hahnemann University.
Paroo meanwhile had further consolidated his Board. Alfred W.
Martinelli, Chairman of the Board, was an excellent businessman
and widely respected. He was no Snyder, however, and Hahnemann
as usual had little ability to extend its credit line to the extent
needed to compete with the other health systems. Indeed, it was
reportedly $20 million in debt.

Paroo was now in an entirely different frame of mind. He had
divorced his wife and acquired unanticipated financial obligations.
He needed more security. In the end, it seemed quite clear to the
Board that Hahnemann University would not survive in the era of
rapid expansion and high financing of health services. This was
not actually certain, but Paroo chose to put it that way. HUHS
would have been wise to "shrink into profitability" and thus avoid
the financial disaster that was to eventuate in just a few years.

When actual negotiations started, it soon became obvious that
it was not just between AHERF and Hahnemann. Sherif had made
a prior commitment to MCP that nothing would be done unless
it had the complete, enthusiastic support of MCP. That was not
Paroo's idea, but he had no choice. He was now only the beggar at
the table. MCP made sure that it would be in complete charge of
the merged schools and health system. Only loyal MCP executives

and Department Chairmen would have key appointments. MCP, the formally docile Women's Medical College, planned a hostile takeover lock, stock, and barrel of Hahnemann University. In the opinion of the MCP elite, it was just a decaying institution. They indicated to Sherif that only they could swing the deal with the approval and blessing of the American Association of Medical Colleges, AAMC. This venerable organization would actually be happy to approve any merger that would reduce the number of medical schools and hopefully decrease enrollment of medical students at the same time. Sherif greatly enjoyed the situation. Considering himself an underdog who had made good despite all odds, he relished taking over the "Big Guy." There is a strong suspicion that tacit agreements were made that Cohen would be the nominal head, Ross would be the Dean, and Kaye would manage the hospitals and the health system. Of course, there was no doubt that Sherif would run everything. Paroo would be retained and put in charge of something that looked important in exchange for his support. Wolman, the HU Dean, received the same consideration; the merger, which relieved them of the financial pressures of the moment, pleased Martinelli and the HU board. Martinelli was genuinely convinced that it was a good, sound business venture and would insure the future of HUHS. No one can blame him for that view. Look what it had done for MCPHS! After much bickering and minor delays, the deal to merge HUHS with MCPHU was consummated in 1994, just six years after Sherif had invaded the Philadelphia healthcare market.

The news of the merger did not seem so bad at first. Quite a few faculty even thought that it was a fortunate event. They were already in the process of trying to ingratiate themselves with the new administration. Attitudes quickly changed when it became obvious that the main campus and directions would come from Queen Lane. The new name, "Allegheny University of the Health Sciences," was installed with expensive signage on Broad, Vine, and 15th Streets. Sherif, Ross, and their cohorts moved into the executive offices on the nineteenth floor of the Hahnemann College Building. Sherif soon held a general faculty meeting that set the style and pace for how the place would be run. He strode in with his entourage with a measured, assertive step. All that was missing was the three cornered hat or the Nazi swastika. Without benefit of notes or podium, he spelled out that he would run the place and make the combined institution the best medical education, research, and service organization in the nation. All that was required was absolute allegiance to him.

Almost as an afterthought, he asked if there were any questions. One emboldened full-time clinical person asked if salaries would be brought in line with those of major medical centers. His prompt reply was accompanied by a contemptuous stare: Only those who are productive and loyal to the institution will get top salaries. That ended the meeting.

A period of the most reckless expansion, spending, and mismanagement now began. Eminent scientists were hired at their own price. Whole floors were remodeled for their use. Three separate libraries were established when one could suffice. A shuttle bus service between the two campuses was installed. These turned out to be minor extravagances and probably could be justified. It would be more difficult to explain why Sherif needed an executive jet to travel between Pittsburgh and Philadelphia. Then there were the insurance deals involving a business vacation at the Cayman Islands and loans at low interest to finance his luxurious home. Looking back, all this could perhaps be overlooked if the management of the combined institutions had produced a positive bottom line.

In retrospect, it is easy to assign the reasons for Allegheny's financial disaster, but the details are obscure. Management and records were all out of Pittsburgh and mixed with those of AHERF. Moreover, the Board of AHERF appeared to function in a secretive manner, and there were not the usual checks and balances customary in an organization that is non-profit and eligible to receive public funds. Sherif was apparently allowed to buy and spend as he wished. His brilliant success in Pittsburgh and his recognition by the AAMC and other accrediting organizations gave him an aura that he could do no wrong. It was a time of growing prosperity, and other health-education systems in Philadelphia were also expanding.

Without doubt, the greatest error was the purchase of private medical practices in an effort to insure referrals to the university hospital. At the peak of this frenzy to acquire a referral base, it was reported that 270 practices were bought. If this were a true figure, it would involve a commitment of at least $100 million. To accomplish this coup, Sherif employed a mysterious character, Harvey Levy, who apparently had phenomenal success in buying private practices and running them successfully as a maverick health system. Levy was a businessman who liked to speculate and knew how to deal with doctors who felt they were working too hard for their money. For the first year, Levy would propose to the doctor a deal that appeared as a half-time job at full-time pay. Methods would be found later to squeeze the practice into profitability. This venture was a catastrophic failure. The majority of doctors involved promptly relaxed efforts to build up and retain their practices since they had full-time pay no matter whether they saw few or many patients. This was now a nine-to-five job with at least one day off for golf and vacations in Florida and Hawaii. Levy's prior success in this business was not duplicated for Allegheny. How could Levy and his staff of only a few people run the business and operative details of so many practices?

Medical practice is mainly person-to-person interaction and cannot be efficiently run by remote management. Physicians soon became frustrated and disgusted, and they tried to get out of their contracts as they watched their practices deteriorate. As a method of gaining referrals to the university hospitals, it was a disastrous failure. It actually reduced referrals from the usual historical sources while it produced little itself for the vast amount of money invested. In their aggressive venture, Sherif and Levy caused the competing institutions also to buy up practices that they did not need and at unreasonable high prices, thus inflating the market. UPHS bought up as many practices as did MCPHUHS, which created very severe financial loss that contributed to the demise of Kelley, the CEO. JUHS that did not buy any private practices was the only health system to do well financially. The failure of operating private practices by central healthcare organizations is confirmed by the subsequent mad rush to get out of the contracts by all concerned. There is little disagreement that Allegheny's unwise splurge into private practice was one of the major factors in the financial disaster that followed. Unfortunately, there were other glaring errors of management.

One would suppose that Sherif, one of the most respected hospital and health system CEOs in the nation, would know how to collect bills. Yet the astounding fact, revealed after the bankruptcy, was that Hahnemann Hospital collected only somewhat less than 20 percent of billing. It is known that hospital collections are notoriously deficient, especially in inner city hospitals that serve a large proportion of indigent patients. However, 20 percent is ridiculous. Before Allegheny took over, Hahnemann Hospital was collecting over 80 percent of its bills. One of the main defects in the billing system was that everything that involved finances had to be worked through Pittsburgh. The system was so cumbersome that the local people who had the responsibility did not know what was happening to their bills. Ultimate blame rests on the Board of Allegheny that wasn't watching the finances. The Board allowed Sherif to spend as he liked and pull the wool over its eyes as his extravagances led to growing deficits.

I got a flavor of how Sherif controlled and protected his Board when a rumor circulated that a former middle management employee who had been released from Hahnemann was on the Board of AHERF. The faculty was concerned so I volunteered to verify this position, as there was no published list of AHERF board members. I called Sherif's office and got his secretary, who was quite gracious. I told her that I would like a list of AHERF board members. She replied, "I cannot release that information. Mr. Abdelhak needs first to know why you need this information." This was a surprise to me since AHERF, as a non-profit organization that received public money, could not legally have a secret board. Certainly as a member of the faculty, former officer of Hahnemann University, and a financial contributor to AHERF, I had a every right to know who was on the board. Not wishing to make a scene, I replied, "Don't disturb Mr. Abdelhak. I simply want to know if a certain Mr. John Doe is a member of the board. At the moment, I do not need to know who are the other members of the board." She answered immediately, "He is not a member." That ended the conversation, but I was left with some wonderment about Sherif's sensitivity about who was on his board. This episode reinforced my suspicion that Sherif controlled his board very tightly, and this was how he was able to operate in his own style without any checks and balances.

Sherif's style also included a very high salary for himself and his people. In 1995 his salary and benefits were $1,216,757—certainly the highest recompense for CEOs of university health systems in Pennsylvania. Kelley, CEO of UPHS received $871,220, while Paul C. Brucker, CEO of the JUHS, incidentally the most profitable university health system, received the relatively modest sum of $479,240. Sherif rewarded his trusted people very well. Donald Kaye, CEO of MCPHU Hospital System, received $759,136. David W. McConnell, Chief Financial Officer, received $711,665. Even Ross, the Provost, received $659,043, which seemed excessive considering the comparable salaries of academic officers of other university medical schools. In view of the fact that health systems were suffering a recession in1995 and beginning to lay off workers, these salaries raised markedly from previous years were an authentic demonstration of the greed of the leaders of the health business, especially Allegheny. All the institutions were non-profit at the time. They paid minimal wages to workers, avoided taxes, received state and federal money, and raised charity money from the public.

It does seem apparent that morally and ethically these executives were exceeding the bounds of what might be considered normal behavior in the management of a medical university. Indeed, I am not addressing illegal actions. Such greed is entirely acceptable and even admired in profit-oriented big business. Had Sherif and his ilk been successful and not degenerated into bankruptcy, they might still be in power today. But mismanagement and misuse of moneys intended for education, the advance of knowledge, and the elimination of disease can never be considered morally correct behavior, and it distinctly borders on the criminal.

Sherif aggrandized and advertised his buildup of the AHERF empire by a development department of vast proportions. He hired the best available personnel and supported their programs enthusiastically. It was rumored that at one time as many as forty people were working on various projects. This flurry of activity reached a peak in 1997-98. Daily full-page newspaper ads appeared, accompanied by radio and television news items about the amazing advances and treatments occurring in the schools, hospitals, and clinics of AHERF. Even a tabloid type newspaper entitled "Allegheny News" was published. The September 8, 1997, issue contained three sections, each eight pages long, with general news of the eastern and western areas and a focus on clinical care. It was well done but obviously very expensive to produce and distribute.

Fund raising was another important function of the development department. No effort was spared to extract the maximum amount of donated moneys from alumni, faculty, staff, suppliers, friends, and the general public. There were the usual special meetings, gala affairs, and personalized appeals. How successful this was will never be accurately known. For 1997 a figure was rumored of $43 million. If true, with all the money in the bank this was an impressive figure. But anyone who has tried to raise money for a university health system knows that a lot of pledges are never collected, and some moneys would not have come in without expensive fund raising. Still, for an institution that barely raised a $1 million in yearly outside charity funds, this was a distinct improvement. It was only a drop in the bucket, however, compared to Sherif's appetite for spending money. As it turned out, this figure had to be optimistic because no such money was found when the books were examined at bankruptcy.

In a mad buying frenzy in 1996, Allegheny bought the Graduate Health System, including Graduate Hospital itself, Graduate Hospital on City Avenue, Parkview, Rancocas, and Mount Sinai Hospitals. All these hospitals were obviously facing financial disaster. Why else would they want to sell out to the hated Allegheny outfit? Graduate Hospital had a long, distinguished history. It was originally affiliated with the University of Pennsylvania. After World War II, Graduate Hospital served brilliantly as the main clinical teaching resource of the popular Graduate School of the University of Pennsylvania. In the late 1980s, it formed an effective health system that was competitive with the university hospitals. After profitable expansion, it now found itself with too many employees and facilities for its declining business. Mount Sinai was also a Philadelphia icon, having served for many years as the southern division of the Albert Einstein Hospital Health System. After years of neglect and decay, it was now desperate for someone to rescue it. Parkview and Rancocas were smaller community hospitals that had become redundant in the atmosphere of high tech medicine.

It did not take long for Sherif and his mastermind Kaye to realize that they were in deep financial trouble. Seventeen hundred employees were laid off on October 13, 1997. Mount Sinai Hospital was closed. To appease his conscience and allay fears of creditors, Sherif announced that he would take 20 percent pay cut. Instead, records in 1997 show that he received a 13 percent increase. Despite an outward show of flamboyance and optimism, creditors and banks were becoming increasingly anxious.

Over the next six months the situation only got worse as Allegheny fell further behind in paying its debts, and the banks were not lending any more money. In March 1998, it was announced that Vanguard Health Systems of Nashville was considering buying six hospitals from Allegheny. The deal fell through when Vanguard more seriously investigated Allegheny's financial operations in the Philadelphia region. Among other shady financial transactions, there was an indication that Allegheny was dipping into restricted funds in order to pay off some urgent debts. Now the banks and creditors became extremely nervous. Loans were called. Merchants refused to deliver unless the existing bills were paid. Just a month later on April 27, Allegheny repaid an $89 million loan by a consortium of four banks, headed by Mellon Bank. There was a strong suspicion that Mellon Bank executives who sat on the Allegheny Board had engineered this payment in anticipation of the imminent collapse of Allegheny.

Inevitably, Sherif was fired on June 5, 1998. AHERF appointed Anthony Sanzo, supposedly Sherif's protégé, to manage affairs. Sanzo's job was to salvage what he could but mainly to protect whatever assets remained that rightly belonged to Allegheny Hospital and its health system in the Pittsburgh area. AHERF's fear was that the Philadelphia fiasco would destroy the reputation and operation of Allegheny Health System in Pittsburgh. At the same time, he had only rubber bands and stick paste to fix the Philadelphia operation. The sale of the six hospitals to Vanguard was still alive and might have been able to stave off outright bankruptcy, at least temporarily. Kaye, the CEO and President of Allegheny's nine hospitals and Philadelphia health system, also resigned. Allegheny did not bother to replace him. As expected, it did not take long for Vanguard to bow out of the deal to buy the hospitals.

As cash became extremely scarce, the eight hospitals, the private practices, and the medical university filed for Chapter 11 on July 21, 1998. In size and monetary value, this was by far the largest healthcare bankruptcy. Estimates range from $1.3 to 1.6 billion. Unfortunately, it also involved the medical university because the hospitals and the schools were all incorporated under a single corporation.

The rumor factory had been active, of course, and everyone anticipated the collapse of AHERF. Students especially, who had such a big investment in a medical career, would now find themselves out on the street or competing to get into a medical school all over again. Patients were scheduled for crucial procedures, physicians were unable to function, and executives did not know what to do except shut down. Consternation, anger, frustration, and despair dominated the scene. As always seems to happen in such situations, some clear minded, dedicated individuals suddenly arise as leaders to steer a path towards survival. They were all MCP faculty, which is understandable because practically all Hahnemann faculty of any stature had been fired or bought out. It would appear that the heroes of the day were altruistic, but there was a suspicion that there was some financial incentive to perform their tasks. Notwithstanding, they did what they had to do, and the end result that there wasn't even a one-hour lapse in the operation of the hospitals or the university. Federal, state and city politicians and executives were contacted, and the proper arrangements were made to insure the protection of federal grants, state subsidies, and city contracts. The AAMC continued accreditation, and other medical schools promised to accept students if the collapse were to occur. The Board of Trustees rediscovered itself and reorganized. It named Dorothy Brown as President. A long time member of the Hahnemann Board and former president of Rosemont College, she lent an air of reliability to the future of the institution. Salaries were paid, healthcare and education delivered, and research performed—without benefit of the great leaders who just a few days earlier had been considered indispensable.

The natural consequence of disaster is attack by scavengers and desertion by all who can escape advantageously. Physicians who had good practices soon found other local institutions more attractive. They left and took their patients with them. Professors who had grants soon found other employment. The great Cardiovascular Institute was dissolved and its considerable grant moneys raised through private efforts were dissipated by the AHERF financial manipulations. This was a severe body blow because Hahnemann's success was largely due to its superior reputation and performance in cardiovascular diseases. Associated with a relaxation of state control of advanced cardiac treatment facilities, many community hospitals quickly installed catheter laboratories and cardiac by-pass surgical suites to cash in on this lucrative business. From being first in cardiac procedures, Hahnemann fell to fourth position in the Philadelphia area. Orthopedics was also decimated with the collapse of Graduate Hospital. All in all, it was quite obvious that unless some substantial financial relief came along soon, Hahnemann Hospital would have to close. The medical school would probably be able to stagger along as a kind of two-year school.

Relief came in the form of a buyout of the eight hospitals and the university by the Tenet Healthcare Corporation of San Diego, California, a for-profit corporation. The total cash deal was for $345 million dollars, far less than what Vanguard had offered before the bankruptcy. It did little for the estimated eighty thousand creditors. If other assets were not found, the creditors would get no more than five cents on the dollar. Even worse, Sherif and his cohorts had dipped very heavily into restricted funds that included endowments to the various hospitals and grants for research and education in university departments. The only funds he did not touch were those that could not be easily purloined—government grants. I lost about $75,000, part of a fund that my colleagues and I raised from friends and relatives to support research and education in the Department of Pharmacology. Other faculty lost greater sums of restricted money. Although some have sued AHERF, it is extremely unlikely that any of this money will ever be recovered.

As a for-profit corporation, Tenet was certain to run the hospitals on a for-profit basis that, incidentally, may eventually become the standard for all hospitals. When it came to the medical university, Tenet got cold feet attempting to apply its business expertise to managing this complex, unfamiliar assortment of prima donnas. With typical acumen, the decision was "Let's get someone else to run it. We will use it as part of our charitable contribution to the community, meanwhile utilizing it for our healthcare delivery operation and image."

Manual Stamatakis suddenly appeared at this time. A businessperson with political connections, he happened to be on the boards of both Allegheny and Drexel Universities. It developed that Drexel University was employed to manage the defunct Allegheny University of the Health Sciences. It was a sweet deal for Drexel because the terms released to the public seemed liberal in favor of Drexel. The big inducement was a $50 million no-strings-attached contribution to the Drexel University Endowment Fund. Then there was a $30 million yearly operating fund. With reasonable business and academic institution management skills, Drexel

University should lose no money in this enterprise. The main advantage of the deal to Drexel, however, was the acquisition of access to tremendous biological and medical science and expertise that had NIH funding in excess of $50 million.

Drexel was established in 1891 as an Institute of Art, Science and Industry. In the next few years, it was one of the first to educate librarians. By 1914, it had developed Schools of Engineering, Domestic Science and Arts, Secretarial, and an Evening School. Drexel distinguished itself as one of the first higher educational institutions to establish and foster co-operative education. The name was changed by 1936 to Drexel Institute of Technology, which better reflected its functions and purposes. Climbing the academic ladder, Drexel became a University in 1969. As computer science and technology became available, Drexel took advantage. Even in the early 1980s, every student at Drexel was required to have access to a microcomputer. A long held ambition was the desire to exploit the very promising field of biomedical engineering. Drexel established schools of Biomedical Engineering, Science and Health Systems and Environmental Science, Engineering and Policy in the late 1990s. It also established research agreements with Thomas Jefferson University in order to supply access to the biological sciences. It can therefore be appreciated that, at this time and situation in Drexel's development, a merger with a well-established medical university would be decidedly advantageous, especially if it could be done at no expense to Drexel. The president of Drexel, Constantine Papadakis, glowed with ecstasy and issued this public statement:

"MCP Hahnemann is an acknowledged leader in medical education innovation, as is Drexel in engineering and science. The beneficiaries of the Drexel/ MCP Hahnemann collaboration will be the students and faculties of both institutions as well as the people of greater Philadelphia and the Commonwealth of Pennsylvania."

With this optimistic statement, apparently supported by Drexel Board Chairman Chuck Pennoni and Trustee Manuel Stamatakis, in the fall of 1998 Drexel undertook the task of the management and

Later a law school estab

consolidation of two bankrupt medical schools along with
subsidiary schools and educational programs. The intriguing
element was the combination of Tenet, a for-profit healthcare
industry, with a non-profit educational institution. Drexel would
have little or nothing to do with the running of the hospitals and
other health related services. This was a large area for conflict
because medical education is completely based on actual contact
and practice of the student with the sick patient. The best medical
schools have the superior clinical facilities, and this attracts the
best students and the most talented physicians. Advanced education
of residents and fellows is also a function of the medical school.
Selection of department chairmen and service chiefs is done jointly,
and there also is an overlap in the financing of clinical departments.
Experienced administrators of academic health centers soon learn
the common path to successful operation: "Keep the hospital beds
full and the clinics busy." This becomes the dictum of every person
in the medical school or the hospital whether it's the president,
dean, professor, nurse, or porter.

Drexel fortunately had assets that would be useful in running
the complexities of a medical university. Frank Bachich, Drexel's
chief financial officer, had been the chief financial of HU in the
1980s, so he was very well acquainted with financial management
of a medical educational establishment. When I was the Dean in
the early 1970s, I hired him as an assistant and watched his rise
over the years into a mature, conscientious, and resourceful financial
officer. Drexel had been a leader in adopting computer technology
and should be able to update the MCPHU system. Long interested
in developing superior engineering medical technology, Drexel now
had the opportunity to integrate medical-biological research and
development with engineering know-how, which would be a great
incentive. Finally Drexel's experience in organizing educational
programs, appeasing accrediting bodies, and qualifying from a
technical school into a university should make the usual academic
details a cinch to manage.

A main problem of the merger with Drexel would be financial.
In any merger, one party inevitably must absorb the other. All

Also Drexel had a large endowment
± $400 million

three institutions had marginal financial histories. None had the endowment or borrowing capacity to float a comparative medical center to University of Pennsylvania or Jefferson. Of the three, Drexel under the leadership of President Papadakis showed a credible capacity to raise money from the community and its alumni. It was doubtful, however, that Drexel could raise money for a medical center. The hospitals, clinics, practices, and all the buildings were owned and run by Tenet on a for-profit basis. MCPHU had a practice plan but the income from was small compared to the Tenet operation. Thus Drexel had little contact with grateful patients and others who would be likely to donate to a health oriented program. Still, with ingenuity it could work

A main attraction for Drexel was the potential to receive and control federal research funds. As much as $100 million would be possible. Such moneys would buy a lot of professors, administrators, and technicians, besides adding high-class equipment and supplies. Overhead costs paid by the government might amount to as much as another $50 million. It sounds like a sinecure. Unfortunately, I know of no university that has been able to work grants for a real profit that could be used for teaching and to lower tuition. The greatest detrimental effect of big grants is to cause a rise in salaries, including those of administrators, which cannot be maintained unless new and bigger grants are secured in subsequent years. The grant business in universities is inherently a pyramid scheme. In addition the University must raise comparable funds from the community to support the research operation. More serious is the withdrawal of government funds in times of economic setback, placing the university into economic jeopardy.

EPILOGUE

"All is for the best in the best of all possible worlds."

From *Candide* by Voltaire

After many months of negotiation, the Trustees of Drexel University announced on April 25, 2002, that they approved the agreement with Tenet to merge MCP Hahnemann into Drexel University. Tenet retained full ownership and management of all the hospitals, which would continue to be affiliated with Drexel. Although MCP Hahnemann University would continue to operate as a fully accredited four-year medical school with a practice plan for its full-time clinical professors, it lost control and management of its main clinical facility, Hahnemann Hospital. MCP Hahnemann University in effect became a two-year medical school, although recognized as a fully accredited four-year medical school, with an advantageous affiliation with a commercial corporation that has successful experience in buying and operating hospitals for profit.

There was nothing new about this. It had already happened in about a dozen medical schools in the country, some far better endowed than MCP Hahnemann. Both Jefferson and the University of Pennsylvania had sufficient endowments to continue to maintain a full interest in their main campus hospital, although the latter was wavering towards complete separation. It will be interesting to observe how the merger of three educational schools, each with marginal endowments and scant state support, will affect the competition for students, research money, and clinical practice. Among the staff and faculty of MCP Hahnemann, there was considerable optimism that the merger would result in benefits to education, research, and even to delivery of healthcare. Naturally, all were concerned with what would happen in regard to their own careers, both from a professional and financial viewpoint.

From my viewpoint as an individual who had a relationship with the institution for over fifty years, the events that have culminated in the merger were astonishing, baffling, bizarre, and irrational. Medical education has been and will continue to be primarily an apprenticeship program. Medical research requires clinical facilities. Medical care cannot be delivered without licensed physicians, a hospital, and clinics. In brief, the clinical facilities are the medical school. Without them there is no laboratory and no instructional material. This is especially important because the basic sciences no longer have laboratory instruction and the medical student gets little hands-on experience before his clinical instruction years. High quality of the hospital and clinical services attract superior faculty, staff, residents, and students. Separation of the medical school from the operation of the clinical services means a loss of control of the clinical faculty. Drexel has the challenge to manage a situation that no university has been able to control entirely and successfully to date. The moneys involved in the clinical operation overshadow by far the research and educational functions. Soon the university finds itself using its endowment to pay the large salaries of clinicians and executives who have little if any involvement in education and research and certainly not in the main mission of an academic university.

The years since I retired in 1986 have been an era of extraordinary expansion of medical science, technology, and ability to deliver health services. The costs of surgery and medical treatments, research, and medical education have risen at a faster rate than the growth of the economy. It is inevitable that bankruptcy of the system will occur and cause an increase of the rationing of medical services and maybe even of research. Meanwhile, academic medical centers have had corresponding growth in size and complexity. It is interesting and pertinent to note that the relative position of the

Philadelphia academic centers to each other and to those in other states has not appreciably changed over the years. UPMC remains in the first or second position in the nation, competing with Johns Hopkins Medical Center. Indeed the Philadelphia area placed fourth in the nation in NIH moneys received in 2001 for research and edged out Baltimore, which dropped to fifth position. Boston was first, followed by New York and San Diego. The actual figures for the main Philadelphia centers were: UPMC #2 at $334 million; JUMC # 44 at $74.7 million; TUMC #73 at $28.8 million; and MCPHMC #90 at $15.8 million. In Philadelphia, saturated with fine medical centers, each can only grow by acquiring business from its competitors. The MCPHMC medical school now graduates over 250 medical doctors a year, making it one of the largest in the nation. Its endowment, however, remains miniscule, and it cannot grow unless it raises the cash to hire the talent and provide the facility in which they can work. Hopefully, the combination of the three inadequately financed schools can ride the crest of a wave and float on to greater achievement.

Like Panglos, the philosopher in Voltaire's satiric novel *Candide*, I regard the events that have led to the merger with incredible optimism. Takeover by Allegheny and MCP, bankruptcy, buyout by Tenet, Drexel's hiring to run the university, and finally solvency and merger with Drexel—perhaps it was all to the best in the incredible machinations in the operation of a complex society.

As I write this at the age of eighty-six, I hope that my mind is sufficiently balanced to perceive the events of my life with proper introspection. None will disagree that I have been very fortunate to survive the calamities that strike everyone in a long life. I was also lucky to have been associated with a medical school that gave me the opportunity to develop into a mature teacher and researcher and later into an executive. Hahnemann Medical College and Hospital never held me back, even though it did not rank in the top echelon. I'm proud to have had the opportunity to contribute to the development of the present facility and the reorganization into a university of the medical sciences. What a wonderful group of dedicated people it was my opportunity to work with. It is impossible to mention by name all the wonderful students, professors, and executives, but I love them all, including the ones who gave me much trouble.

Dec.2003

Acknowledgement

Martha Jablow did a great job of copyediting. Barbara Williams helped with references and illustrations.

Copyright 2013
age

Born 1916
3 1

15 yrs older than I am — CR: 84
15
99 !

NOTES AND REFERENCES

Chapter I (1916-1935)

New York City at the turn of the century (1900) was inundated with immigrants. Housing was in short supply and people crowded into tenements. The city was much involved with early labor problems, World War I, and into the post-war Roaring Twenties. The nature of the environment into which I was born is reflected in these references:

Byron, Joseph. *New York Life at the Turn of the Century in Photographs*. Dover Publications, 1985.

Harris, Bill, *The History of New York City*. Portland House, 1989. (*See Chapters 10 and 11 in particular.*)

Allen, Oliver E. New York, New York: *A History of the World's Most Exhilarating and Challenging City*. Atheneum Publishing. 1991.

Charles A. Lindbergh had an enormous influence on young people in the 1920s and 1930s, perhaps as great as that of the Space Age today:

Berg, A. Scott. *Lindbergh*. G.P. Putnam's Sons, 1998.

Brooklyn with its population of over three million and its industry is really a city unto itself. At one time it was considered the bedroom of New York City. Almost anyone you met either lived in Brooklyn or had relatives and friends who spent part of their lives there. During the time

I spent in Brooklyn, the Long Island College of Medicine was the sole medical school serving the borough and thus had enormous clinical facilities available for its students. Some of the social atmosphere and living conditions are captured in the following reference:

Frommer, M. K. and H. Frommer. *It Happened in Brooklyn.* Harcourt Brace and Company, 1993.

Chapter II (1936-1941)

The Long Island College of Medicine as it existed in 1909 is described briefly in the Flexner Report. In 1936 the major changes were that the hospital and the medical school were separate corporations. An important new facility was added, known as the Polak Building, which contained student laboratories in the basic sciences. It is fair to say that the school was fairly comparable in organization and structure with other private medical schools of the late 1930s that were not a part of an established university.

Flexner, Abraham. *The Flexner Report: Medical Education in the United States and Canada*, 1910. Science & Health Publications, 1740 N. Street, N.W., Washington, DC 20036 (*See p. 266*).

During my medical school attendance, I published the following papers:

DiPalma, J.R. and J.R. Johnson "A Substitute for Cargile Membrane in the Construction of Brodie Bellows," *Science*, 88:113. 1938.

Johnson, J.R. and J.R. DiPalma "Intramyocardial Pressure and its Relation to Aortic Blood Pressure," *Amer. J. Psysiol.* 125:224. 1939.

DiPalma, J.R. "A Simple Artery Clip." *Science*, 92:44. 1940.

DiPalma, J. R., S.R.M. Reynolds, and F.I. Foster. "Measurement of the Sensitivity of the Smallest Blood Vessels in Human Skin: Responses to Graded Mechanical Stimulation in Normal Men," *J. Clin. Invest.*: 20, 333. 1941.

As pertains to my relationship with Dr. Crawford, the work on the shock syndrome, referred to below, was actually performed in 1942 and published in 1943 during my internship:

DiPalma, J.R. "The Circulation in the Skin in the Shock Syndrome: Comparison of Simple Prognostic Features of Clinical Value," *J.A.M.A.* 123: 684. 1943.

Chapter III (1942-1944)

Kings County Hospital in Brooklyn was one of the New York City hospitals, comparable to the famous and much older Bellevue Hospital in Manhattan. From the late 1930s it was a magnificent structure capable of housing 2,000 patients and replete with all the medical services of the era. There were about 125 interns and residents divided into an open division run by independent attending physicians and a closed service operated by attending physicians on the faculty of the Long Island College of Medicine. There was supposed to be better teaching on the closed service but actually there were more similarities than differences.

The following six papers were actually done during the year 1941-1942 which I spent in the Department of Physiology after graduation from medical school:

Reynolds, S.R.M., J.B. Hamilton, J.R. DiPalma, G. R. Hubert and F.I. Foster. "Dermovascular Actions of Certain Steroid Hormones in Castrate, Eunochoid and Normal Men," *J. Clin. Endo.* II, 228. 1942.

Reynolds, S.R.M. and J.R. DiPalma. "Dermovascular Changes during the Menstrual Cycle: Failure to Find a Cyclic Variation in Contractile or Dilating Capacities of the Capillaries of the Skin," *J. Clin.Endo.* II,226. 1942.

DiPalma, J.R. and F. I. Foster. "The Segmental and Aging Variations of Reactive Hyperemia in Human Skin," *Amer. Heart J.*: Vol. 24, No. 3, pp. 332-344. 1942.

DiPalma, J. R., S.M.R. Reynolds and F. I. Foster. "The Quantitative Measurement of Reactive Hyperemia in the Human Skin:

Individual and Seasonal Variations," *Am. Heart J. 23* 377. 1942.

DiPalma, J.R. "Quantitative Alterations in the Hyperemia Responses to Local Ischemia of the Smallest Blood Vessels of the Human Skin Following Systemic Anoxemia, Hypercapnia, Acidosis, and Alkalosis," *J. Exp. Med. 76*, 401. 1942.

Milberg, I. L. and J.R. DiPalma. "The Effects of Certain Vehicles and of Salt Solutions upon Reactive Hyperemia in the Skin: Application in a Case of Lichen Rubon Planus," *J. Invest.Derm. 5*, 403. 1942.

I finally got the work on blood volume, in which I used the dye Evans Blue, published in 1944:

DiPalma, J.R. and P. E. Kendall: "The Relationship between Blood Volume and Blood Specific Gravity in the Recovery from Cardiac Decompensation," *J. of Lab. & Clinical Med.*, Vol. 29, No. 4, pp. 390-397. 1944.

Chapter IV (1944-1950)

Despite the rigors of private practice, I managed to turn out quite a bit of research; although some of it was clinical, most was quite fundamental in nature:

DiPalma, J. R. and N. B. Dreyer. "Failure of Thiourea to Alter the Autonomic Responses of Intact Animals," *Endocrinol., 36*, 236. 1945.

DiPalma, J.R. and J.J. MacGovern. "Disadvantages of Thiouracil Treatments of Angina Pectoris," *Amer. Heart J.* Vol. *32*, No. 4, pp. 494-503, 1946.

DiPalma, J.R. "Objective and Clinical Study of the Tongue," *Arch. Int. Med. 78*, 405. 1946.

Gubner, R., J.R. DiPalma, and E. Moore. "Specific Dynamic Action as a Means of Augmenting Peripheral Blood Flow," *Amer. J. Med.* 213, 46-52. 1947.

DiPalma, J.R. and J.J. Lambert. "Importance of the Methoxy Group in Antifibrillatory Compounds," *Science*, Vol. 107, No. 2768, pp. 66-68. 1948.

The Thorndike Laboratory, one of the great medical research laboratories, was first headed by George Minot, then William Castle, and eventually by Maxwell Finland. A biography of Finland describes the laboratory's history and development up to the 1980s:

Robbins, Frederick C. *Maxwell Finland http://stills.nap.edu/html/ biomems/mfinland.html*

The next two papers were actually the result of work done during my fellowship at Harvard in 1946:

Greenwood, W. F., A.C. Barger, J.R. DiPalma, J. Stokes, III, and L. H. Smith. "Factors Affecting the Appearance and Persistence of Visible Cutaneous Reactive Hyperemia in Man," *J. of Clinical Investigation*, Vol. XXVII, No. 2, pp. 187-197, 1948.

Barger, A.C., W. F. Greenwood, J. R. DiPalma, J. Stokes, III, and L. H. Smith. Venous Pressure and Cutaneous Reactive Hyperemia in Exhausting Exercise and Certain Other Circulatory Stresses," *J. of Applied Physiology*, Vol.2, No. 2. 1949.

The following two papers were the culmination of four years' work on antifibrillatory compounds:

DiPalma, J.R., J. E. Schultz, R.A. Reiss, and J. J. Lambert, "Pharmacological Study and Clinical Use of an Alphafagarine Like Compound (N-Methyl)—N-(3,4 Dimethoxy Benzyl)— Beta—(4 Methoxyphenyl) Ethylamine-HC1," *J. Pharmacol. & Exp. Therap.* 98. 1950.

DiPalma, J. R., J.J. Lambert, R.A., Reiss, and J.E. Schultz, "Relationship of Chemical Structure to Antifibrillatory Potency of Certain Alphafagarine Like Compounds," *J.Pharmacol.* 98, 251. 1950.

A fundamental review paper summarizing my work on antifibrillatory drugs:

DiPalma, J.R., and J. E. Schultz. "Antifibrillatory Drugs," *Med. 29*, 123. 1950.

Chapter V (1951-1960)

For those who have no real concept of homeopathy, I recommend the original work of Samuel Hahnemann, Organon of Medicine, 6th edition. It is translated into English by Jost Kunzli, M.D., Alain Naude and Peter Pendleton, published by J.P. Tarcher, Inc., Los Angeles (1982) and distributed by Houghton Mifflin Co., Boston. A modern version of Samuel Hahnemann and his contributions is contained in the following references:

Cook, Trevor M., *Samuel Hahnemann, The Founder of Homeopathic Medicine.* Wellingborough, Northamptonshire, England: Thorsons Publishers Ltd. 1981.

Vithoulkas, G., *The Science of Homeopathy*, New York: Grove Press, Inc., 1980.

An excellent authoratative history of Hahnemann Medical College has been written by Naomi Rogers, a professional medical historian. She specializes in alternative medical therapies. The book contains accurate information about the development of the college covering the years 1948 to 1998:

Rogers, N. *An Alternate Path: The Making and Remaking of Hahnemann Medical College of Philadelphia.* New Brunswick, NJ and London: Rutgers University Press, 1998.

The early history (the first 50 years, 1848-1898) of Hahnemann Medical College was extensively written about by Thomas Lindsley Bradford:

Bradford, T.L., *History of the Homeopathic College of Philadelphia.* Philadelphia: Boernicke and Tafel, 1898.

Another brief work was written by William Pearson who was Dean from 1921 to 1942:

Pearson, Wm. *The Hahnemann Monthly*, 82 (1947): 413.

A superior source of historical information about Hahnemann Medical College and its faculty can be accessed at Drexel University College of Medicine, Archives and Special Collections and Women in Medicine and Homeopathy, Philadelphia, PA (hereafter referred to as the Hahnemann Archives).
   Warburg technology made possible the study of metabolism of organs isolated from the body, such as liver slices. It was a great advance in the understanding of the biochemistry of the body and the biochemical action of drugs and vitamins. The following two papers explain what Otto Warburg's technology was and give some details about the 1931 Nobel Prize winner:

Warburg, O. [Otto Warburg: a biographical essay (author's transl)]. [Japanese] [Biography. Historical Article. Journal Article] *Seikagaku—Journal of Japanese Biochemical Society, 51 (3): 139-60, 1979 Mar.*

Warburg, O. Geissler AW. Lorenz S. [The production of normal metabolism from neoplastic metabolism by the addition of vitamin B1]. [German] [Journal Article] *Zeitchrift fur Naturforschung—Teil B—Anorganische Chemie, Organische Chemie, Biochemie, Biophysik, Biologie.* 25 (5): 559, 1970 May.

I was in Philadelphia when the following four articles were published, but the work was performed in Brooklyn the previous year. (These were the days when scientists made their own apparatus.)

DiPalma, J.R., and E.E. Suckling, "Square Wave Stimulator for Cardiac Research, Radio-Electronic Engineering," Ed. of *Radio and Television News, 46,* 14-226, 1951.

DiPalma, J. R. and A.V. Moscatello, "Excitability and Refractory Period of Isolated Heart Muscle of the Cat," *Amer. J. of Physiology*, Vol. 164, No. 3, 1951.

DiPalma, J.R. and A. V. Moscatello, "Analysis of the Actions of Acetylcholine, Atropine, Epinephrine and Quinidine on Heart Muscle of the Cat," *J. Phamacol. & Exp. Therap.* Vol. 101, No. 3, 1951.

Acierno, L., F. Burno, F.Burstein and J.R. DiPalma, "Actions of Adenosine Triphosphate on the Isolated Cat Atrium and their Antagonism by Acetylcholine," *J. of Pharmacol. & Exp. Therap.* Vol. 104, No. 3, 1952.

I wrote my first book chapter. Then I attempted to show that Hahnemann had a very fine course in Pharmacology:

DiPalma, J.R., "Diagnosis and Therapy of Cardiac Arrythmias," *Clinical Cardiology*, pp. 823-906; F.C. Massey, Ed., Williams, Wilkins Co, Baltimore, MD 1953.

DiPalma, J.R., "The Teaching of Pharmacology," *J. Med. Educa.* 28, 1953.

The two publications above are probably what secured me the chance to write a chapter in Victor Drill's new outstanding text of phamacology (below):

DiPalma, J. R., "Cardiac Depressants," *Pharmacology in Medicine*, V. Drill, Ed. McGraw-Hill, NY. 1954.

Burno and Burstein, my first two summer fellows, get their names on a scientific paper:

Burno, F., F. Burstein, and J. R. DiPalma, "Comparison of Antifibillatory Potency of Certain Antimalarial Drugs with Quinidine and Procaine Amide," *Cir. Res.* II, 414, 1954.

I get back to trying to find the ideal antifibrillatory drug:

DiPalma, J.R., "The Pharmacology of N-(4-methoxybenzyl)-Isoquinolium chloride WIN 2173 with Particular Reference to its Cardiac Effect," *J. Pharmacol.* 113, 125, 1955.

I get to give a name lecture:

DiPalma, J.R. "The Treatment of Cardiac Arrhythmias" (the A. Walter Suiter Lecture), New York State Medical Society, *N.Y. State M. J.* 56, 2503, 1956.

I revised my chapter in the second edition of Drill's text of pharmacology:

DiPalma, J.R. "Cardiac Depressants," *Pharmacology in Medicine*, V. Drill, Ed., 2d edition, McGraw-Hill, NY. 1958.

Back to some research:

DiPalma, J.R. and P. Hitchcock, "Neuromuscular and Ganglionic Blocking Action of Thiamine and its Derivatives," *Anesthesiology*, *19*, 762, 1958.

DiPalma, J. R., "The Delay in Transmission of the Atrial Impulse to the Ventricle," *Angiology*, 9, 219, 1958.

DiPalma, J. R., "Refractory Period and Latency of the Premature Ventricular Systole," *Angiology* II, 126, 1960.

Another book chapter:

DiPalma, J.R. "The Place and Use of Digitalis Glycosides in Congestive Heart Failure in Edema," *Mechanisms and Management*, Ed. J.H. Moyer and M. Fuchs, W.E. Saunders, Philadelphia and London, 1960.

Chapter VI (1961-1967)

Hahnemann Medical College had a wonderful set of By-laws. They were written at the request of the Liaison Committee of Medical Education (LCME) of the AMA-AAMC in the early 1940s by John C. Scott, the chairman of the Department of Physiology. They allowed the dean an executive position but balanced this with a system of faculty governance that was very democratic. This was in contrast to the autocratic governance of former deans. Dean Kellow took advantage of these By-laws to run the school in a very successful manner:

By-laws of the Hahnemann Medical College of Philadelphia (Copy of June 25, 1963). (Hahnemann Archives).

All kinds of information about medical schools is available from:

Association of American Medical Colleges
2450 N Street, N.W.
Washington, D. C. 20037
Phone: 202-828-0416
Fax: 202-828-1123
Website: *www.aamc.org*

The Department of Pharmacology's work on 2-PAM Cl was not published in the scientific literature. Reports of this work are at the Army Chemical Center, Edgewood, MD. Pralidoxine Chloride is the trade name of 2-PAM Cl, now an FDA-approved drug marketed for the therapy of anticholinesterase drugs overdose and accidental poisoning with certain insecticides. It is available only as an injectible for oral prophlylactic use not practical for civilian use. See prescription books such as:

"Facts and Comparisons," published by *Facts and Comparisons*, 111 West Post Plaza, Suite 300, St. Louis, MO 63146 (Loose leaf binder, revised monthly, or yearly bound editions)

When the studies were declassified, an important publication resulted:

Calesnick, B., Christensen, J., Richter, M., "Human Toxicity of Various Oximes," *Arch. Environ. Health*, 15; 599-608, Nov. 1967.

Work on the Venus Flytrap, Dianaea Muscipula, were published in Science:

DiPalma, J.R., Mohl, R. and W. Best, Jr.: "Action Potential and Contaction of *Dianaea Muscipula* (Venus Flytrap)," *Science*, 133; 878, 1961.

Balotin, N.M. and J. R. DiPalma: "Spontaneous Electrical activity of *Dianaea Muscipula*," *Science* 138; 1338, 1962.

DiPalma, J.R., McMichael, R., and DiPalma, M. : "A Touch Receptor of *Dianaea Muscipula* (Venus Flytrap)," *Science*, 152; 539, 1966.

Some more general articles on carnivorous plants:

Heslop-Harrison, Y. "Carnivorous Plants," *Scientific American*, 238: 104-116, 1978.

Lloyd, F. E. *The Carnivorous Plants*, Ronald, New York, 1960.

Alikham, E. "How Does the Venus Flytrap Digest Flies?" *Scientific American*, 287; 134, Dec., 2002.

During the period of my tenure in Academe, I had graduate students under my guidance who produced meritorious research:

Comer, M. S. and J. R. DiPalma, "TM10 Activity in Cholinergic Compounds," *Arch.Int. Pharmacodyn.* CSSSI., 368, 1961.

Rosenthale, M.E. and J.R. DiPalma, "Acute Tolerance to Norepinephrine in Dogs," *J. Pharmacol. 126*, 336, 1962.

Coppola, J.A. and J.R. DiPalma, "Histamine as a Factor in Tolerance to Levarterenol," *Am.J. Physiol. 202*, 114, 1962.

Rosenthale, M.E. and J.R. DiPalma, "Norepinephrine Storage and Acute Tolerance," *Arch. Int. Pharmacodyn. 146*, 529, 1963.

Zarro, V.J. and J.R. DiPalma, "A Preparation of the Spinal Cat by an Anterior Approach," *J. Pharm. Pharmacol.* 16, 427, 1967.

Zarro, V. J. and J.R. DiPalma, "The Sympathomimetic Effects of 2-Pyridine Aldoxine Methylchloride (2-PAM cl), *J. Pharmacol. 147*, 153, 1965.

DiGregorio, J., and J.R.DiPalma, "Some Pharmacological Actions of 2 Phenylquinoline Methiodide," *Brit. J. Pharmacol.*, 30:531-40, 1967.

Choi, Y.S. and J.R. DiPalma, "Studies on the Interaction of Norepinephrine with Some Other Drugs on the Aortic Strip of the Rabbit," *Arch.Int. Pharmacodyn*, 205: 11-22, 1973.

An interesting note about the above paper is that R. F. Furchgott who was awarded the Nobel Prize in 1999 devised the aortic strip preparation. Skillful work with this preparation led to the discovery of nitric oxide as a very important signaling agent in the body. Indeed, the discovery of the use of ViagraÒ in male impotence may be traced to the aortic strip preparation.

Growing orchids has increased in popularity and practicality since I first started in 1960. Plants and supplies can be obtained in most local nurseries and even The Home Depot. Information about local societies, books and publications is best obtained from The American Orchid Society, 16700 AOS Lane, Delray Beach, FL 33446; phone: 561-404-2000.

Despite many committee assignments and family obligations, I managed to do some original research and to write perhaps too many book chapters:

DiPalma, J. R., "Antihypertension Agents which Affect Catecholamine Release," *Hypertension, Recent Advances*, A.N. Brest and J. J. Moyer, Ed., pp.393, Lea & Fegiger, Phila., 1961.

DiPalma, J.R., "A Study of Cardiac Ischemia Produced by Temporary Coronary Artery Ligation," *Angiology 12*, 564, 1961.

DiPalma, J. R. "The Pharmacology of Coronary Vasodilators," pp. 328-331, *Coronary Heart Disease, W. Likoff and J. H. Moyer. Symposium*, 1962.

DiPalma, J. R. "The Basic Pharmacologic Principles Underlying the Use of Sedatives and Tanquilizers," *Clin. Ped. 2*, 225, 1963.

DiPalma, J. R. "Animal Techniques for Evaluating Sympathomimetic and Para-sympathomimetic Drugs," *Animal and Clinical Pharmacological Techniques in Drug Evaluation*, Nodine, J. H. and P.E. Siegler, Ed., 105-109, Year Book Medical Publisher, Chicago, 1964.

DiPalma, J. R. "Animal Techniques for Evaluating Digitalis and its Derivatives," *Animal and Clinical Pharmacological Techniques in Drug Evaluation,* Nodine, J. H. and P.E. Siegler, Ed., 154-159, Year Book Medical Publisher, Chicago, 1964.

DiPalma, J. R. "The Pharmacology of Coronary Vasodilators (Cardiovascular briefs)," *Penn. Med. J. 67*, 42, 1964.

I not only edited Drill's Phamacology in Medicine, but I also wrote six of the chapters:

DiPalma, J. R., Ed., *Drilll's Pharmacology in Medicine*, 2nd Edition (1488 pages) McGraw-Hill, N.Y., 1965.

DiPalma, J. R., "Introduction and Brief History of Drill's Pharmacology in Medicine," 3d Ed., pp. 1-6, J.R. DiPalma, Ed., McGraw-Hill, N.Y. 1965.

DiPalma, J. R. "Drugs in Epilepsy and Hyperkinetic States," *Drill's Phamacology in Medicine,* 3d Ed., pp. 232-245, McGraw-Hill, N.Y. 1965.

DiPalma, J. R. "Drugs Depressing Cardiac Muscle," *Drill's Phamacology in Medicine*, 3d Ed., pp. 624-635, McGraw-Hill, N.Y. 1965.

DiPalma, J. R., "Digestants and Drugs Useful in Gallbladder Disease," *Drill's Phamacology in Medicine,* 3d Ed., pp. 760-762, McGraw-Hill, N.Y. 1965.

DiPalma, J. R. "Chemotherapy of Protozoan, Infections, Malaria," *Drill's Phamacology in Medicine*, 3d Ed., pp. 1376-1391, McGraw-Hill, N.Y. 1965.

DiPalma, J. R. "Prescription Writing and Useful Tables," *Drill's Phamacology in Medicine,* 3d Ed., pp. 1443-1460, McGraw-Hill, N.Y. 1965.

DiPalma, J. R. "New Inotropic and Chronotropic Drugs,"

Mechanisms and Therapy of Cardiac Arrythmias, Dreifus, L.,
Ed., Hahnemann Symposium, Grune & Stratton, N.Y. 1966.
DiPalma, J. R. "Introduction to Cancer Chemotherapeutic Drugs,"
Cancer Chemotherapy, Hahnemann Symposium, Grune &
Stratton, N. Y., 1967.

Chapter VII (1968-1972)

*I wish I had been able to read this book, published in 1981, before
I got into the deaning business in 1967:*

Van Cleve Morris, *Deaning, Middle Management in Academe*,
University of Illinois Press: Urbana, Chicago, London, 1981.

*Besides being interesting, informative and amusing about the life
and functions of a Dean, it has a most valuable table in the Appendix
C on criteria for evaluating a dean (pp. 169-179).*

*Governance and finance dominate the management of any large
institution, especially medical schools. A very comprehensive and well-
organized book was written by William G. Rothstein (below). Covering
the period between 1750 and 1980, it describes the history and operative
methods of medical schools, especially those after 1950. Replete with
many tables and over 1,000 references, it is a must read for any serious
effort to understand medical school operation:*

Rothstein, W. G., *American Medical Schools and the Practice of Medicine,
A History*. Oxford University Press, Oxford and New York, 1987.

*The following references describe important factors in the operation
of medical schools in the 1970s:*

Siegel, Bernard. "Medical Service Plan in Academic Medical
Centers," *Journal of Medical Education,* 53: 794-95, 1978.
Petersdorf, R. G. "Faculty Practice Income—Implications for Faculty
Morale and Performance," *Clinical Research* 21: 914, 1973.
Magraw, R. M. "Perspectives from the New Schools—The Costs

and Financing of Medical Education," *New England Journal of Medicine*, 289, 561, 1973.

Deitrich, J. E. and Benson, R.C., *Medical Schools in the United States at Mid Century*, McGraw-Hill, New York, 1953.

Lippard, V. W. *A Half-Century of American Medical Education, 1900-1970*, Josiah Macy, Jr. Foundation, One Rockefeller Plaza, New York, NY 10020, 1974.

As Hahnemann grew in size and stature with a College of Allied Sciences and a Graduate School, it began to think University status. Since our sister institution, Jefferson, had also acquired it, we were trying to compete. Accordingly, a top-notch committee to plan and make recommendations was appointed. Its report in full was dated April 29, 1968. Incidentally, one of the committee's recommendations was not to form an undergraduate component, but to affiliate or merge with another established institution. Prophetically, among the prime prospects was the Drexel Institute of Technology. Both institutions did become universities, and 34 years after this report did actually merge in 2002.

The new president of Hahnemann, Wharton Schober, had an extraordinary capacity for creating bad publicity for himself and the institution. In the main, it was due to his indiscretions but also it was magnified by a mad desire to be in the press whether the story was good or bad. The following references from newspapers and magazines are highly descriptive of the man and his adventures:

"What's Festering at Hahnemann?" *Philadelphia Magazine*, Vol. 64, No. 11, p. 118, Nov. 1973.

"Addict's Death Blamed on Drug Treatment" by Karl Abraham, *The Philadelphia Bulletin*, May 17, 1972.

These and many other journal articles may be accessed in the Hahnemann Archives.

Shober's publicity team also tried desperately to create good publicity:

"Cheyney, Hahnemann Link Forces to Produce More Black Doctors," *The Philadelphia Tribune*, Dec. 29, 1970.

"Physician's Assistant: The Newest Breed of Medic," *The Philadelphia Inquirer*, Sept. 10, 1972.

"Stars Hope and Ellington Sparkle at Hahnemann Gala," *The Philadelphia Inquirer*, Dec. 10, 1973.

The carbon dioxide therapy (CDT) of mental disorders was first mentioned in the medical literature in 1929. It did not make any significant impression and was abandoned until revived by Meduna in the 1950s:

Meduna, L. J., "Carbon Dioxide Treatment, A Review" J. *Clin. & Exper. Psycopath*. 15: 235-254, July, Sept. 1954.

A reliable and respected investigator, Meduna concluded after careful clinical investigation that CDT was not for general use. CDT again disappeared from approved use until LaVerne revived it in the 1970s:

LaVerne, A. A. "Carbon Dioxide Therapy (CDT) of Addictions," *Behavioral Neuropsychiatry*. 45(11-12, 1-6): 13-22, Feb-Sept. 1973.

LaVerne, A.A., "Carbon Dioxide therapy, healing, and air pollution: A more effective rapid coma technic for psychiatric disorders," *Behavioral Neuropsychiatry* 2 (3): 6-25, Jun-Jul., 1970.

LaVerne's work on CDT was considered promotional rather than careful unbiased clinical investigation by most reviewers. Today CDT is not even mentioned in the leading textbooks of neuropsychiatry.

The poison pen letters were supposedly sent by the "Faculty of Nine." Despite much detective work, no one even specifically identified who actually sent the letters. They were ingeniously written and very effective in weakening Shober's power and influence. Modern versions of poison pen letters are articles planted in the scandal journals and press. Most of the letters are in the Hahnemann Archives.

Stephen L. DeFelice, M.D., whom I met at Walter Reed Army Institute of Research (WRAIR) is a most interesting character. He is best known for the development of carnitine as a useful drug, invention of the word "nutraceutical," and the establishment of the Foundation for Innovation in Medicine (FIM):

DeFelice, S. L., *The Carnitine Defense*, Rodale; distributed by St. Martin's Press, 1999.

During this period of my life as an executive, I could not manage to do serious research (bench work). However, determined to keep up my professional pursuits, I did manage to keep a full schedule of teaching pharmacology and maintaining a publishing record in my main interest in promoting clinical pharmacology. Together with Benjamin Calesnick, I started a journal in clinical pharmacology:

Seminars in Drug Treatment, Edited by Joseph R. DiPalma and Benjamin Calesnick; Henry M. Straton, Inc., New York, NY, June 1971-July 1973.

Published quarterly, it went through two volumes. Praised by the critics, it failed because of lack of sales. My venture into articles on clinical pharmacology in an established journal (American Family Physician) was more successful. The first of 62 of these articles were re-published in book form:

DiPalma, J.R., Editor. *Practical Pharmacology for Prescribers*. Medical Economics Company, Book Division, Oradell, NJ, 1979.

The rest of the 283 articles have been collated and bound in book form.

DiPalma, J. R. *Collected Papers in Clinical Pharmacology*. 2001 (Hahnemann Archives.)

Some general and research articles during this period include:

Winkelman, A.C. and DiPalma, J.R., "Drug Treatment of Parkinsonism," *Sem. In Drug Treatment*. 1, 10-62, 1971.

DiPalma, J.R. "Clinical Phamacology as a Specialty," *J. Clin. Pharmacology*, 12: 399-402, 1972.

Hitner, H., DiGregorio, J., DiPalma, J.R., "Structure Activity Relationship for 2—phenylquinoline methiodide analogues." *Arch. Int. Pharmacodyn.* 200: 273-80, 1972.

Hitner, H., DiGregorio, J., DiPalma, J.R., "Ganglionic and Adrenergic Effects of 2—Phenylquinoline Methiodide Analogues," *Arch. Int. Pharmacodyn.* 206: 264-71, 1973.

Chapter VIII (1973-1976)

On May 30, 1973, Shober put out a modest publicity piece entitled "Hahnemann's Destiny" (Hahnemann Archives). Brief, but very optimistic, it predicted great advances to be made by his regime. A much more elaborate blurb was published later in that year:

"Hahnemann Today," December, 1973 (Hahnemann Archives).

It predicted great advances. However, Shober's press was still bad, a carryover of the misadventures of the previous year:

"Alumni, Faculty Assail Hahnemann President," *Philadelphia Daily News*, Jan. 22, 1973.

This was the result of the very unpopular move by Shober to oust the existing alumni group and form an entirely new one more congenial to the president.

"Alumni Group is Ousted by Trustees in Smoldering Dispute at Hahnemann." *The Philadelphia Bulletin*, Dec. 12, 1972.

Shober's idea of creating good press was to hold a large, impressive celebration of Hahnemann's successes:

"Stars Hope and Ellington Sparkle at Hahnemann Gala," *The Philadelphia Inquirer*, Dec. 10, 1973.

By the next year, Shober managed to get more favorable press:

"Shober Proving He's the Man for Top Job at Hahnemann," *The Philadelphia Bulletin,* Nov. 3, 1974.

The visits of the Liaison Committee of the AMA-AAMC-LC were more detailed and accurate estimations of the institution's progress. In 1970, one year before Shober took office, a scheduled visit rated the institution as generally quite good and allowed a revisit in seven years, the maximum allowed. In 1973, the faculty requested a special visit of the Liaison Committee in an effort to get rid of Shober. This time the committee found much to the faculty's surprise that the institution had made a considerable advancement of its goals. However, the AMA-AAMC-LC only allowed a revisit of three years with a small increase in enrollment. I made a factual summary of the findings of the two visits:

"Summary of Accreditation Visit Departmental Findings, December 1970. Estimate of Achievements Accomplished to Date," (June, 1973). (Hahnemann Archives).

The actual surveys of the AMA-AAMC-LC, November 1970-73, may be accessed in the Hahnemann Archives. Briefly described are the Wilkes-Barre, Lehigh, and Gannon University programs:

Rogers, Naomi, *An Alternate Path.* Rutgers University Press, New Brunswick, NJ, pp. 248-249, 1998.

The Physicians' Assistant Program was started at Hahnemann in 1972. Publicity regarding this event:

"Physicians' Assistants: The Newest Breed of Medic," *The Philadelphia Inquirer,* Sept. 10, 1972.

A joint program with Cheney College was very helpful in advancing Hahnemann's efforts to encourage blacks to enter medical and health fields:

"Cheney, Hahnemann Link Forces to Produce More Black Doctors."
The Philadelphia Tribune, Dec. 29, 1970.

To Shober's credit, he encouraged faculty planning and discussion. I was commissioned to plan and execute a faculty retreat on the subject of how Hahnemann Medical School should be governed and organized. Over a period of two days, a panel of deans of the Philadelphia medical schools and selected faculty discussed in detail such subjects as departmental structure in relationship to governance, constructive relationships among volunteer, full-time and basic science faculty, responsibilities of the Institution in the planning and delivery of health care in the community, among other pertinent subjects. The Deans discussed the structure and functions of the Board of Trustees, including the controversial subject of membership of faculty and students:

"Proceedings of the Faculty Retreat on the Organization and Governance of Hahnemann Medical College and Hospital," Nov. 18-19, 1972, Marriott Motor Hotel, Philadelphia, PA, Compiled and edited by Frederick W. Pairent, Ph.D. (Hahnemann Archives).

Moyer wrote an elaborate report that he sent to the Board of Trustees. It attempted to show that Shober had fired him unjustly:

"Report to the Board of Trustees of Hahnemann Medical College and Hospital of Philadelphia" from John H. Moyer, M.D., Executive Vice President for Academic Affairs, Sept. 27, 1972 (Hahnemann Archives).

Moyer's dispute with the institution and Shober also made the papers:

"Doctor Sues Hospital Officials in Long Dispute at Hahnemann," *The Evening Bulletin*, July 24, 1974.

The Flexner Report of 1910 effectively ended commercially oriented medical schools in America. Federal funds for health service plans accessible to medical schools, starting in 1960, greatly reorganized medical schools toward commercial objectives. Faculty Practice Plans have since grown apace. An excellent article on this subject is:

Macleod, G.K., Schwarz, M.R. "Faculty Practice Plans, Profile and
    Critique," *JAMA*, 256: 58-62, 1986.

I did manage to do some research with the help of graduate student Dave Ritchie:

DiPalma, J.R., Ritchie, D.M., McMichael, R.F. "Cardiovascular
    and Antiarrythmic Effects of Carnitine," *Arch. Int.
    Pharmacodyn* 217 (2) 246-50, 1975.
Richie, D.M, DiPalma, J.R., McMichael, R.F. "Effect of Helium
    on Membrane Resistance," *Arch. Int. Pharmacodyn.* 217 (2)
    302-8, 1975.

Chapter IX (1977-1978)

With the economy receding in the late 1970s and the government cutting funds going to healthcare and education, a severe depression developed in all medical schools. At Hahnemann, it was natural to blame Shober for financial failure. The newspapers made hay of Shober's extravagances, leading to the banks' reluctance to lend any more money to Hahnemann. Realizing his economic difficulties, Shober managed to plant a favorable editorial:

"City Hospitals Aid the Economy," *The Philadelphia Inquirer*, April
    8, 1977.

Mayor Frank Rizzo who had shut down the city hospital, Philadelphia General Hospital, was an interesting character:

Paolantonio S. A., Frank Rizzo, *The Last Big Man in Big City America*,
    Camino Books, Inc., Philadelphia, PA, 1993.

A telling blow toward financial disaster was the resignation of Roger Hunt, CEO of the Hahnemann Hospital:

"Hahnemann Loses Top Executive," *The Evening Bulletin*, May 27, 1977.

Yet despite the financial disaster, Shober's control of the Board of Trustees was so great that he was reelected:

"Hahnemann Reelects Shober; 3 Vice Presidents Have Quit," *The Evening Bulletin,* May 24, 1977.

However when Hahnemann failed to gain a vital loan, Shober was forced to resign by the Board:

"Hahnemann President Quits" *The Philadelphia Daily News*, May 27, 1977.
"Hahnemann Loses Top Executive," *The Evening Bulletin*, May 27, 1977.
"Hahnemann President Steps Down," *The Philadelphia Inquirer*, May 28, 1977.
"Hahnemann Hospital Seeks Loan from 3 Phila.Banks," *The Evening Bulletin*,
June 20, 1977.
"Hahnemann and Banks Meet on Loan," *The Evening Bulletin*, June 22, 1977.

Hahnemann's Board now turned to the faculty to put up collateral for the desperately needed loan. William Likoff, hastily elected as president, was of inestimable help. Most of the existing Board subsequently resigned. A handsome portrait of Likoff is on the cover of "Modern Medicine" as well as a short biography of his medical achievements.

"Contemporaries, William Likoff, M.D." *Modern Medicine*, 36:12, 16, May 6, 1978.

Another factor contributing to Schober's demise was his questionable involvement with U.S. Representatives Daniel J. Flood and Joshua Eilberg in obtaining a special grant from the Feds and to float a municipal bond for the construction of the new Hahnemann Hospital. The first inkling of trouble was the cancellation of a money-raising fete for Representative Flood:

"Hahnemann Drops Fete for Rep. Flood," *The Evening Bulletin*, March 31, 1977.

Later there was an FBI investigation of a Hahnemann Hospital contract for construction:

"FBI Probes Hahnemann Contract," *Sunday Bulletin*, Dec. 18, 1977.

The whole matter was summarized, including the involvement of U.S. Attorney David Marston, in an ingeniously entitled article, "Phillygate."

"Phillygate: Hahnemann Hospital Focus of Marston Furor," *American Medical News*, Jan. 30, 1978.

In November, 1978, the newspapers announced that Shober was indicted for banking and mail fraud. He was eventually cleared of a charge of bribery of Rep. Flood by the U.S. Government.

"Shober is Acquitted of Bribery: Still Faces Mail Fraud Charges," *The Evening Bulletin*, Nov. 2, 1978.

Shober's machinations in the last day of his tenure are well described and documented in Naomi Rogers' history of Hahnemann (see pages 263-269). Some years later, Shober wrote his own story of his experiences at Hahnemann and his eventual indictment and clearance of all charges:

Shober, W. "First Person, Absence of Redress," *Princeton Alumni Weekly*, Feb. 22, 1982.

The above articles may be accessed in the Hahnemann Archives.
The financial crisis was partially alleviated by a decision, blamed on me, to raise tuition drastically from $6,100 to $10,000 per annum. The other Deans of the Philadelphia medical promptly raised their tuition a similar amount.

"Hahnemann Hikes Med School Costs," *Philadelphia Daily News*, Jan. 24, 1978.

Besides my articles in "American Family Physician" and work on my pharmacology textbook, I did manage to write other significant articles and do a little research:

Di Palma, J.R., and Richie, D. M., "Vitamin Toxicity," *Ann. Rev. Pharmacol.* 17: 133-148, 1977.
Richie, D.M., DiPalma, J. R., McMichael, R. F. "Helium Effect on Isolated Nerve Activity," *Arch Int. Pharmacodyn* 231: 57-62, 1978.

Chapter X (1979-1982)

Likoff finally managed to get a decent chairman of the board to lead the repair of Shober's tenure. A good picture of Charles Kennedy Cox is in an interview by the Inquirer:

"Trouble Spot: New Chairman Takes on the Hahnemann Challenge," *The Philadelphia Inquirer*, January 10, 1979.

Changes in financing and purposes of medical schools cause the LCME to revise its periodic bulletin, especially to conform to commercial functions:

"Functions and Structure of a Medical School, 1973, compared to Functions and Structure of a Medical School, 1985," (Hahnemann Archives).

The elements of change led the General Professional Education of the Physician (GPRP) Report of the AAMC and an extensive study by the Commonwealth Fund:

"Physicians for the Twenty-First Century," Association of American Medical Colleges, Washington, D.C., 1984.

"Prescription for Change: Report of the Task Force on Academic Health Centers. To preserve the functions of academic health centers for the future." The Commonwealth Fund, NY, NY, 1985.

Molecular biology did not become a dominant concept until the 1950s and 1960s. An excellent explanation of the origins of this now all-pervasive field is

Astbring, W. T., *Adventures in Molecular Biology.* The Harvey Lectures, Series XLVI, 3-44. Charles C. Thomas, Springfield, IL.

Steve DeFelice's ebullient character is best illustrated by his recent book:

DeFelice, S. L. *Old Italian, Neighborhood Values*, 2002, 1st Books Library. *www.1stbooks.com* 1-800-839-8690

A brochure issued by Fidia Research Laboratories describes the pharmacology and clinical usefulness of the ganglioside GM_1 Cronassial®:

"Dossier of Cronassial, Fedia Research Laboratories," Abano Terme (Padua), Italy, 1980 (Hahnemann Archives).

An account of the establishment of a neurological research institute at Georgetown University Medical School is:

"Italian Company Seeks Foothold in U.S. Science," *The Scientist*, Vol. 4, #1, January 8, 1990 (Hahnemann Archives).

Enthusiastic about gangliosides, I wrote a general article for Italian consumption. Fortunately, it made only very mild clinical claims:

DiPalma, J.R. "Gangliosidi: Ruolo biologico nel sisterna nervoso e implicazioni Terapeutiche." *Farmaci*, 6/7: 382-388, 1981.

There are many research articles on gangliosides. Our brief contribution was:

Kalia, M., DiPalma, J.R., "Ganglioside-Induced Acceleration of Axonal Transport Following Nerve Crush Injury in the Rat," *Neuroscience Letters*, 34: 1-5, 1982.

Bert Brown became president on Feb. l, 1983, eight months after I stepped down as Dean. His plan for the development of the University is presented in an annual report:

"Hahnemann University, Annual Report, 1982-1983" (Hahnemann Archives).

An excellent picture of Brown is on the cover of an alumni magazine. Also in this issue, the National Health Constitutional Convention is described in three separate articles:

Alumni, A Magazine for the Graduates of Hahnemann, Winter, 1984, 10-12, 13-14, 15-17 (Hahnemann Archives).

Brown accepted the committee's recommendation of Iqbal Paroo, M.H.A., as CEO of the Hospital in 1984. A brief resume is in the bulletin:

Hahnemann University, Winter, 1986 (Hahnemann Archives).

A more extensive biography is in Chapter XIII and in:

Hahnemann University, Summer, 1988, 11-19 (Hahnemann Archives).

Paroo's inaugural address in the same issue of "Hahnemann University" is very prophetic of what happened to Hahnemann University in the 1990s.

A brief biography of John R. Beljan, M.D., the newly appointed dean is in:

"New Dean of Medicine," *Alumni,* Winter, 1984, 8-9 (Hahnemann Archives).

Victor Herbert at the time of his appointment was carrying on a campaign to debunk the vitamin and nutrition hustlers:

Herbert, V., *Nutrition Cultism*, Stickley, Philadelphia, 1981.

Ironically, with the advent of "alternative therapy" nutritional therapy became popular and the word "nutraceutical" was coined.

During the final years of my deanship, I was more involved in politics and the growing duties required of a rapidly developing organization. I did manage to write some significant articles of academic interest:

DiPalma, J. R., and McMichael, R. "The Interaction of Vitamins with Cancer Chemotherapy." *Ca-A Cancer Journal for Clinicians.* The American Cancer Society, 29: 280-286, 1979.

DiPalma, J.R. "Peripheral Vascular Changes During Exercise in Therapeutics through Exercise," Editors: D. Lowenthal, K. Bharadwaja, and W.W. Oaks. Grune and Stratton, N.Y. 69-77, 1979.

DiPalma, J.R. "Practical Pharmacology for Prescribers," *Medical Economics*, Oradell, NJ, 338 pp. 1979.

Edward Hemwall was the last graduate student under my direction:

Hemwell, E. and J.R. DiPalma, "Cardiovascular Effects of Indapamide on Frog Hearts and Open Chest Cats." *Arch.Int. Pharmacodyn and Therap.* 248: 225-237, 1980.

I was much interested in getting specialty boards in clinical pharmacology:

DiPalma, J.R., "The Case for Boards in Clinical Pharmacology," *JAMA*, 243: 1918-1920, 1980.
DiPalma, J.R., "Role of the Clinical Pharmacologist in Meeting the Educational Needs of the Primary Care Physician," *Jour. Clin. Pharmacology*, 18: 254-257, 1981.

I was very honored to give a talk on vitamins before the New York Academy of Medicine, which resulted in this article:

DiPalma, J.R. and McMichael, R. "Assessing the Value of Mega-nutrients in Disease," *Bull., N.Y. Acad. Med.* 58: 254-62, 1982.

My interest in gangliosides led naturally to an application to neuropathies:

DiPalma, J.R., "Therapy of Diabetic Peripheral Neuropathy," *Geriatrics*, 37: 43-46, 1982.

Chapter XI (1982-1986)

The deplorable status of continuing education at Hahnemann in the 1980s was described in one page of a report by the evaluation team of the Middle States Association of Colleges and Schools:

Letter and report addressed to Bertram S. Brown, M.D., and signed by Matther F. McNulty, Jr., Sc.D., Chancellor, The Medical Center, Georgetown University, May 17, 1983, pp.10, 25 (Hahnemann Archives).

A more favorable description of the School of Continuing Education is in Hahnemann Medical College Bulletin, 1980-1982 (Hahnemann Archives). In the 1990s, continuing education was rejuvenated practically single-handedly by Allen B. Schwartz. M.D. and continues to grow in scope and excellence into the new century.

Philadelphia General Hospital, "Old Blockley," was our best affiliation, but it was closed by Mayor Rizzo in 1977. A description may be accessed at http://www.phila.gov/health/history/parts/part_5.htm

An affiliation developed between Hahnemann and Health East (parent company of Lehigh Valley Hospital Center and Allentown Hospital) in the spring of 1986, culminating two years' work by Brodsky and myself. The relationship was described in:

Degrees and Stitches. 10 No. 11, June 6, 1986 (Hahnemann Archives).

Some of the other valuable affiliations of this era were:
Crozer Chester Medical Center, Chester, PA, Medical Education Director James Clark, M.D. (We shared surgical residents with this center and later it was designated as a clinical teaching campus.); Monmouth Medical Center, Long Branch, N.J., Medical Education Director William S. Vaun, M.D., and Robert Packer Hospital and Guthrie Clinic, Sayre, PA, Paul C. Royce, M.D., Medical Education Director. A rough estimate would indicate that approximately 50 percent of clinical medical education was accomplished at affiliates.

Chapter XII (1986-2000)

I was asked by McGraw-Hill to edit and revise its PreTest in Pharmacology (an exam preparatory series for the National Board exams). This was a popular series and I went on to edit and revise it for the next ten years.

DiPalma, J. R., Barbieri, E.J, DiGregorio, G.J., Ferko, P.A., Sterling, G.H., *PreTest in Pharmacology*, Fourth Edition, 1986, Fifth Edition, 1988, Sixth Edition, 1991, Seventh Edition, 1993, Eighth Edition, 1996, McGraw-Hill, New York and London.

The last two editions of the text in pharmacology were:

DiPalma, J.R., DiGregorio, G.J., *Basic Pharmacology in Medicine*, Third Edition, McGraw-Hill, New York, NY, 1990.

DiPalma, J.R., DiGregorio, G. J., Barbieri, E.J., Fesko, A.P., *Basic Pharmacology in Medicine,* Fourth Edition, Medical Surveillance, Inc., P.O.Box 1629, West Chester, PA, 1994.

Dr. Likoff died on July 3, 1987. He was one of Hahnemann's most extraordinary alumni. I wrote a memorial piece which I hope does him justice and honor:

DiPalma, J.R., "In Memorium: William Likoff, 1912-1987," *Clin. Cardio.* 10, 550-551, 1987.

My interest in carnitine resulted in a review article:

DiPalma, J.R., "Carnitine Deficiency," *American Family Physician*, 38: 243-251, 1988 (63 references).

Previous work which showed that nutritional substances at a higher dose or route of administration could cause pharmacological effects resulted in an invitation to do a paper for the Annual Review of Nutrition:

DiPalma, J.R., Thayer, W.S., "Niacin as a Drug," *Ann. Rev. Nutr.*, 11: 169-87, 1991.

A final article on low back pain control was written by invitation at the request of Martin Savitz, M.D., an alumnus who was guest editor of a special issue of the Mount Sinai Journal of Medicine:

DiPalma, J.R., DiGregorio, G.J., "Management of Low Back Pain by Drug Therapy," *Mount Sinai Journal of Medicine* 58: 101-109, 1991.

During the 1980s and 1990s, vast changes in the economics and commercial operation of medical services occurred. Arnold Relman, M.D., editor of the New England Journal of Medicine became the spokesman of these changes:

Relman, A.S. "Here Come the Women." *New Eng. J. Med.* 302:1252-3, 1980.

Relman, A.S., "Will Profit Takers Change the Face of Medicine?" *Patient Care 15*: 244-5, 249, 252. 1981.

Relman, A.S. "The Future of Medical Practice," *Health Affairs*, 2: 5-19; Summer 1983.

Relman, A.S. "Two Views in the Debate over Commercialized Medicine," *Technology Review* 87: 10-15, 1984.

Relman, A.S. "What's Happening to Our Health Care System?" *Bulletin, American Academy of Arts and Sciences,* 39" 11-29, 1986.

Relman, A. S. "The Changing Climate of Medical Practice," *New Eng. J. Med.* 316: 333-4, 1987.

Relman, A.S. "Practicing Medicine in the New Business Climate," *New Eng. J. Med.* 316: 1150-1, 1987.

Relman, A.S. "Salaried Physicians and Economic Incentives," *New Eng. J. Med.* 319:784, 1988.

Relman, A.S. *"American Medicine at the Crossroads: Signs from Canada,"* New Eng. J. Med. 320:590-1, 1989.

Relman, A.S. "The Corporatization of the United States Healthcare System," *Connecticut Medicine*, 62: 97-8, 1998.

Relman's reporting and analysis are excellent but the main problem to be addressed is how to deliver maximum health care at affordable cost without excessive rationing and exploitation by profit-seeking entrepreneurs and commercial combines. Specifically, what is quality medical care?

Couch, J.B., M.D., J.D., Editor, *Health Care Quality Management for the 21ˢᵗ Century*, (27 contributors) American College of Medical Quality, Venice, FL 1991.

Chapter XIII

The best sources of information concerning the bankruptcy of Allegheny Health, Education and Research Foundation include:

Burns, L.R., Cacciamani, J., Clement, J., and Aquino, W. "The Fall of the House of AHERF: The Allegheny Bankruptcy." *Health Affairs*, Jan.-Feb., 2000, The People-to-People Health Foundation, Inc.

Stark, K., Gammage, J. "Sherif Abdelhak, The Man Who Bankrupted Allegheny," *The Philadelphia Inquirer Magazine*, Part I, July 18 Part II, July 25, 1999.

The AHERF empire building in many ways resembles a pyramid scheme that has come to be known as a Ponzi operation. An excellent story of the life of Charles Ponzi is:

Darby, M. "In Ponzi We Trust," *Smithsonian*. Washington: Dec., 1998, 29; 134-149.

To understand the sequence of events which led to the bankruptcy, a summary of dates and happenings is useful:

__1988__: AHERF buys MCP Hospital and the MCP Medical School and establishes itself as a health center in Philadelphia.

__1991__: AHERF expands by taking over St. Christopher's Hospital for Children in Philadelphia, Warminster General in Bucks County, and Rolling Hills Hospital in Elkins Park.

__1994__: AHERF purchases Hahnemann Hospital and Hahnemann University Medical School and merges these with MCP and the other hospitals.

__1996__: AHERF purchases the Graduate Health System, composed of Graduate, Parkview, Rancocas and Mt. Sinai Hospitals.

__1997__: This was the peak year of AHERF expansion. Although an expansive mood was continued, the empire was beginning to crumble. Mt. Sinai Hospital, a venerable Philadelphia hospital, was closed and 1,700 employees laid off. The extravagant plan to buy up private practices was cut after buying the practices of 274 primary care doctors and 36 specialists. Harvey Levy, a highly paid executive and buddy of Abdelhak, was attenuated:

"A Top Official Leaving Allegheny," *The Philadelphia Inquirer*, May 13, 1998.

The bosses of the area health systems paid themselves very well and Abedelhak led all the rest with a salary well over $1 million in 1995 with generous perks on the side:

"Despite Lean Times at Area Hospitals, Top Executives Get More Raises," *The Philadelphia Inquirer,* Jan. 19, 1997.

After years of operation in the Philadelphia area, AHERF put out a glowing report to its board of trustees extolling the financial, operational, and educational achievements:

Abdelhak, S. S., Sanzo, A.M., Ross, L.L., Kaye, D., Bland, C., Chakurda, T.C. "A Report to the Board of Trustees, Academic and Fiscal Year 1994" (Hahnemann Archives).

Even more expansive was an expensive 120-page brochure put out December 10, 1997, extolling the accomplishments in health care by the AHERF empire. It was accompanied by a letter signed by William P. Snyder, III, Chair of the Board. Pictures of leading executives and neat charts reflect a very successful enterprise:

"Report to the Board," Allegheny Health, Education and Research Foundation, 1997 (Hahnemann Archives).

At enormous cost, AHERF published a full-length newspaper of three sections, totaling 24 pages, which was widely distributed over the entire state, but largely in the Pittsburgh and Philadelphia areas:

"Allegheny News," The Publication of the Allegheny Health, Education and Research Foundation, Vol. 1., No. 4, Sept.8, 1997 (Hahnemann Archives*).*

1998, March: The financial deficit growing daily and now unable to borrow money, the Ponzi-like Abdelhak empire began to crumble. Allegheny desperately sought to survive by selling off its assets to Vanguard Health Systems. However, the sale fell through once Allegheny's shaky financial structure was revealed.

1998, April: It was later revealed that Allegheny had repaid an $87 million loan to a four bank consortium which was led by Mellon Bank. Naturally, creditors felt that the Mellon combine received preferential treatment. Mellon executives were on the Allegheny Board:

"Allegheny Repaid Mellon $87Million," *The Philadelphia Inquirer*, July 23, 1998.
"Bankruptcy and Sale for Allegheny," *The Philadelphia Inquirer*, July 21, 1998.
"Health System Reveals It's $1.3 Billion in Debt," *The Philadelphia Inquirer*, July 21, 1998.
"Allegheny Tells Judge Payroll in Jeopardy," *The Philadelphia Inquirer*, July 22, 1998.

1998, June: Finally, Abdelhak is fired:

"President Out at Allegheny Health System," *The Philadelphia Inquirer*, June 6, 1998.
"Allegheny CEO's Growth Strategy Proves 'Paper Thin,'" *The Philadelphia Inquirer*, June 7, 1998.

1998, July: MCP Hahnemann University, eight of Allegheny's Philadelphia area hospitals and several hundred doctors' practices file for Chapter 11. The bankruptcy of a health-education combine is the largest in the nation estimated to have cost $1.3 billion. Who was to blame?

"Just Who was Minding the Allegheny Store?" *The Philadelphia Inquirer*, July 12, 1998.

Fortunately, Congress backed $4 million in tuition loans, thus enabling the medical school to continue to operate. The students were much relieved:

"Congress Aids Allegheny Med School," *The Philadelphia Inquirer*, July 17, 1998.

Several health industry entrepreneurs were eyeing the Allegheny hospitals. Vanguard Health Systems was the most interested:

"Vanguard Health Bids for All of Allegheny," *The Philadelphia Inquirer*, July 18, 1998.

"Bankruptcy and Sale for Allegheny," *The Philadelphia Inquirer*, July 21, 1998.

"Profit-driven Hospitals Knock on Region's Door," *The Philadelphia Inquirer*, July 26, 1998.

1998, August: Too late Allegheny found that owning doctors' practices was a huge waste of money:

"Seeking to Shed Doctors' Practices," *The Philadelphia Inquirer*, August 2, 1998.

Harvey Levy who bought doctors' practices for Allegheny tried to start a new network with a different health center:

"Trying to Revise His 'Dream' of a Physician Network," *The Philadelphia Inquirer*, Aug. 9, 1998.

"Hospital to Move Against Ex-Exec; Allegheny Will Seek to Ban Ex-Exec," *The Philadelphia Inquirer*, Aug. 14, 1998.

When in financial trouble, "rob Peter to pay Paul" is the usual practice:

"Allegheny Leaders Shifted Millions from Endowments," *The Philadelphia Inquirer*, Aug. 16, 1998.

"Allegheny to Study Restricted Fund Use," *The Philadelphia Inquirer*, Aug. 18, 1998.

An attempt was made to recover the generous perks from the well-paid executives:

"Allegheny Asks Execs to Return $6 Million," *The Philadelphia Inquirer*, Aug. 28, 1998.

1998, September: Mayor Edward G. Rendell tried to form a coalition that would buy and run the hospitals:

"Mayor Has Purchase Idea for Allegheny," *The Philadelphia Inquirer*, Sept. 5, 1998.

Dedicated faculty and key members of the Board made an effort to save the University. Acting President Dorothy McKenna Brown and recently appointed Dean Barbara Atkinson were actively engaged in this movement:

"Allegheny People Seek Plan to Save Their University," *The Philadelphia Inquirer*, Sept. 6, 1998.

The Allegheny debacle shook the whole country's health system and especially New York with its many hospitals and medical schools:

"Philadelphia Shaken by Collapse of a Health Care Giant," *The New York Times*, Aug. 22, 1998.

September 1998 was an extremely troubled period as the bidders tried to shake down Allegheny and Allegheny aimed to cover up the full extent of the disaster. Meanwhile, there were widespread cutbacks. Worried faculty were avidly seeking other jobs.

"Children's May Bid for One Hospital; New Allegheny Bidder Emerges," *The Philadelphia Inquirer*, Sept. 18, 1998.

"Attorney General Wants a Closer Look at Allegheny Finances; State Files to Become Allegheny Creditor," *The Philadelphia Inquirer*, Sept. 19, 1998.

"Money Missing at Allegheny; Research Projects Jeopardized," *The Philadelphia Inquirer*, Sept. 20, 1998.

"The Fate of Eight Allegheny Hospitals Awaits an Auction: Going, Going . . . Gone in 9 Days," *The Philadelphia Inquirer*, Sept. 22, 1998.

"Professors Denounce the Cutbacks; Many of the Faculty at Allegheny Told They Won't Have Jobs," *The Philadelphia Inquirer*, Sept. 24, 1998.

"Allegheny Bids Due; Tenet Interest in Doubt," *The Philadelphia Inquirer*, Sept. 25, 1998.

"Two Allegheny Bidders Back Off," *The Philadelphia Inquirer*, Sept. 26, 1998. "A Muddier Picture for Allegheny; Amid Skittish Bidders and Deterioration of the Health Systems, 'It's Not a Good Situation,'" *The Philadelphia Inquirer*, Sept. 27, 1998.

"Allegheny Bid is Cut On Eve of Deadline; Vanguard Health System Cited Deteriorating Finances; Bidder Reduces $460 Million Offer," *The Philadelphia Inquirer*, Sept. 30, 1998.

"Tenet Agrees to Rescue Allegheny; The Offer: $345 Million to Buy Eight Hospitals," *The Philadelphia Inquirer*, Sept. 30, 1998.

Tenet's offer also included the buyout of MCP Hahnemann University. Tenet's intention, as a non-profit corporation, was to let the University remain a non-profit institution and be managed for a two-year period by Drexel University. U.S. Bankruptcy Court Judge M. Bruce McCullough tentatively approved the sale with the proviso that details be worked out by the October deadline. Tenet's projected takeover created great excitement and worry for the future, as reflected in the following Philadelphia Inquirer articles on Sept. 30, 1998. The headlines tell the story:

"Tenet's Presence in Philadelphia Prompts Frown on Bond Ratings"
"Med School Could Boost Drexel's Image; At the Least, a Change for the Better, Workers Say"
"Tenet's 'Soft' Image Does Not Mollify All"
"Large or Small, Creditors Get Little"

Further Inquirer articles define the Tenet takeover, including:

"Allegheny Employees Will Keep Their Jobs for Now, Tenet Says," *The Philadelphia Inquirer*, Oct. 1, 1998.

A period now followed of pleadings that led to a final settlement:

"Allegheny Inquiries Aren't Over; Fisher Said State Will Pursue Misuse of Allegheny Funds," *The Philadelphia Inquirer*, Oct. 1, 1998. *(Mike Fisher was Pennsylvania Attorney General at the time.)*

"Tenet Healthcare Says It is Aware of Its Challenge," *The Philadelphia Inquirer*, Oct. 4, 1998.

"Allegheny To Cut At Least 70 from Doctor Network Before Sale to Tenet," *The Philadelphia Inquirer*, Oct. 13, 1998.

"Drexel Says It Will Not Run Med School," *The Philadelphia Inquirer*, Oct. 14, 1998.

"Tenet Granted a Delay in Allegheny Purchase," *The Philadelphia Inquirer*, Oct. 20, 1998.

"Allegheny Served With Subpoenas," *The Philadelphia Inquirer*, Oct. 20, 1998.

"Gearing Up in Case Allegheny Falls; Other Area Hospitals are Trying to Plan for a Larger Patient Load," *The Philadelphia Inquirer*, Oct. 22, 1998.

"Drexel is Pressed to Reverse Vote in Allegheny Deal; Creditors Would Give Money if University Agrees to Run Allegheny's Schools; Politicians Are Lobbying," *The Philadelphia Inquirer*, Oct. 22, 1998.

"Ridge to Urge Drexel Board to Manage Allegheny University," *The Philadelphia Inquirer*, Oct. 24, 1998. *(Tom Ridge was Governor of Pennsylvania at the time.)*

"Demise of Allegheny Could Have Some Benefits (Decrease in Hospital Beds)," *The Philadelphia Inquirer*, Oct. 25, 1998.

"Drexel Takes Allegheny Med School," *The Philadelphia Inquirer*, Oct. 27, 1998.

Now Drexel was all smiles, having swung a deal that promised to be advantageous in all respects—financial, educational, and fitting in with Drexel's ambition to excel in medical technology and engineering, as illustrated by the Fall 1998 Alumni Bulletin cover picture of Drexel Board Chairman Chuck Pennoni, Trustee Manuel Stamatakis, and President Papadakis:

"Drexel," The Alumni Magazine of Drexel University, 9/No. 3, Fall, 1998 (Hahnemann Archives).

Drexel University did successfully manage the MCP Hahnemann Medical University from 1998 to 2002 with the aid of supporting funds from Tenet. In June 2002, a final merger was achieved and MCP Hahnemann University of the Medical Sciences became Drexel University College of Medicine, Drexel University College of Nursing and Health Professions, and Drexel University School of Public Health. The merger was advertised in the newspapers and the internal public relations newsletter, Drexel Newspaper:

Advertisements in *The Philadelphia Inquirer*, June 12, 2002, p.B12, and June 25, 2002, p. E10.
Advertisement in *Physician's News Digest*, June, 2002, #15, *www.physiciansnews.com*
"President's Message: It's Now Official," *Drexel Newspaper*, Newsletter 3, No. 5, July/August, 2002.

Abdelhak was the only person who served time for the Allegheny debacle. He was arrested in March 2000 for spending more than $50 million of restricted medical endowments and using the system's dwindling cash to make secret political contributions and renovate his son's high school locker room. His preliminary hearing lasted more than one year, and most charges were thrown out or whittled down. In late August 2002, Abdelhak pleaded no contest to one misdemeanor count of spending restricted endowment funds. He began serving a sentence of 11 ½ to 23 months on Sept. 3, 2002, at the Penn Pavilion work-release facility in New Brighton, near Pittsburgh. During this work—release period, he volunteered at a church for two months and took off nearly one-third of his time—three weeks and three days—to get unspecified medical treatment, which later was reported to be for coronary heart disease. Abdelhak was paroled after serving three months and six days:

"Paying Debt to Society via Church," By Karl Stark, *The Philadelphia Inquirer*, Feb 16, 2003

# # #

CDT for addictions ?

Carbon Dioxide Therapy

Breathe CO_2

Made in the USA
Lexington, KY
07 June 2013